Government Procedures and Operations

snova
New York

Government Procedures and Operations

COVID-19 in Nursing Homes: Impact, Transmission and Prevention
Fred C. Wallace (Editor)
2023. ISBN: 979-8-88697-673-1 (Hardcover)
2023. ISBN: 979-8-88697-683-0 (eBook)

The Significance of the COVID Pandemic in Nursing Homes
John S. Gill (Editor)
2023. ISBN: 979-8-88697-660-1 (Hardcover)
2023. ISBN: 979-8-88697-682-3 (eBook)

Putting an End to Surprise Medical Billing
Danial E. Tackett (Editor)
2022. ISBN: 979-8-88697-296-2 (Hardcover)
2022. ISBN: 979-8-88697-327-3 (eBook)

Abortion Rights, Access, and Legislative Response
Jorge P. Sandford (Editor)
2022. ISBN: 979-8-88697-258-0 (Softcover)
2022. ISBN: 979-8-88697-294-8 (eBook)

Review of Capitol Police Procedures During the Capitol Attack
Rafael B. Phillips (Editor)
2022. ISBN: 979-8-88697-260-3 (Hardcover)
2022. ISBN: 978-1-53617-478-6 (eBook)

More information about this series can be found at
https://novapublishers.com/product-category/series/government-procedures-and-operations/

Charles M. Edmond
Editor

Marijuana

Health Issues, Hazards and Usage

snova
New York

NOTICE TO THE READER

The Publisher has taken reasonable care in the preparation of this book but makes no expressed or implied warranty of any kind and assumes no responsibility for any errors or omissions. No liability is assumed for incidental or consequential damages in connection with or arising out of information contained in this book. The Publisher shall not be liable for any special, consequential, or exemplary damages resulting, in whole or in part, from the readers' use of, or reliance upon, this material. Any parts of this book based on government reports are so indicated and copyright is claimed for those parts to the extent applicable to compilations of such works.

Independent verification should be sought for any data, advice or recommendations contained in this book. In addition, no responsibility is assumed by the Publisher for any injury and/or damage to persons or property arising from any methods, products, instructions, ideas or otherwise contained in this publication.

This publication is designed to provide accurate and authoritative information with regards to the subject matter covered herein. It is sold with the clear understanding that the Publisher is not engaged in rendering legal or any other professional services. If legal or any other expert assistance is required, the services of a competent person should be sought. FROM A DECLARATION OF PARTICIPANTS JOINTLY ADOPTED BY A COMMITTEE OF THE AMERICAN BAR ASSOCIATION AND A COMMITTEE OF PUBLISHERS.

Library of Congress Cataloging-in-Publication Data

ISBN: 979-8-88697-869-8

Published by Nova Science Publishers, Inc. † New York

Contents

Preface

An estimated 43.5 million Americans used marijuana in the last year. Despite growing acceptance and accessibility of this drug and its derivatives, we lack definitive evidence on the short- and long-term health implications of marijuana use. Marijuana use among youth and young adults is a major public health concern. As policy and legalization efforts evolve and the availability of legal marijuana increases, communities and families need guidance surrounding marijuana use.

Chapter 1

Marijuana and America's Health: Questions and Issues for Policy Makers*

Senate Caucus on International Narcotics Control

Wednesday, October 23, 2019
U.S. Senate, *Washington, DC.*

The hearing was convened, pursuant to notice, at 3:22 p.m., in 215 Dirksen Senate Office Building. Senator John Cornyn, Chairman, presiding.

Members Present: Senator Dianne Feinstein, Co-Chairman and Senator Jacky Rosen.

The CHAIRMAN. Good afternoon. I would first like to begin this hearing by thanking our witnesses, and thanks to my Co-Chair, Senator Feinstein. We have been looking for a forum to have a hearing like this. As in so many areas, it seems like we are putting the cart ahead of the horse, and we would now really like to hear from the experts about what they can tell us about the public health consequences of marijuana use in the country.

So far this year we have centered our efforts on prevention of addictive substances from entering the country and infiltrating our communities, but now we want to talk about something a little different.

As you know, a 2018 Report by the Substance Abuse and Mental Health Services Administration found that an estimated 43.5 million Americans used marijuana in the last year. The percentage of the population 12 years of age

* This is an edited, reformatted and augmented version of Hearing before the Senate Caucus on International Narcotics Control, United States Senate, One Hundred Sixteenth Congress, First Session, Publication No. S. HRG. 116–252, dated October 23, 2019.

In: Marijuana
Editor: Charles M. Edmond
ISBN: 979-8-88697-869-8

and older currently using marijuana has increased in recent years from under 7 percent in 2010 to more than 10 percent in 2018.

And while marijuana is still a prohibited drug under federal law, more than 90 percent of the states allow for some medical use of marijuana in some capacity, and 10 states and the District of Columbia now allow for the recreational use of marijuana.

Despite growing acceptance and accessibility of this drug and its derivatives, I believe we lack definitive evidence on the short- and long-term health implications of marijuana use. That is especially true for vulnerable populations like adolescents, pregnant women, and people suffering from mental health issues.

Earlier this year, our Surgeon General, one of our witnesses here today, issued an Advisory that highlighted the risks of marijuana use for pregnant and nursing women and adolescents.

I remain concerned about the lack of evidence regarding health risks of these groups, as well as the general population. And it may be helpful at some point for the witnesses to discuss what type of evidence that the medical community considers conclusive, or at least solid enough to make a policy determination on. Because there seems to be a lot of folk myths and other idiosyncratic ideas that really have not gone through the sort of peer review and published requirements that most scientific evidence has to go through in order to be accepted by policymakers.

In 2017, the National Academy of Sciences, Engineering, and Medicine published one of the most comprehensive studies on the research of the health effects of recreational and therapeutic use of marijuana and cannabis-derived products.

It included nearly a hundred conclusions. They found conclusive or substantial evidence that cannabis or cannabanoids, but not necessarily marijuana or marijuana-derived cannabanoids, are an effective treatment for chronic pain, chemotherapy-induced nausea and vomiting. However, they found insufficient or no evidence regarding potential therapeutic effects of cannabis or cannabanoids for a variety of health conditions considered.

Additionally, they found substantial evidence that marijuana use had increased the risk of motor vehicle crashes, the development of schizophrenia, and other psychoses, and complications in pregnancy like lower birth weight.

It is critical for people like Senator Feinstein and I and other policymakers to understand the public safety implications of increased marijuana use before we dive into the admittedly complex and difficult job of changing federal policy.

In 2018, the Food and Drug Administration approved the first drug with an active ingredient derived from marijuana to treat rare, severe forms of epilepsy. It was only after rigorous studies and a thorough review by the FDA that physicians can have confidence in the safety, efficacy, and consistency of that drug. All this is to say that there are so many questions that still need to be answered.

Surgeon General, Dr. Volkow, and the experts on our second panel will help shed light on what science tells us about the public health risks of marijuana and what we still need to learn.

I look forward to hearing the testimony and discussing how we can work to prevent youth access to marijuana, and properly evaluate the safety and efficacy of any therapies that may utilize marijuana and cannabinoids.

Let me now turn the floor over to my Co-Chairman, Senator Feinstein, for any opening remarks she would care to make.

Co-Chairman FEINSTEIN. Thanks very much, Mr. Chairman. As you know, I enjoy very much working with you, so this is a pleasure.

The point of today's hearing is to better understand marijuana's impact on public health, and so I thank you very much for holding it.

One thing I have learned is that marijuana is much more complex than I thought. It apparently contains hundreds of different compounds, all of which produce different effects. I am told that much of what we know about marijuana is anecdotal, which of course is problematic for us in terms of making policy. It is problematic for medical professionals in knowing how to treat it. And it is problematic for consumers when they use it.

I am told this is due in part to the fact that marijuana's status as a Schedule One Drug makes it difficult to research. It is my belief that science should inform our policy, and that is why I, along with Senator Grassley and others, introduced the Cannabidiol and Marijuana Research Expansion Act which would remove barriers to research.

The NIH recently increased the number of grants awarded to study marijuana, and I hope it will continue to do so. This will enable marijuana's potential therapeutic benefits really to be more understood as they are explored.

It is important that we learn more about appropriate dosing and delivery mechanisms. It is important that we learn how marijuana components interact with other medications, how long-term use impacts the body. It is my understanding that the limited existing research has found varying degrees of evidence that components of marijuana may effectively treat conditions like intractable epilepsy, chemotherapy-induced nausea. I know that for a fact from family issues. And, vomiting. Muscle spasticity, chronic pain, and short-term sleep disturbances.

The Food and Drug Administration has approved four marijuana-derived drugs to treat many of these illnesses. Despite the potential benefits, it is equally important to understand its adverse effects.

For instance, studies show that marijuana can have a negative impact on the developing brain—this is one thing I hope to hear a little more about—including decreased cognitive abilities, loss of IQ, and increased risk of psychosis.

I am going to end here, Mr. Chairman, in the interests of seeing—of listening to our panel, and I will put my remarks in the record. Thank you.

The CHAIRMAN. Thank you, Senator.

Our first witness is Vice Admiral Jerome Adams who serves as the 20th Surgeon General of the United States. During his tenure as Surgeon General, Dr. Adams has created several initiatives to tackle our Nation's most pressing health issues, including the opioid epidemic, oral health and the links between community health and both economic prosperity and national security.

The Surgeon General issued an Advisory in August of this year on the potential health effects of marijuana use for adolescent brain development and use by pregnant mothers.

Our second witness on the first panel is Dr. Nora Volkow, who has served as Director of the National Institute of Drug Abuse, or NIDA, since May 2003. That is quite a run. As a research psychiatrist and scientist, Dr. Volkow pioneered the use of brain imaging to investigate the toxic effects and addictive properties of abusable drugs.

If I could ask each of you to limit your opening statement to about five minutes, and then we will make your complete statement part of the record, and then we can engage in some questions and answers, that would be great.

So let me turn to you, Dr. Adams, to start, please.

Statement of Jerome Adams, M.D., Surgeon General of the United States

Dr. ADAMS. Thank you very much, Chairman Cornyn, Co-Chairwoman Feinstein, and members of the Caucus. I appreciate the opportunity to share my recent marijuana advisory with you and to join national experts to discuss a complex issue that I feel demands our attention and our action.

As you mentioned, in August 2019 I issued a Surgeon General's Advisory on Marijuana Use in the Developing Brain, emphasizing the importance of protecting our Nation from the health risks of marijuana use in adolescence and during pregnancy.

I did this in response to alarming rates of marijuana use among pregnant women and young people, widespread and growing access to increasingly potent marijuana through legalization at the state level, and mounting evidence that marijuana use poses a risk to healthy brain development and to public health.

As Surgeon General I have visited with communities and clinicians in places like California and Colorado, Georgia and Texas, Nevada and Oklahoma. And as a former state health commissioner myself, I have spoken with health department leaders across the country, my friends, many of them reluctant overseers of an enormous and poorly informed national public health experiment.

Over and over I hear great and escalating concern about the rapid normalization of marijuana use, and the impact that a false perception of its safety is having on our communities, and specifically our young people and our moms-to-be.

As you mentioned, sir, as of today 33 states and the District of Columbia have legalized marijuana in some way. I will say it again: We are conducting a massive public health experiment on our citizenry. And with greater legalization, young people are reporting a decline in perceived harmfulness of the drug. In 2018, only a third of adolescents said they thought weekly marijuana use was harmful.

Marijuana is now the third most commonly used elicit substance in adolescents, behind alcohol and e-cigarettes. Last year, over 9 million 12- to 25-year-olds reported marijuana use, and each day 3,700 adolescents become new marijuana users.

Unfortunately, the scary truth is that while the perceived harm of marijuana is decreasing, the potential for harm is actually increasing due to widespread access, increased potency, and multiple forms.

Marijuana is now everywhere, especially in states that have legalized. And it can be smoked, drunk, eaten, and baked. As I like to say, this ain't your mama's marijuana. Not enough people know that today's marijuana is far more potent than in days passed. The amount of THC has increased three-fold in commonly cultivated plants over the last few decades, and dispensary products are often much stronger. Edible oils and waxes can deliver unpredictable concentrations of THC often of 70 percent or more. This is important because the higher the THC concentration, the higher the risk to our young people.

Across the country we have seen increased emergency department visits for psychosis and for nonfatal overdose. The earlier and more often a person uses marijuana, especially at these higher THC levels, the greater the peril.

Nearly one in five people who begin marijuana usage during adolescence will become addicted. Yes, you can become addicted to marijuana.

Science tells us frequent marijuana usage during adolescence can impair a child's attention, memory, and decisionmaking, and young people who regularly use marijuana are more likely to show a decline in IQ in school performance, are more likely to drop out, and are even more likely to attempt suicide.

In pregnant women, marijuana is actually the most commonly used elicit substance. Between 2002 and 2017, marijuana use among pregnant women doubled. Marijuana usage during pregnancy can not only affect the baby's brain, but also can result in lower birth weight, a marker for early death and disability. And that is why that is so important.

The Colorado PRAM study revealed a 50 percent increase in low birth weight in marijuana-using moms. THC is transmitted via breast milk, meaning the risk continues even after delivery.

And finally, marijuana and tobacco smoke share some of the same harmful components, so no one should smoke either product around the baby.

We already know a lot about the harms and potential harms of marijuana use on the developing brain, but I will be the first to admit we need to know more. We need to better understand the long-term health consequences of prenatal and youth exposure to marijuana, as well as strategies to decrease harms.

But I want you to hear me say this: We know enough now to deliver sound guidance to protect the future of our Nation's youth. My Advisory includes resources to help parents, teachers, clinicians, and others safeguard our youth from harm, but it will take all of us using the best evidence and communicating it clearly to ensure a healthy future for our young people.

This Advisory was carefully written based on the best currently available science, with input from NIDA, SAMPHSA, CDC, FDA, ACOG, AAP, and others. So please go to surgeongeneral.gov and share it.

I will finish by saying my bottom line to you today is this: No amount of marijuana use during pregnancy or adolescence is known to be safe. Therefore, communities must consider and should not minimize the short- and long-term public health impacts of marijuana use.

Thank you again for the opportunity to share this important information, and for your support in promoting healthy fetal and adolescent development to protect the youth of America. And I look forward to your questions.

The CHAIRMAN. Thank you, Doctor. Dr. Volkow.

Statement of Nora Volkow, Ph.D., Director, National Institute of Drug Abuse, North Bethesda, Maryland

Dr. VOLKOW. Good afternoon. Thanks very much for having me here, Chairman Cornyn and Co-Chairman Feinstein, and for holding this hearing on marijuana.

It is an opportunity for us to bring to you what we are funding at the National Institute on Drug Abuse and what type of research we are funding to try to clarify the effects of marijuana in the young brain.

As you mentioned, in 2018 there were 43.5 million people who reported use of marijuana in the past year, making it the most commonly used illicit drug in the United States, and its use is increasing.

Marijuana exerts its effects by activating cannabinoid receptors which are part of our endogenous cannabinoid system that modulates multiple physiological processes in our brains and bodies. This system emerges early in gestation when it plays a critical role in helping to orchestrate brain development, which is why exposure to marijuana during early development can impact the function of the brain later in life.

THC, the component of marijuana responsible for its intoxicating and addictive effects, freely crosses the placenta. Fetal exposure is associated with significant negative outcomes, including fetal growth restriction, lower birth weight, and preterm delivery.

Research is ongoing to clarify the mechanisms through which it contributes to these effects, and to investigate the effects of marijuana to the fetal brain when used by itself or when combined with teratogenic drugs such as alcohol and nicotine.

Adolescents, whose brains are also undergoing major developmental changes, are also particularly vulnerable to the negative effects of marijuana. Clinical studies of THC exposure during adolescence have shown greater sequence sensitivity to the rewarding effects of other drugs, which could be one reason why dosages of marijuana at a young age are more vulnerable to addiction later in life, not just to marijuana but to also to other drugs.

Epidemiological studies have found repeatedly that kids who regularly consume marijuana have lower academic achievements and a higher risk of dropping out school. Brain imaging studies have shown that frequent marijuana use during adolescents is associated with structural and functional changes in areas of the brain necessary for attention, memory, emotions, and motivation, which might account for the adverse cognitive and behavioral effects associated with youth marijuana use.

The association between marijuana use and mental illness is another area of major concern, particularly in light of the higher content of THC in today's marijuana. Serious mental illnesses and suicide are on the rise in our country. And while multiple factors are likely contributing to this rise, it is imperative to understand if exposure to high potency cannabis in adolescence is one of them.

High potency marijuana can trigger acute psychotic episodes, which is one of the main causes for emergency department visits associated with cannabis use, which are also rising.

While most of these episodes are short lasting, they can become chronic. Multiple studies, though not all, have associated adolescent marijuana use with an overall risk for the early onset of chronic psychosis such as schizophrenia.

Adolescent marijuana use is also associated with increased risk of suicidal behavior. Many of the studies done to assess the effects of adolescent marijuana use have been criticized because of certain limitations. For example, some of them may have not controlled for other factors that affect adolescent brain development. Some may have had insufficient sample sizes. Most of them were conducted at the time when THC content in marijuana was much lower.

To address this shortcoming, NIDA is leading two major studies. Study one is the Adolescent Brain Cognitive Development, or ABCD study, which is the largest long-term study of brain development in child health in the United States. The study has recruited over 11,000 children, aged 9 to 10, who will be followed into early adulthood to investigate how the brain develops, and how its development is affected by substance use, including marijuana.

The other one, which complements the ABCD study, is A Healthy Brain Child Development, or HBCD study, which is part of the NIH initiative and is currently in its pilot phase. This study would establish a large cohort of pregnant women and their infants to assess the child's brain cognitive and emotional development longitudinally over the course of the first 10 years of their lives. Findings will help researchers develop standards for normal brain development in childhood and to characterize the long-term impact of prenatal and postnatal drug exposures.

Ensuring normal brain development is fundamental for achieving a person's full potential, which is why we owe it to the future generations to protect them from the potentially disruptive effects of cannabids to their brains and well being.

Thank you very much, and I look forward to your questions.

The CHAIRMAN. Thank you very much, both of you.

I am struck, Dr. Adams, by your description as a poorly informed national health experiment with regard to marijuana. And of course part of what we are trying to do today is have a better informed discussion about this national health experiment.

I see some parallels, perhaps—and I would be interested in your commentary on this—to what we learned about tobacco decades in the past. I even went back, with my staff's help, and found some advertisements by the tobacco industry where they would tout the health benefits of smoking. And not only were those not proven using the sort of peer-reviewed evidence, scholarship that we would expect, but there was not disclosure of the negative, the detriment to health—things like addiction to nicotine, lung cancer, cardiovascular disease, and the like.

And I feel like there are some parallels, perhaps, here in the way we are wading into this debate. Do you think that is analogous, Dr. Adams, and Dr. Volkow? Or is it different?

Dr. ADAMS. Well, sir, thank you for saying that. Because as the Surgeon General, I want every policy decision to have as much science infused into it as possible. And you are correct.

We have seen this play before. We have seen it with a number of substances. Once upon a time, cocaine was thought to be an effective medicine and harmless. Once upon a time, opioids were thought to be good for whatever ails you, and to not have any harmful effects and no higher dosage limit.

And not that I am in any way, shape, or form comparing marijuana to those substances, but from a policy point of view I think the lesson we should have learned was that we have to make sure the science is leading the policy, and that the tail is not wagging the dog. And many of the indications that people are using marijuana for are unproven. We are overstating the benefits and, in my opinion, we are downplaying the risks. And that is why I put out my Advisory, because one risk we cannot afford to ignore is the risk to our pregnant women and our young people, our Nation's future.

The CHAIRMAN. Dr. Volkow.

Dr. VOLKOW. Yes, I will completely agree, and I do want to state also the other aspect that we are learning with the use of marijuana at very high content, is we are finding out medical negative effects that we did not know existed. For example, a perfect example is the iferamesic syndrome where people that take high content THC chronically develop a syndrome where they cannot stop vomiting, with very, very intense abdominal pain.

This was not described until 2006. And again, we have never seen it because we did not get exposed to this type of marijuana. So my concern relates to the fact that if we are not looking at something, particularly as we for example are discussing the use of marijuana in pregnancy, if we do not evaluate the outcome in these infants, we will not be able to understand what could be potentially very negative effects.

And that is illustrated also with tobacco. In nicotine we did not know that smoking during pregnancy could have such negative effects until we studied it.

Dr. ADAMS. And I am so glad you have someone on the second panel who is an expert on MVAs. There is this big misbelief out there that marijuana makes you a better driver, but the Colorado data shows us that MVAs went up, fatal MVAs went up in Colorado involving marijuana usage.

And again going back to young people, I have got a teenager who is about to drive. The chips are already stacked against him. And we know that, just statistically speaking. The last thing we want is for these young people to think that marijuana use is safe or, Heaven forbid, that it actually will make them a better and more relaxed driver and lose even more of our teenagers on the roads now than what we already are.

The CHAIRMAN. I know much of your testimony so far has focused on adolescents, pregnant women, and people with other conditions that would maybe make them more vulnerable, but are you suggesting, by inference, that marijuana consumption for a consenting adult who is otherwise healthy is harm-free?

Dr. ADAMS. Well, as Surgeon General of the United States, the first thing I would say is absolutely not. There are plenty of substances out there which adults can partake of that are not only not harm-free, but which my office has a long history of trying to rein the horse back in on.

You mentioned tobacco. Alcohol is one of the top killers of folks in our country. I think that again we need to learn from our mistakes and be careful about normalization of behavior.

One of the other dangers about marijuana usage is that we do not know what we do not know. And so we do not want to conduct this experiment on our citizenry. And that is adults and young people. But we know enough about young people to take action now, and that is why I focused my efforts and my attention in that space at this point in time.

But again, sir, I do not want anyone to mistake what I am saying as implying that these products are considered safe for general adult usage.

The CHAIRMAN. Let me ask you about the research, because you have both referred to studies that have been done. Are there impediments, legal or otherwise, to the study of the health effects of marijuana in place?

Dr. ADAMS. I will start off just by saying that Secretary Azar, the President, and I, have all stated publicly we need to make it easier to do research.

The CHAIRMAN. What do we need to do to make that happen?

Dr. ADAMS. Well, HHS is partnering with DEA. We are going around the country and talking to folks to find out barriers that exist to research. One of the things that has been announced within the past month was DEA making more strains of marijuana available so that folks can test more than just the—from the one facility in Mississippi, where you could typically get strains from.

But Dr. Volkow is an expert in this area, and NIDA is intimately involved in the research process. So I would turn it over to her.

Dr. VOLKOW. Part of the problem relies on the fact that marijuana is a Schedule One. And if you want to do research on a Schedule One, you have to get a DEA registration that can take, if you are lucky, one year to obtain, and that delays the process enormously.

And every time that you make a change in your protocol, that also has to be submitted, and you have to wait for that to be approved. So it is a very lengthy, on the ability to get the research going. And then once you are going, right now the only source for marijuana that is available in our country is that that we provide through a contract to Missouri to a farm in Missouri.

So if you as a researcher are interested in a particular strain of marijuana, you come to us at NIDA, it is probably unlikely that we have it and we will have to cultivate it. So the process also is very slow there.

And finally, to the other component that makes it very difficult is that we are interested in understanding what people are taking out there. I mean, in the states they are legalizing marijuana and there are these dispensaries. And the varieties are very distinct.

And so we do not know the difference between this or that. This product is being sold telling that it has this characteristic. We cannot fund research that relates to products that are actually being bought through these dispensaries because it is illegal.

So we have been working for the past, I would say, several years with DEA to try to come up with an accommodation that would allow researchers to streamline the process so that they can work on an understanding both potentially negative but also potentially therapeutic effects of cannabids.

The CHAIRMAN. Well I know Senator Feinstein mentioned some legislation that she is working on with Senator Grassley on the impediments to research, but that is perhaps something that we could work on together.

Co-Chairman FEINSTEIN. Great. I would love it. Thank you.

Dr. ADAMS. Can I give a shout-out to Senator Feinstein? I am not allowed——

The CHAIRMAN. Absolutely.

Dr. ADAMS. I am not allowed to endorse or comment on pending legislation, but I was doing my homework. And you and Senator Grassley made a statement in the introduction of your legislation. You said medical treatment should be based on sound science, and for those who are sick that there are safe medications that have been proven effective.

I could not agree with that more. And I think it is very important that folks such as yourself are acknowledging that and spreading that word.

Co-Chairman FEINSTEIN. Thank you.

The CHAIRMAN. Senator Feinstein.

Co-Chairman FEINSTEIN. Thanks very much, Mr. Chairman.

And thank you—[coughing], excuse me, I have a little throat problem.

Dr. ADAMS. I am a doctor. I can help you with that. [Laughter.]

Co-Chairman FEINSTEIN. I may come to you.

As I understand, investigations are ongoing. To date, nearly 1,500 lung injuries have been associated with the use of e-cigarettes and vaping products, with 33 confirmed deaths.

THC has been present in most of the tested samples of these cases. Here is the question: Do we have enough research to understand the potential impacts of using e-cigarettes and vaping devices to consume marijuana products? What is the situation? And what happens to the lung when you use it?

Dr. ADAMS. Thank you for that question. This is something I am terribly concerned about, and that HHS is really mounting an all-hands-on-deck response to.

We have stood up our Emergency Operations Center at CDC. We are working with state and local health departments to get information in as quickly as possible. And you summarized it correctly, ma'am. A large number of these cases have been associated with vaping THC, particularly THC that has been obtained through the black market, if you will.

Co-Chairman FEINSTEIN. Explain what happens when you do this.

Dr. ADAMS. Ma'am, well as an anestheologist I can tell you, God did not mean for much of anything besides oxygen to go into your lungs. And when you aerosolize oil and then suck it into your lungs and let it re-accumulate on the lining of your lungs, it can cause all sorts of bad things to happen.

And I will also tell you, one of the big problems is we do not know what is in these pods. A lot of them are made on the black market, and the ones that are even made through, quote, "legitimate sources" we do not know all that is contained in them. And it is why last December I put out a Surgeon General's Advisory warning about the epidemic rise in vaping among young people, a 78 percent increase in vaping among students. And I pointed out at the time that a third of young people who were vaping had reported vaping marijuana.

So I would say to you, before I turn it over to Dr. Volkow that, number one, the FDA and the CDC advised against vaping products containing THC.

Number two, we advised not to modify or add any substances such as THC or other oils to products purchased in stores.

And finally, no amount of marijuana usage during pregnancy or adolescence, no matter how it enters the body, is known to be safe. And no pregnant woman or young person should be vaping.

Dr. Volkow?

Co-Chairman FEINSTEIN. Could I ask you a question? Have autopsies been done on the lungs of the 33 confirmed deaths? Do we know what happens to the lungs?

Dr. ADAMS. Ma'am, what I would say is that—and again, I used to run a state department of health in Indiana. And one of the challenges is that these investigations start at a local level, and a lot of times the decisions about which samples are going to be collected, and which autopsies are going to be done are made before the state department of health is even alerted.

And then the CDC finds out after that. So one of the big things that we are trying to help people understand is that we have to have a high index of suspicion. We have got to ask the right questions. And we should be doing an autopsy on all of these cases.

Co-Chairman FEINSTEIN. So autopsies have not been done?

Dr. ADAMS. On some of them, but not all of them, ma'am.

Co-Chairman FEINSTEIN. On some of them?

Dr. ADAMS. Yes.

Co-Chairman FEINSTEIN. Well what has been learned from the autopsies? What happens to the lungs?

Dr. ADAMS. We know that there is damage to the cells of the lungs, to the tissues of the lungs. There is a lot of misinformation out there. Some of these cases had been reported to be associated with Vitamin E, and that was the case for some but it actually looks—it is an inflammatory injury. It is almost—I am trying to think of a good comparison—but again, it is as if a cell——

Co-Chairman FEINSTEIN. Enough to cause death?

Dr. ADAMS. Oh, absolutely, ma'am. Lymphoid pneumonia has been found in some of these folks. But in other folks, it is as if the cells and the tissue were being eaten away. Again, you are putting toxic materials into the lungs that were never meant to be inhaled.

Dr. Volkow.

Dr. VOLKOW. Yeah, just basically in medical school they teach you that you should never, ever allow lipids to get into the lungs because they produce a very massive inflammatory reaction. So that's—and since you require the lungs to function properly for oxygen to be transferred, this is probably one of the reasons why it has had such negative effects.

But I think it is also highlighting how we are approving these technologies in ways without recognizing what their negative effects are. And you are highlighting the acute effects. But, for example, we do not know what may be the effects on the function of the lung long term in those cases that you do not see this acute presentation.

Co-Chairman FEINSTEIN. Well let me ask this question. Are vaping devices well enough known? Do they bring on death——

Dr. VOLKOW. Well, that——

Co-Chairman FEINSTEIN [continuing]. As it goes into the lungs? If you use—I do not know how to ask this question. If you use a vaping device, are you more apt to die?

Dr. VOLKOW. Not necessarily. You are using a device that has quality control. And, for example, one of the things that we have done at NIDA is to develop a standard electronic cigarette that can be used to determine whether, for people that cannot stop smoking, that use of these vaping devices can help them actually be able to protect them from the negative effects of combustible tobacco.

So provided that you have standards of quality control, both the device as well as the cartridges that you are using and the content of nicotine and the products, this device could be given as a therapeutic option for those that cannot stop smoking.

Dr. ADAMS. And can I answer that question in another way, ma'am?

Co-Chairman FEINSTEIN. Yes.

Dr. ADAMS. Even the people who are advocates for e-cigarettes and vaping devices describe them as "harm reduction." Less harm does not mean harmless. No young person, no pregnant woman, no person who is not currently smoking, should even entertain using these devices. Because, again, you are taking substances that are in an unknown pod, and you are vaporizing them and taking them back into the lungs. And whether that is marijuana, or anything else out there, again we do not know what we do not know. But we know that those substances were never intended to go into your lungs, and they can be toxic.

Co-Chairman FEINSTEIN. Yes. I have particular concern about marijuana use by very young children. And the fact that—reports have shown that it results in a decline in IQ, in poor school performance, and higher rates of school absences.

How prevalent is this?

Dr. ADAMS. Let me take that at the 30,000-foot level, and then kick it to Dr. Volkow. It is important for us to understand, and a lot of folks say, well, I have smoked a joint, or I smoked marijuana back in the '80s, back in the '70s. The potency is much, much higher. A higher THC content equals more danger.

Number two, not everyone is going to have the same effect. Every person is different. And so some people—as we know, some people smoke for five years and get lung cancer, and some people smoke for 50 years and do not get lung cancer.

But if you are talking about a child, you want to give that child— I have three young kids—the best chance at life.

Co-Chairman FEINSTEIN. Yes.

Dr. ADAMS. And we know that on a population level that the cumulative effects of having an entire population, 9 million young people using marijuana products is going to be a net negative for our country.

But do you want to get into specifics, Dr. Volkow?

Dr. VOLKOW. Yeah, I will just point out, I mean it is not surprising in a way because this endogenous cannabinoid system, one of the things that it does, it modulates the activation of neuronal networks. So when you are hyper-stimulated, it brings it down. When you are hyper-inhibited, it brings it up to create that certain window of optimal function. So if you are taking marijuana, in a way you are filtering many of those stimuli. And your development is dependent on those stimuli to actually create the final architecture.

Co-Chairman FEINSTEIN. How does marijuana impact school performance? What does it do to the brain?

Dr. VOLKOW. The simplest one, it interferes with memory and learning. Someone that is stoned cannot remember. And that is not just adolescents, that is any adult.

Co-Chairman FEINSTEIN. I did not know that.

Dr. VOLKOW. And as a result of that, if you are a student and your job is to learn, and marijuana stays in the body for a long time, you are going to have a long-lasting effect in your capacity to memorize and you will fail school.

And that is without addressing the possibility that——

Co-Chairman FEINSTEIN. Is the memory loss permanent?

Dr. VOLKOW. That is a question that there is controversy. There is some evidence that there is long-lasting impairment in memory and attention by some studies, and others show that after several months it recovers.

And we don't—that is one of the reasons why we are doing the ABCD study, to actually, unequivocally determine if long-term use of marijuana will produce a long-lasting or irreversible change in memory, attention, and other process of cognition.

Co-Chairman FEINSTEIN. Wow. Is it because marijuana today is stronger, the THC factor?

Dr. VOLKOW. That is not going to help at all. The content is much, much higher. And the higher the content—it is actually three-fold higher overall, and——

Co-Chairman FEINSTEIN. Wait, wait, wait. I am not trying to— three times higher than when?

Dr. VOLKOW. Than 2002.

Co-Chairman FEINSTEIN. Really?

Dr. VOLKOW. Yes.

Dr. ADAMS. Ma'am, there was a study that looked at marijuana from 1995 till 2014, and they saw that marijuana in 1995 the average strains were about 4.5 percent THC. The average strains in 2014 were about 12 percent. So that is where we get the three times number. But it is important to remember now that dispensaries have marijuana that is testing at about 20, 25 percent. So that would be five times stronger than 1995.

And then when you put it into oils and waxes, you can get 70, 80, 90 percent THC. So I hate comparisons, but something that I say to folks that tends to resonate is, that is like the difference between having a light beer in 1995 and drinking a pint of vodka today. It is literally that much of a difference in concentration.

Co-Chairman FEINSTEIN. I do not think people know that.

Dr. ADAMS. I do not think they do either, ma'am.

Co-Chairman FEINSTEIN. How do we get that out?

Dr. ADAMS. Well, again, the Surgeon General Advisory. We need you all to help share it at surgeongeneral.gov. Please let people know this ain't your mother's marijuana.

Dr. VOLKOW. And the other problem that is confounded is that when you go and buy a product, you do not actually know what the content of 9 THC is. And this particularly becomes problematic when you get an edible. You get the chocolate and you do not know the content, and so you do not know how much to take of it.

And one of the reasons why people end up in emergency room admission with a psychotic episode is because the content is so high.

Co-Chairman FEINSTEIN. Well, now how big a problem is this?

Dr. VOLKOW. In terms of emergency department——

Co-Chairman FEINSTEIN. No, the high content of hallucinogenic quality in marijuana today versus 10—excuse me, 10, 15 years ago?

Dr. VOLKOW. It is very problematic. And studies have consistently shown, for example, that investigate the negative effects of marijuana that the higher the content of 9–THC the greater the likelihood that you will have a psychotic episode. The greater the likelihood, actually, the risks associated with schizophrenia——

Co-Chairman FEINSTEIN. Which changes the nature of beliefs about marijuana. Because most people that I know believe it is relatively harmless. And what you are saying is, it is not today; that it is much stronger, and that it is much more volatile.

Dr. ADAMS. Exactly. And Dr. Volkow is an expert and speaks on the effects on the individual, and she has, again, spoken of her wonderful brain imaging studies. I tend to look at the population level. And the metrics we look at are motor vehicle accidents going up. Emergency department admissions going up.

Co-Chairman FEINSTEIN. For marijuana use? You can prove that?

Dr. ADAMS. Yes, ma'am. The emergency department admissions have gone up for accidental ingestions and for people showing up with psychosis. We are seeing all sorts of untoward effects from marijuana usage, again particularly in young people. But real concerning population health trends related to marijuana usage.

Co-Chairman FEINSTEIN. Could you provide us with some information? We may want to put out a paper as a result of this, and that might be one of the things that we would discuss.

The CHAIRMAN. Well I know that has been one of the functions of this Caucus in the past, is to issue reports or papers on different topics, and certainly that is something we ought to consider doing.

Co-Chairman FEINSTEIN. Because I have young people in my family and, you know, you think it is all nothing. Hopefully they do not use it, but they sure can talk about it. So I think if I am understanding what you are saying, the potential danger of marijuana has gone up rather dramatically in the last 10, 15 years?

Dr. ADAMS. The potential danger has gone up, while the perceived harm of the product has gone down. And what I was quoting in my opening statement was NISDA data that looks at—that surveys young people from SAMPHSA. SAMPHSA data that surveys young people and asks them their perception of the dangers of marijuana. And their perceptions of danger are going down, particularly in states that have legalized, because they see it all around them. While the actual risk, both from a scientific point of view and on a population health level, is going up.

Co-Chairman FEINSTEIN. What has California done?

Dr. ADAMS. Well, you have got someone from the California Cannabis Research Commission who is going to be on the second panel.

Co-Chairman FEINSTEIN. Oh, good.

Dr. ADAMS. And I have been out there. I visited U.C. Davis. I have visited U.C.S.D. I have been to the L.A. County Health Department. I will tell you that all of the health officials I have spoken to are terribly concerned about the spike in pregnant women who are using.

We have seen a doubling in pregnant women who report using marijuana, and they are concerned about the number of young people. It is causing disciplinary problems in schools, and we do not know what the long-term health effects are going to be. So in your State, ma'am, we are very concerned.

Co-Chairman FEINSTEIN. So just quickly, how is it more concentrated, more volatile, than it used to be?

Dr. VOLKOW. The plant itself. I mean, like in biology you can determine the content of the active ingredients by breeding up varieties that have higher content. And that is how they have come up with plants that have higher and higher content, manipulating it. And now, with the use of resins, you can extract the active ingredient and put it in a cartridge——

Co-Chairman FEINSTEIN. Oh, dear.

Dr. VOLKOW [continuing]. And that gives you even higher content. So this is just basically genetic, what the agricultural business has been doing to try to improve on the quality of the plants.

Co-Chairman FEINSTEIN. So we should not regard it as "harmless"?

Dr. VOLKOW. Oh, it is not harmless at all. And when you were asking about your own state, there were actually showing me that one of the emergency departments in one of the main hospitals in San Diego where they basically will have an eight-fold increase in emergency admissions from the cannabis over a period of eight years. Eight-fold. It is gigantic.

Co-Chairman FEINSTEIN. This is not just vaping——

Dr. VOLKOW. This is not just vaping——

Co-Chairman FEINSTEIN. Oh, I thought you said——

Dr. VOLKOW [continuing]. And smoking, and edibles, and every single way of administering cannabis.

Co-Chairman FEINSTEIN. So if a mother uses this strong stuff while she is pregnant, will that impact——

Dr. VOLKOW. She can become psychotic herself. High-content THC, what people do not realize is high-content marijuana with very high THC can trigger an acute psychotic episode. And that leads you to the emergency department. It is a horrible experience.

Co-Chairman FEINSTEIN. What if she is pregnant? What does it do to the unborn child?

Dr. VOLKOW. Well, you have there, on top of the negative effects to the mother, the fact that the marijuana will go into the fetus and affect the brain of the fetus. The fetus cannot complain, right?

Co-Chairman FEINSTEIN. Right.

Dr. VOLKOW. But it is going to very likely be interfering. Imagine that there is this very precise process by which your brain determines when this neuron migrates here, when this neuron divides, when this neuron interconnects with another, and that is modulated by your own endogenous cannabinoid system.

When you artificially stimulate that system, you are basically disrupting all of that perfect orchestration. That is why we have so much concern about the use of marijuana among pregnant women, children, and adolescents.

Co-Chairman FEINSTEIN. Can a baby be born addicted to marijuana?

Dr. VOLKOW. I do not know of any description of a baby having been born addicted to marijuana. But what we do know is that babies can be born sedated because of the use of marijuana, particularly during the last trimester.

But the condition of a baby that is born addicted, that has not been something that has been documented.

Dr. ADAMS. And ma'am, something that again I was just in your state two weeks ago talking about were the infant mortality rates. We know one of the predictors of infant mortality is low birth weight. Well I was shocked when I saw the Colorado PRAMS data that showed that women who smoke marijuana have a 50 percent increased chance of having a baby born at low birth weight.

And so that is another thing that people do not think about when they are prescribing marijuana to women who are pregnant or could be becoming pregnant.

Co-Chairman FEINSTEIN. Thank you.

The CHAIRMAN. Well, unfortunately we are going to have to stop there with the first panel, because we obviously have a lot of questions and we want to continue the conversation, but we want to get to the second panel, too.

So thank you, Dr. Adams, Dr. Volkow, for your contribution. And, believe me, we want to continue the conversation. Because as you can see, Senator Feinstein and I, and I am sure our other colleagues who could not be here today, have a lot of questions. And I think the American people deserve the facts, which is what we are trying to get to here.

So thank you very much, and we will invite the second panel to come forward and get situated, and we will get started in just a second.

Dr. ADAMS. And, Senator, we are happy to submit any information you need about the harms of marijuana usage that we have collected. Please share my Advisory, surgeongeneral.gov. We need to get the word out to folks that this is not some harmless product out there.

The CHAIRMAN. We will do that, sir. Thank you.

Dr. VOLKOW. And thanks for doing the hearing.

The CHAIRMAN. Thank you.

(Pause.)

Well thank you very much. Our second panel includes experts who have conducted research on various aspects of public health and marijuana use.

First, Dr. Robert Fitzgerald, who currently serves as a Professor in the Department of Pathology at the University of California-San Diego, where he is also the Director of the Toxicology Laboratory, Director of the Toxicology Laboratory, and Associate Director of the Clinical Chemistry Laboratory. He is Board Certified in Toxicology and Clinical Chemistry by the American Board of Clinical Chemistry, and his research, Senator Feinstein, focuses on marijuana-impaired driving. I know you had questions about that.

Dr. Staci Gruber is Director of the Cognitive and Clinical Neural Imaging Core and the Marijuana Investigations for the Neuroscientific Discovery Program, otherwise called the MIND Program, both housed at the Harvard-affiliated Psychiatric Hospital in Belmont, Massachusetts' McLean Hospital. She is also an Associate Professor of Psychiatry at Harvard Medical School. Her research focuses on cognitive development and the effects of marijuana's major constituent compounds.

Dr. Sean Hennessy is Professor of Epidemiology in Bio Statistics at the University of Pennsylvania's Perelman School of Medicine. Dr. Hennessy conducts research in the field of pharmacoepidemiology. That is a mouthful. Which is the study of the health effects of drugs and other medical products in populations. Dr. Hennessy is the past Scientific Chair and past President of the International Society for Pharmacoepidemiology and has served as the FDA's Drug Safety and Risk Management Advisory—served on that committee, the Drug Safety and Risk Management Advisory Committee for the FDA. Dr. Hennessy contributed to the National Academies of Science's 2017 Study on Marijuana's Health Effects.

And finally, Dr. Madeline Meier is the Assistant Professor of Psychology at Arizona State University and Post-Doctoral Fellow, with support from the Duke University Trans Disciplinary Prevention Research Center. Her research interests involve adolescent marijuana use, as well as the health effects of marijuana concentrates. So obviously there is a lot of interest in what you have to say.

If I could first recognize Dr. Fitzgerald and ask each of you maybe to speak for about five minutes, and then maybe be open to some questions. Your written remarks will be made part of the record, without further ado.

So, Dr. Fitzgerald.

Statement of Robert Fitzgerald, Ph.D., Professor of Pathology, University of California–San Diego, California

Dr. FITZGERALD. Thank you, Senator, Senator Feinstein. It is a pleasure to be here today to discuss issues related to marijuana and driving.

As a way of brief introduction, my first job out of graduate school was as a forensic toxicologist from the State of Virginia where I helped work with the medical examiner to determine the cause and manner of death in medical examiner's cases.

At the ME's office, I saw the devastating effects of driving under the influence on a routine basis. I also had the opportunity to work with both state and local law officers, along with prosecution and defense, to present scientific data in courts of law.

Currently I am a clinical toxicologist at UC–San Diego where my research focuses on developing analytical methods to measure concentrations of THC and metabolites following recent marijuana exposure.

I am part of a large team of investigators at the University of California-San Diego's Center for Medical Cannabis Research focused on understanding both beneficial and detrimental effects of cannabis on human health. We recently completed enrolling subjects in one of the largest studies to date looking at the effect of smoked marijuana on driving performance, and are in the initial stages of analyzing this data.

The relationship between marijuana use and driving impairment is complex because of the unique pharmacokinetics—that is the time course in the body, and pharmacodynamics—that is its physiological effects—of THC.

With ethanol there is a clear relationship between amount consumed, blood concentrations, and effect on driving. With marijuana, these types of relationships are much more complex.

The relationship between blood THC concentrations and crash risk has not been established. But there is a clear understanding that THC impairs driving performance. The question that remains is how to best identify drivers who are impaired by marijuana. There are no perfect solutions, and legislative directives must balance keeping our roadways safe with due process.

The problems with determining the relationship between concentrations of THC and impairment is that levels of THC vary widely depending on the route of administration, the time of sampling after dosing, and the characteristics of the individual consuming.

Generally, smoked marijuana causes effects that start shortly after inhalation and last for about three hours. While subjects who eat marijuana start feeling effects about an hour later, and can have effects up to eight hours later.

Unlike alcohol, which is cleared within 24 hours of drinking, THC and several metabolites accumulate in the body with repeated dosing. So frequent users have baseline concentrations of THC that exceed the per se limits in many states.

After smoking, THC concentrations in blood change rapidly. And our studies have documented the poor relationship between concentrations of THC and measures of impairment. Studies like this led the National Safety Council to put out a Position Statement in 2017 that reads: "It is further concluded that, due to rapid changes in blood THC concentrations over time, there is no minimum safe threshold blood concentration below which a driver can be considered to have been unaffected while driving following recent marijuana use. Consequently, there is no scientific basis for the adoption of THC per se laws for driving."

This statement was also supported by the International Association of Chiefs of Police. Despite these position statements, 18 states currently have some form of per se statutes.

How do we keep our roads safe? In California, prosecution of driving under the influence of drugs is currently based on officer observations combined with toxicology testing. This practice will likely continue for the foreseeable future.

Since there is no reasonable expectation that THC or a metabolite of THC will be useful for per se impairment, an alternative approach would be to develop methods that identify recent use. The biological specimens that could be used to determine if a driver has recently used marijuana are blood, breath, and oral fluid.

The primary advantage of breath and oral fluid over blood is that they can be collected at the roadside at the time of a traffic stop, as opposed to blood which typically takes about 90 minutes to collect.

This is an important consideration because, unlike ethanol, concentrations of THC fall by more than 90 percent in that short time frame. There is a variety of ongoing efforts to identify recent-use markers.

In respect to my time limit, I would like to close my initial statement by mentioning two items that I think this Caucus needs to be aware of so they can help shape appropriate regulations.

Due to federal restrictions, investigators cannot study the cannabis products our population is exposed to. As Dr. Adams indicated, we have unleashed a massive experiment that is sort of uncontrolled in our population, and our most powerful resources, our research community, has limited ability to study that.

This is a critically important public health issue that needs to be changed. Currently there is no standardized data collection for driving under the influence of drugs. Without good data, it is difficult to develop good policy.

I hope my testimony was helpful and look forward to answering questions. Thank you.

The CHAIRMAN. Thank you very much. Dr. Gruber.

Statement of Staci Gruber, Ph.D., Professor of Psychiatry, Harvard Medical School, Boston, Massachusetts

Dr. GRUBER. Thank you, Senator Cornyn and Senator Feinstein, and members of the Caucus who may tune in later to see this——

Co-Chairman FEINSTEIN. Could you speak directly into the microphone?

Dr. GRUBER. Certainly. Is that better?

Co-Chairman Feinstein. Yes.

Dr. GRUBER. I should be better at this.

So as you have heard, and as we know, the Nation is in the midst of a green rush, and marijuana or cannabis headlines flood news outlets daily. Yet it is often difficult for people to read through study findings and make sense of what we know and what we do not.

Despite the fact that 33 states have fully legalized medical marijuana, and another 15 have limited medical marijuana laws, leaving only 2 states without access, nearly all of what we know about the impact of marijuana comes from studies of recreational marijuana users.

These studies typically focus on those with chronic, heavy marijuana use. Data across studies is somewhat inconsistent, but generally reflect differences between those who use marijuana and those who do not spanning a number of areas that we have heard allusions to already, including cognitive performance. Domains most commonly affected include memory and executive functioning. For example, the ability to inhibit inappropriate responses, or to use feedback to change one's behavior. These are reportedly impacted by marijuana use.

Earlier onset of marijuana use, as well as higher frequency and magnitude of use, are also associated with greater difficulty on these tasks. And studies of brain structure and function have also reported deficits or differences between marijuana users and non-users, specifically as among early onset or adolescent users of marijuana.

This is not surprising. As you heard from Dr. Volkow, we know that during adolescence the brain is neuro-developmentally vulnerable. That is, it is under construction. It is sensitive not just to marijuana but to other substances—alcohol, illness, injury.

Another concern that we have heard a lot about today is the rising potency of marijuana products. Particularly problematic for youth, our most vulnerable consumer group, THC, the primary intoxicating compound of the plant has increased 300 percent, or more than three-fold, in flower products since 1995. And these novel concentrate products that we have also heard illusions to, Dabs, Shatter, Wax, you have heard these terms, THC levels of these products go at least up to and sometimes north of 90 percent. Cannabidiol, or CBD, may mitigate some of the negative effects that we see from THC, but it is virtually undetectable in recreational products today. Thus far there have been no studies that have directly assessed the impact of potency or novel versus conventional products in either recreational consumers or medical patients.

It is also important to remember that not all marijuana use is the same. And our recreational marijuana consumers are not the same as our medical marijuana patients.

For example, their goal of use is wholly different. Our recreational marijuana consumers—I have spent nearly 30 years with these folks—their goal is to change their current state of being, or to get high. Our medical marijuana patients are not interested in getting high. They use to alleviate symptoms. They say things like I want to sleep through the night. I would like to be able to take a drive with my son. I want to go for a walk with my kids.

As a result, their product choices are often different. Recreational consumers often choose products very high in THC. Our medical patients choose products that may be high in THC but often contain other compounds, things like cannabidiol or other non-intoxicating compounds.

Cannabis and cannabinoids have demonstrated therapeutic potential for a number of indications. We heard reference to the 2017 National Academy's report noting conclusive or substantial evidence that cannabis or cannabinoids were effective for, quote, "the big three, chronic pain, nausea and vomiting as a function of chemotherapy, and muscle spasticity as a function of MS.

We also know that epadadialexis or purified CBD extract was approved for pediatric onset intractable seizure disorders. But despite the fact that medical cannabis has been legal since 1996, data regarding the impact of medical marijuana treatment is severely limited. Preliminary evidence from the very first longitudinal studies of medical marijuana patients demonstrate improvements in some areas of cognitive performance, including areas noted to be impaired in those with recreational use.

We also see improvements in clinical state, better sleep, decreased pain, and notable reductions in the use of conventional medications including opioids, so important in the midst of this crisis.

When it comes to marijuana, one size does not fit all. We have a single term, marijuana, and we often hear it used to refer to anything like the whole plant or individual compounds from the plant, intoxicating or not, which mean very different things.

Current regulations around marijuana limit the type and scope of research projects we can do. And, contrary to popular belief, we cannot currently study the impact of products that patients and consumers are actually using via clinical trial models, significantly reducing external or ecologic validity.

Further, as Dr. Volkow testified, the Schedule One status of marijuana leads to a number of obstacles in conducting research. Policy at this point has clearly outpaced science. And as the Nation has warmed toward both the use of medical and recreational marijuana, the need for empirically sound data is critical in order to maximize benefit and reduce harm.

Regardless of how you feel about marijuana, science and not emotion or rhetoric must be our guide. We have a responsibility to provide the best and most accurate data to our medical marijuana patients, our recreational consumers, our health care providers, and the general public so they can make the best, most informed decisions about marijuana use.

At this point, I would thank you for your ongoing efforts and being willing to help move things forward. Thank you.

The CHAIRMAN. Thank you, Dr. Gruber. Dr. Hennessy.

Statement of Sean Hennessy, Pharm.D., Ph.D., Professor of Epidemiology, University of Pennsylvania Perelman School of Medicine, Philadelphia, Pennsylvania

Dr. HENNESSY: Good afternoon, Senators. My name is Sean Hennessy and I am a Pharmacist Epidemiologist at the University of Pennsylvania. I was a member of the 16-person committee that wrote this 468-page report entitled "The Health Effects of Cannabis and Cannabinoids" that the National Academics of Science, Engineering, and Medicine released in January 2017.

The report is a comprehensive review and synthesis of the thenexisting literature about the potential health effects, both therapeutic and harmful, of cannabis and cannabis-derived products.

The report lists nearly 100 different conclusions about these effects. It also discusses four barriers to conducting research on cannabis and makes four recommendations on how to address research gaps.

I would like to summarize this report as 6–4–4. Six health effects with high-level evidence. Four challenges to conducting research. And four recommendations to moving forward. So among the highest levels of evidence about the health effects of cannabis we made the following conclusions.

One, cannabis use prior to driving appears to increase the risk of motor vehicle crashes, as we have heard about today.

Two, in states where cannabis is legal, there is an increased risk of unintentional cannabis overdose in children.

Three, pregnant women who smoke cannabis increase the risk that their baby will be born with lower birth weight.

Four, initiating cannabis use at a younger age is a risk factor for developing problematic cannabis use later in life.

Five, long-term cannabis smoking increases the risk of chronic breathing problems. And six, some people with chronic pain or muscle spasm from multiple sclerosis can obtain relief of their symptoms using cannabis-based products.

Most of the studies for these uses examined orally administered cannabis extracts, rather than smoked cannabis. The report also identified the following four challenges to conducting research on the health effects of cannabis.

One, there are specific regulatory barriers, including the classification of cannabis as a Schedule One substance that impede research.

Two, it is difficult for researchers to gain access to the quantity, quality, and type of cannabis product that they need to conduct research.

Three, it is difficult to obtain funding to support cannabis research. And four, improvement and standardization in research methods are needed.

Finally, the report makes the following four recommendations: One, public health agencies and other groups should fund a national cannabis research agenda.

Two, agencies of the U.S. Department of Health and Human Services should convene a workshop to develop a set of federal standards and benchmarks to guide high-quality research on cannabis.

Three, federal, state, and local health authorities should fund improvements to the public health surveillance system.

And four, the CDC, NIH, FDA, and others should convene a committee to characterize regulatory barriers and propose strategies to develop the resources and infrastructure that are needed to conduct cannabis research.

I thank you for your attention and the opportunity to discuss these important issues, and look forward to answering your questions.

The CHAIRMAN. Thank you, Dr. Hennessy. Dr. Meier.

Statement of Madeline Meier, Ph.D., Assistant Professor of Psychology, Arizona State University, Tempe, Arizona

Dr. MEIER. Good afternoon, Mr. Chairman and Senator Feinstein.

Co-Chairman FEINSTEIN. Could you speak directly into the mike? It is hard to hear.

Dr. MEIER. Thank you for inviting me to contribute to my knowledge about cannabis effects on cognitive functioning.

The most comprehensive study of cannabis use in cognitive functioning was published by our group in 2012. Today I am going to describe that 2012 study and explain the findings, why they are important, and what additional research is needed.

We have studied the association between persistent cannabis use over time and change in IQ from childhood to adulthood. And we asked whether cannabis effects on IQ were concentrated among adolescent onset cannabis users. That is, cannabis users who began using before age 18.

Data came from the Dunedin Study, which is a study of 1,000 children born in 1972 and '73 in Dunedin, New Zealand, and followed from birth to age 38, with 96 percent of the sample taking part in the study at age 38.

IQ was tested at age 13, before anybody in the cohort had started using cannabis, and again at age 38 after some members of the cohort had been using cannabis for years. We found that persistent cannabis use from ages 18 to 38 was associated with decline in IQ. And this decline in IQ was concentrated among adolescent onset persistent cannabis users. These are cannabis users who began using cannabis before age 18 and continued using for many years thereafter.

Specifically, individuals who began using cannabis in adolescence before age 18, and used it for years showed an average 8 point IQ decline from childhood to adulthood. However, individuals who used cannabis short-term in adolescence showed only weak evidence of IQ decline.

Further, individuals who began using cannabis in adulthood sometime after age 18 did not show decline in IQ even when they used persistently.

Quitting or reducing cannabis use did not fully restore intellectual functioning. Decline in IQ could not be explained by alcohol or other drug use, or by reduced years of education among cannabis users.

Decline in IQ could also not be explained by low childhood socioeconomic status or poor childhood self-regulation. Friends and relatives reported noticing more attention and memory problems in everyday life among the persistent cannabis users. These findings are important for a number of reasons.

First, an especially important feature of this study is that we had IQ test data from both before and after study members started using cannabis. This allowed us to rule out the possibility that IQ deficits in cannabis users predate the onset of cannabis use.

We showed that regardless of their IQ test performance in childhood, adolescent onset persistent cannabis users performed worse than nonusers, and worse than adult onset cannabis users on IQ tests in adulthood.

Second, the eight-point IQ decline we observed among cannabis users who began using cannabis in adolescence and continued using for many years is non-trivial. For example, an average person has an IQ of 100, placing them in the 50th percentile for intelligence, compared to same-age peers. If this average person loses 8 IQ points, they drop from the 50th to the 29th percentile for intelligence.

Third, IQ is a predictor of a person's access to a college education, their lifelong total income, their access to a good job, and their performance on the job. Individuals who lose 8 IQ points may be disadvantaged relative to their same-age peers in many important aspects of life. In fact, the adolescent onset persistent cannabis users from our 2012 study ended up in occupations that were less prestigious, less skilled, and less well paid than their parents' occupations.

Finally, only about 2 percent of the sample became those adolescent onset persistent cannabis users. Thus, any effect of cannabis on IQ is confined to a relatively small segment of the population. Nonetheless, findings are concerning given that fewer adolescents today believe that regular cannabis use presents a serious health risk.

Additional research is needed to answer the following questions:

One, what are the mechanisms underlying cannabis-related IQ decline?

Two, what are the parameters of cannabis use that determine the magnitude and persistence of cognitive deficits? These are things like frequency, duration, quantity of use, and potency.

Three, does cognitive functioning recover with abstinence?

Four, are there individual differences in susceptibility to cannabis-related cognitive deficits?

To answer these questions, we need large-scale longitudinal studies to follow use from before to well after cannabis initiation, and to combine cognitive testing with brain imaging to better understand the mechanisms that might underlie cannabis-related decline in IQ.

The Adolescent Brain and Cognitive Development Study was launched in part to meet this need. Thank you.

The CHAIRMAN. Thank you, Dr. Meier.

Welcome, Senator Rosen. Thank you for joining us. Let me start with a five-minute round of questioning.

Dr. Gruber, just a point of clarification. We heard from the previous panel that THC concentrations in recreational marijuana have at least tripled. But I see in your paper you say that you believe it has quadrupled from 1995 to 2017. Is that correct?

Dr. GRUBER. I think the prior panel referenced the paper that was published——

I think the prior panel referenced the paper that was——

Co-Chairman FEINSTEIN. Louder, please? I'm sorry.

Dr. GRUBER. Sure. Is that better? I think the prior panel referenced the publication from 2014——

The CHAIRMAN. Oh, okay.

Dr. GRUBER. At that time, the difference from '95 to 2014 was about three times.

The CHAIRMAN. Three times?

Dr. GRUBER. Right now, the average potency across the Nation from government-seized products is about 17 percent. That is contrasted to about just under 4 percent in 1995.

The Chairman. Okay, so that is significant. You think the best information is it has quadrupled in concentration?

Dr. GRUBER. I would say in terms of national averages for THC, that is right.

The CHAIRMAN. But——

Dr. GRUBER. Those were recreational products.

The CHAIRMAN. But you also point out—and this is really the point I wanted to get to—is that there are concentrates, other products that have been created. You mentioned things like Dabs, the colloquial name for concentrated oil, created by extracting THC from flower-based marijuana products, Shatter Wax, Butter, and others, that all have a significantly higher concentration potency compared to conventional marijuana products as high as 80 percent more concentrated. Is that correct?

Dr. GRUBER. Or higher, absolutely right. This is the recreational market that is very focused on increased THC because if the goal of use is to become intoxicated, or to change your current state of being, you are looking for products that will deliver that bigger bang for the buck, if you will. So these products are very, very popular and becoming more popular across the Nation in the recreational market.

The CHAIRMAN. Well it strikes me as significant. If you smoke it, it is about four times more powerful than it was in 1995. But you can take it in a concentrated form that could be 80 percent of traditional marijuana product.

Dr. GRUBER. Exactly. THC is significantly higher, as we heard from our first panel, significantly higher these days than in prior years.

The CHAIRMAN. Well I can imagine just from a scientific standpoint trying to figure out what the dosing is, and what the effect of a dose is very difficult given the range of ways that people can get access to the active ingredient.

Dr. GRUBER. Mode of use is very important in terms of onset of effects and duration of effects. Absolutely true. Especially important for our medical cannabis patients.

The CHAIRMAN. Dr. Fitzgerald, you have done a lot of work, you said, in terms of its impact on impaired drivers. Would it be fair to say that the concentration of THC and whether it is consumed from recreational use of smoking marijuana compared to these concentrates? Does it have a—is there a correlation between the concentration of the product that you consume and the level of impairment for drivers?

Dr. FITZGERALD. So I think that is one of the issues that Dr. Adams brought up, as well, is that we have not even been able to study the Dabs and the concentrates. It is not possible to do those studies, currently.

The CHAIRMAN. But those are not standardized products? I mean, like you would be able—you cannot compare widgets to widgets, I guess.

Dr. FITZGERALD. Correct.

The CHAIRMAN. Because they are all sort of concocted by whoever makes them, according to their own recipe, and the like.

Dr. FITZGERALD. Several issues there. One, we do not know what is actually in those. They are labeled. California actually does have a reasonably good laboratory system for analyzing plant materials, as well as Dabs and things for pesticides and concentrations of THC. But that is only in the legal market. And the legal market, unfortunately, is a small share of the total market of recreational marijuana.

The CHAIRMAN. As we know, there has been an unfortunate increase in suicides in the country, a lot of concerns about our Veterans in particular, but not just Veterans. It is just young people and others who end up taking their life.

I wonder, do you find any correlation between self-medication of people with underlying mental health disorders that get exacerbated by the use of marijuana or some of these concentrated products?

I do not know who would be the most appropriate person to ask. If you have an opinion, please jump in.

Dr. GRUBER. I have an opinion, since I work in a psychiatric hospital and have been seeing the patients for about 30 years.

The CHAIRMAN. It sounds to me like you are qualified.

Dr. GRUBER. Maybe, I don't know. It's under debate. I can tell you that there are many, many patient populations that derive real benefit from using cannabis or cannabinoid-based products. And the potential risk for individuals with undiagnosed conditions or disorders—you know, where we hear about these individuals who are using and not necessarily disclosing, or they are self-medicating. One of the important things to be mindful of is that it is not necessarily the cannabis. But we have to be mindful of what is driving the cannabis use.

Individuals who have different types of conditions, as I mentioned, often get benefit from use. But it is very, very important to watch these people over time and to look at the impact versus, you know, sort of a cross-sectional assessment, in a longitudinal fashion.

No doubt some individuals with differing conditions have their conditions exacerbated by cannabis use. That is why it is so important to be able to identify the most likely compounds from the plant which may make things worse versus those which may make things better.

In fact there is evidence to suggest some compounds from the plant may actually really positively impact some of these conditions that we see. And this is why so many people are turning toward them. But without real empirically sound data to guide these types of studies, we have limited ability to give them information.

The CHAIRMAN. Well my understanding, my layman's understanding, is that there is some evidence that epilepsy can be treated using THC-related products.

Dr. GRUBER. Cannabidiol.

The CHAIRMAN. Okay. Is there any—what other benefits have you been able to identify based at least on anecdotal information, in the absence of these longitudinal studies? What other benefits do you suspect may be derived from use of marijuana?

Dr. GRUBER. So different compounds from the plant may very well have individualized benefits. We know about cannabidiol. I think this was mentioned in your bill. Cannabidiol has been shown to potentially be efficacious not just for epilepsy, which is now approved by the FDA, Epidialial Schedule Five, but for other conditions. There have been some interesting studies, including preclinical work, in areas like anxiety. A number of different conditions may be positively impacted by cannabidiol. Other compounds may yield, again, therapeutic potential, but we do not have much in the way of long-term studies. And unfortunately, it is very difficult to study these compounds using clinical trial models, sort of the gold standard for deriving empirically sound data, given our current restrictions.

We have an ongoing—we just started a long-term clinical trial, open label to double-blind, of a whole plant full spectrum product for patients with anxiety. This data will be very, very important since so many people turn to things like CBD and they say it is good for this, it is good for this, and it would be great to have empirically sound data to lean on to actually guide patients and care givers.

The CHAIRMAN. I even have a friend who said they put CBD product in their pet food——

Dr. GRUBER. Sure.

The CHAIRMAN [continuing]. So their pet—it relieves their pet of anxiety. So I guess it cures everything.

Dr. GRUBER. I do not know about everything, but there is some data from studies outside of this country, small studies, in terms of cannabidiols' impact on anxiety, some pre-clinical work, and finally some work here. So it certainly begs the question of how much more we need, which in my opinion is a lot more. But we are starting.

The CHAIRMAN. Thank you. Doctor—Doctor Feinstein? Senator Feinstein. [Laughter.]

Co-Chairman FEINSTEIN. Thank you. Thirty-three states and the District of Columbia have legalized marijuana in some form. And each state has its own laws and regulations.

Should we be concerned that the lack of uniformity across states in terms of testing, labeling, packaging, the strength of products that may be sold, how they may be advertised, and how they may be accessed, can lead to consumer confusion? And this could produce unintended acute public health effects, including increased emergency room visits.

In Colorado, for example, there was a three-fold increase in marijuana-related emergency room visits between 2012 and 2016. So here is the question:

Would uniform regulations across states be helpful to ensure consumer safety and reduce public health impacts such as emergency room visits associated with marijuana use? Who would like to go— why don't we just go right down the line. If you have a comment, make it. If you do not, you do not.

Dr. FITZGERALD. Yes, certainly I think California is a model there for the fact that all the state-approved marijuana has actually been through a very sophisticated testing scheme to show its purity, show that it does not have pesticides, show it does not have fungus, and those things. There is some question about the reliability of different laboratories, and it would be nice to have a reference laboratory that everyone else sort of standardizes against. That would be useful to have uniform labeling. And certainly the CDC can be helpful in that regard.

Co-Chairman FEINSTEIN. Thank you.

Dr. GRUBER. I think it is incredibly important to have uniformity.

Co-Chairman FEINSTEIN. I am having trouble hearing you.

Dr. GRUBER. I think it is incredibly important to have uniformity, and even more important to have full disclosure of "what's in your weed"? People have no idea very often what they are getting. So I think it is incredibly important, since states make their own, sort of their own rules and regulations about what is allowed.

In my State of Massachusetts—and I spend a lot of time in California as well—these things are clearly defined in terms of testing for aflatoxins, heavy metals, pesticides, contaminants, yeast, mold——

Co-Chairman FEINSTEIN. So a standard across the United States would be helpful?

Dr. GRUBER. I think having a reference standard would be incredibly important in making sure every state does thorough testing is critical.

Co-Chairman FEINSTEIN. Thank you.

Dr. HENNESSY. I agree. I do not have anything to add.

Co-Chairman FEINSTEIN. Thank you.

Dr. MEIER. I agree, as well, and do not have anything additional to add.

Co-Chairman FEINSTEIN. Okay. What is the most common form of marijuana concentrate being used by adolescents? And how much THC does it contain? Adolescent use is my big concern.

Dr. MEIER. My group just published I believe the first epidemiological study of that. And we found that you can talk about concentrates as a general class, but there are two really different types of concentrates—one that is extracted using a solvent like butane— and those tend to have generally higher concentrations than the other class of concentrates where the THC is extracted using ice, or just rubbing it. And that has still much higher THC content than, for example, marijuana which is the buds of the cannabis plant. And that adolescents are using all of that. But primarily they are using the solvent-extracted——

Co-Chairman FEINSTEIN. They are using the what?

Dr. MEIER. The solvent-extracted concentrates.

Co-Chairman FEINSTEIN. What is that?

Dr. MEIER. Which go by names, various names. Dabs is the generic name to refer to just taking a very small kind of waxy piece of the concentrate. But then there's Butane Hash Oil, or they call it BHO, and it is called that because you extract the concentrate with butane solvent.

It is also called "Honey Oil," "Crumble," lots of different names for it. And while those products look different, one can look like a waxy sticky substance, one can look like butter, they all contain similarly high levels of THC.

Co-Chairman FEINSTEIN. Ah-hah. So are they heavily used by adolescents?

Dr. MEIER. We know from the State of Arizona one in four adolescents have said they have tried concentrates.

Co-Chairman FEINSTEIN. So what would you suggest we do, if anything?

Dr. MEIER. I think we need—my primary concern is educating parents and people like you to recognize what a concentrate is. It does not look like marijuana. It looks very different, and recognizing that that contains very high levels of THC which could pose risks to health.

Co-Chairman FEINSTEIN. Well would you have a standard for this? Does that makes sense? Or should government get involved in this? I think, you know, when you talk about adolescents, you do not want them to die and you do not want them to become addicted.

Dr. MEIER. Correct. We do not want them to become addicted. But we still need to do research on whether adolescents who use concentrates are more likely to become addicted than if they use the lower THC marijuana.

So I think we need more research, because some evidence suggests that it is possible that these concentrates will not have ill effects if adolescents are titrating their use, which means using less when the THC content is high.

Co-Chairman FEINSTEIN. Thank you. Thanks, Mr. Chairman.

The CHAIRMAN. Senator Rosen.

Senator ROSEN. Well thank you. I want to thank Chairman Cornyn, Ranking Member Feinstein, for holding this important hearing. I want to thank all of you for your years of school and research and dedication to this extremely important topic.

I want to talk a little bit about medical marijuana. Although marijuana is legal in Nevada for both medicine and recreational purposes, the research that you are doing is so important for my state's hospitals, providers, schools, parents, law enforcement agencies, anybody that is concerned with the public health impact. And there are approximately in Nevada about 17,000 medical marijuana patients.

So this research that you do really impacts their lives, their ability to seek treatment for their medical conditions. And so with that in mind, I really appreciate the bipartisan approach which has led to this hearing, and I hope the conversation will continue to be research and science based. It is so important that we have these longitudinal studies, epidemiological studies, so on and so forth. It makes a real difference as to how our communities can educate and legislate, if we need to, to do the right thing.

But I want to talk about the potential benefits of medical cannabis in treating our Nation's Veterans. We have over 220,000 Veterans in Nevada. And, let me tell you, I do not have to tell you how much they do struggle. They struggle with chronic pain. They struggle with depression, anxiety, post traumatic stress symptoms, and in too many cases they are becoming addicted to medications prescribed to them—opioids, other things like that.

Our Veterans have given so much to their country, they just want to come back. They want to claim their lives and continue to serve their communities in whatever way is good for them and their families.

And so VA providers are currently prohibited from recommending or prescribing cannabis use. The VA will not reimburse Veterans for medical marijuana prescriptions from any source.

Former VA Secretary David Shulkin, he stated last week he believes the VA should be involved in research and anything that could potentially help Veterans and their wellbeing.

So to Dr. Hennessy, and then anyone else after, you were a member of a committee that conducted rigorous overview of available research on the potential health benefits of cannabis, or therapeutic benefits. It also identifies barriers to research and you made recommendations.

So I would really appreciate your thoughts of how we might use cannabis to help our Veterans through anxiety and depression in those ways, and find alternatives to treat the issues that they are suffering from when they come home.

Dr. HENNESSY. So thank you for your question, Senator. So of the uses that you mentioned, there is randomized trial data supporting the use of cannabis products for chronic pain. And the cannabis products that were studied most often for chronic pain was an oral solution of one-to-one THC to CBD. It was not either smoked or vaped cannabis.

The other indications that you mentioned, anxiety, depression, PTSD, there are not good data from randomized trials that support the efficacy of either whole cannabis or cannabis-derived products for those indications.

Lack of evidence does not mean that the products are not—that none of the constituents of cannabis are not effective. In some cases it merely means that the studies have not been conducted, or not enough of them have been conducted to identify a beneficial effect, if there is one.

Senator ROSEN. But you would support us funding, or lifting the ban on some of the research to find out if we can use these products effectively, Dr. Gruber?

Dr. GRUBER. Yes. And thank you so much for focusing on this issue. We have a program through the MIND program called Serving Those Who Have Served. And it is dedicated to our Veterans. Because so many are already using cannabis of cannabanoids for treatment, many are interested in using it. But we have no real data.

Senator ROSEN. Right.

Dr. GRUBER. So, you know, we come at this as a quasi clinical trial because we cannot administer products that are in the marketplace, given our current federal regulations and restrictions. So we do the best that we can.

But we followed these folks over time, longitudinally. And we need more data like that to be able to really understand the impact. As referred to by Dr. Hennessy, we do not have a ton of data. But certainly lifting anything that would allow greater research efforts to be made I would be in favor of.

Senator ROSEN. Well thank you. I want to—you spoke about chronic pain, and I was fortunate enough to be able to start the Comprehensive Care Caucus, which is focusing on palliative care, people living with a terminal illness or chronic disease, and they need palliative care, although they may not be getting curative care.

And so can you speak to the effects of how we could use cannabis in the palliative care spectrum for those, as I said, living with chronic disease, or living longer with terminal illness, to relieve some of the symptoms that they may be having as a result of their disease?

Dr. HENNESSY. Sure. So one of the symptoms that patients in palliative care experience is chronic pain. And as I mentioned, there are clinical trials showing that oral solutions of cannabis extract are effective for chronic pain.

In terms of other indications for use in the palliative care setting, I think more research is needed to be able to recommend them as effective therapies. We do not want to recommend therapies and offer false hope to people for therapies that end up not being effective. That, in addition, has side effects on their own.

Senator ROSEN. Right. Thank you.

Dr. GRUBER. I think it is also important, just to dovetail on what Dr. Hennessy is saying, to be able to assess the actual products that patients are using, as opposed to just sort of guessing. And the one-to-one ratios of oral solutions, things like Sativex, are not necessarily in the marketplace for our palliative care patients.

Our ongoing longitudinal study at the MIND program actually follows patients with chronic pain as a subgroup, and they demonstrated improvements over time using lots of different products. But this research is really in its infancy, and this is, as far as I know, the only longitudinal study like this in the country.

Senator ROSEN. Right.

Dr. GRUBER. We need a lot more.

Senator ROSEN. Well I applaud all of your work, and I do think that particularly in the medical space trying to find the ways that we can use marijuana, whether for chronic pain, anxiety, terminal disease, PTSD, depression, if we can find ways that make people— help them go better through their lives, then it is definitely worth researching. And I appreciate your hard work. Thank you.

The CHAIRMAN. Thank you, Senator Rosen.

Dr. Gruber, I think I understand what you were telling me earlier. Let me just confirm I got this right. There is a part of marijuana that will make you high. That is THC, right? The active ingredient?

Dr. GRUBER. That is the primary psychoactive compound in the plant, yes.

The CHAIRMAN. Okay, that is a more eloquent way of saying it than I did. And then there are other products from the marijuana plant, or that can be derived from that, like CBD that you think has some medicinal or beneficial effects? But that has little or no THC in it. Correct?

Dr. GRUBER. Correct. Just to clarify, really quick and dirty, cannabis sativa-L, the plant, is comprised of hundreds of compounds. The primary psychoactive compound is THC. That gets you high. The primary non-intoxicating constituent is cannabidiol, shown to have tremendous—at least thought to have tremendous therapeutic benefit.

There are many, many other cannabinoids—canabachromine, canabajeral, tetrahydro canabaren, as well as terpinoids, the essential oils that give cannabis its characteristic scent and flavor profile that have also been touted to have potential beneficial effects. Flavanoids. The plant is incredibly complex. It is not just THC and CBD, although I know that is where we start our discussions, but it is important to remember that alongside THC we have CBD and other players.

The CHAIRMAN. Would it be possible for Congress to de-schedule or to treat CBD and other non-THC products differently than it would THC or psychoactive components of the plant?

Dr. GRUBER. As I understand it, currently under the Controlled Substance Act anything that comes from the plant cannabis sativa with greater than .03 percent THC by weight falls under Schedule One. Anything that comes from industrial—so-called "industrial hemp" legalized in the 2018 Farm Bill, or Hemp Bill, CBD from that source is legal. So that is de-scheduled.

The CHAIRMAN. So Congress has already carved out an exception, basically, for hemp?

Dr. GRUBER. For industrial hemp-derived CBD, ostensibly the DEA will allow those types of research studies to move forward.

The CHAIRMAN. And what differentiates those two, is one has a negligible, if any, THC component.

Dr. GRUBER. That's right.

The CHAIRMAN. And the other product that is a psychoactive one has the THC at a much more concentrated level.

Dr. GRUBER. Much more concentrated levels. Both plants have THC. Industrial hemp maxes out by definition as .03 percent THC by weight. Cannabis sativa-L, when we think of marijuana, we think of that plant that can be bred to have very, very high levels of THC, as well as levels of other cannabanoids. There are differences in the two cultivars.

The CHAIRMAN. Well that is helpful. Thank you, very much. Senator Rosen, do you have anything else you would like to ask? [No response.]

The CHAIRMAN. Well, let me express my gratitude to each of you and our previous panel of witnesses. This is a conversation we should have started a long time ago, but I am glad at least we are starting it now.

And as you can tell, there is a lot we have to learn, Members of Congress, the policymakers, but I think the American people. I think the risks, the health risks of marijuana use have been undersold, and as we heard from the previous panel, but yet there are beneficial uses that do not involve the psychoactive component we have heard that could be enormously helpful.

So this has been very informative and so I thank you for it. Thank you for your participation. We are going to close the hearing now, but we will leave the record open for another week in case any member of the Caucus has written questions they would like to ask to follow on.

But taking Senator Feinstein up on her suggestion, it may be that the Caucus would decide to publish a white paper on what we have learned here, perhaps for the benefit of others, including policymakers like ourselves, and that is something we are going to look into as well.

So we look forward to continuing the conversation with you, and thank you very much for being here.

(Whereupon, at 5:01 p.m., Wednesday, October 23, 2019, the hearing in the above-entitled matter was adjourned.)

[Questions and answers and submissions for the record follow.]

Senate Caucus on International Narcotics Control
Marijuana and American's Health October
23, 2019 Hearing

Questions for the Record

Senator Cornyn:

Dr. Volkow –

Marijuana and Risk of Mental Illness

The Surgeon General's advisory noted the risk for early onset of psychotic disorders, such as schizophrenia that increases with a higher frequency of marijuana use, higher potency of marijuana products, and younger age of use.

- Could you discuss the studies NIDA has initiated or funded that are looking into this increased risk? Is this risk limited to certain psychotic disorders, or does it apply more broadly to mental illness?

Response:
Multiple NIH Institutes and Centers, as well as other federal and non-federal organizations, have supported research examining the link between marijuana and psychosis. Studies have found that having ever used marijuana, compared to never having used marijuana, is associated with double the risk of schizophrenia,[1] while frequent use or use of marijuana with high delta-9 tetrahydrocannabinol (THC) potency is associated with a six-fold increased risk compared to non-users.[23] Research also suggests that marijuana use has the potential to trigger the first symptoms or exacerbate the course of a lasting psychotic illness in some individuals (e.g., those with a genetic vulnerability).[4] In one study of patients in Europe and Brazil who sought treatment for their first psychotic episode, daily marijuana users were at three times greater risk for a psychotic disorder than non-users. Daily users of *high-potency* marijuana were at nearly five times greater risk compared to non-users.[5]

While the research to date shows the strongest link between marijuana and psychosis, there is evidence for an association between marijuana use and other mental health conditions. A comprehensive review of all the data available in 2017 conducted by the National Academies of

[1] van Os J, Bak M, Hanssen M, Bijl RV, de Graaf R, Verdoux H. Cannabis use and psychosis: a longitudinal population based study. Am J. Epidemiol. 2002;156(4):319-327

[2] Andréasson S, Allebeck P, Engström A, Rydberg U. Cannabis and schizophrenia: a longitudinal study of Swedish conscripts. Lancet.

[3] ;2(8574):1483- 1486.

[4] Caspi A, Moffitt TE, Cannon M, et al. Moderation of the effect of adolescent-onset cannabis use on adult psychosis by a functional polymorphism in the catechol-O-methyltransferase gene: longitudinal evidence of a gene × environment interaction. Biol Psychiatry. 2005;57 (10):1117-1127.

[5] Di Forti M, Quattrone D, Freeman TP, et al. The contribution of cannabis use to variation in the incidence of psychotic disorder across Europe (EU-GEI): a multicentre case-control study. Lancet Psychiatry. 2019;6(5):427–436.

Sciences, Engineering, and Medicine, concluded there is a moderate association between cannabis use and suicidal behavior; that among individuals diagnosed with bipolar disorders, near daily cannabis use may be linked to increased symptoms of mania compared to non-users; and that regular cannabis use is likely to increase the risk for developing social anxiety disorder.[6] The report states that cannabis use does not appear to increase the likelihood of developing depression, anxiety disorder (except social anxiety disorder), or posttraumatic stress disorder.

Additional research is needed to delineate the complex relationships between marijuana use and the risk of mental health conditions. NIDA is leading two major studies with significant potential to advance knowledge in these areas. The Adolescent Brain Cognitive Development (ABCD) study is the largest long-term study of brain development and child health in the United States. Over 11,000 children ages 9-10 have been recruited and will be followed into early adulthood to determine how substance use—including marijuana use—and other childhood exposures affect brain and cognitive development and other childhood health outcomes. While a full picture will take years to emerge, this study has already begun to yield significant insights into the links between marijuana and psychosis. For example, earlier this year, ABCD researchers reported that prenatal marijuana exposure after, but not before, maternal knowledge of pregnancy may be associated with a small increase in risk of psychosis during middle childhood.[7] Complementing ABCD is the HEALthy Brain and Child Development (HBCD) Study, which is supported in part by the NIH HEAL (Helping to End Addiction Long-term) Initiative[SM] and is currently in its planning phase. HBCD would establish a large cohort of pregnant women and assess maternal and child outcomes over the course of at least 10 years. Findings will help researchers understand both normal childhood brain development as well as the long-term impact of prenatal and postnatal drug exposure. The National Institute on Mental Health (NIMH) also supports research on the association between marijuana use and mental health conditions. One NIMH study is examining preexisting differences in key components of the endogenous cannabinoid system as potential predictors of first episode psychosis patients.[8]

- Are there studies looking into other health risks of these higher-potency products? Are you able to expand on those?

Response:
It is difficult to conduct research on high-potency products in the United States. Although the NIDA Drug Supply program offers higher potency marijuana for research, the potency of NIDA products does not match that available on the market. Moreover, federally-funded researchers are unable to access dispensary products, so research on those products is limited to observational studies. Those studies are in turn limited by researchers' inability to analyze the composition—

---

[6] The Health Effects of Cannabis and Cannabinoids: The Current State of Evidence and Recommendations for Research. Board on Population Health and Public Health Practice, Health and Medicine Division. The National Academies Press. 2017
[7] Fine JD, Moreau AL, Karcher NR, Agrawal A, Rogers CE, Barch DM, Bogdan R. Association of Prenatal Cannabis Exposure With Psychosis Proneness Among Children in the Adolescent Brain Cognitive Development (ABCD) Study. JAMA Psychiatry. 2019 Jul 1;76(7):762-764.
[8] https://projectreporter.nih.gov/project_info_description.cfm?aid=9765411&icde=47747207

including THC potency—of the products that research participants are using or the dose at which they are using them.

Nevertheless, there have been some studies examining other health risks associated with higherpotency marijuana products. For example, some of the studies examining the impact of high potency products on psychosis mentioned above also examined effects on brain structure, cognition, and metabolism. One study found that frequent use of high-potency marijuana was associated with changes in brain structure that may underlie cognitive changes.[9] Researchers are also studying whether known health effects associated with chronic marijuana use may be more severe in individuals using higher-potency marijuana. These effects include impairments in learning, memory, and attention,[10] as well as effects on insulin sensitivity and metabolism.[11] In addition, through the NIH-supported ABCD study, researchers will be able to examine the effects of marijuana at various levels of potency on brain and cognitive development and a host of other child health outcomes.

Another important outcome of interest is the development of cannabis use disorder (CUD), which takes the form of addiction in severe cases. Recent data suggest that 30 percent of those who use marijuana may have some degree of CUD. The use of higher potency marijuana is associated with increased risk of developing CUD[12] and increased CUD severity.[13] Researchers are also examining how the use of high potency marijuana concentrates, which have become increasingly popular, affect risk for substance use disorder more broadly. A recent study found that relative to adolescent marijuana users who had not used concentrates, those who had were more likely to use other substances and to experience more risk factors and fewer protective factors for substance use problems, raising concerns about high-risk adolescents' exposure to high-THC marijuana.[14]

Researchers are also interested in how the potency of marijuana products may relate to impaired driving. Marijuana significantly impairs judgment, motor coordination, and reaction time, and studies have found a direct relationship between blood THC concentration and impaired driving ability.[15,16,1718] However, the exact nature of the impairment remains unclear and is often complicated by individuals who have used both alcohol and marijuana. NIH is supporting a project that uses a driving simulator and various levels of THC and cannabidiol (CBD) potency to better characterize these effects and the relationship between potency, blood levels, and driving impairment.[19]

---

[9] Rigucci S et al. Effect of high-potency cannabis on corpus callosum microstructure Psychol. Med., 46 (2016), pp. 841-854
[10] https://projectreporter.nih.gov/project_info_description.cfm?aid=9456715&icde=47797167
[11] https://projectreporter.nih.gov/project_info_description.cfm?aid=9740528&icde=47797188
[12] Arterberry BJ et al. Higher average potency across the United States is associated with progression to first cannabis use disorder symptom. Drug and Alcohol Dependence, Volume 195, 1 February 2019, Pages 186-192
[13] Freeman TP, Winstock AR. Examining the profile of high-potency cannabis and its association with severity of cannabis dependence Psychol. Med., 45 (2015), pp. 3181-3189
[14] Meier MH et al. Cannabis Concentrate Use in Adolescents. Pediatrics. August 2019. e20190338; DOI: https://doi.org/10.1542/peds.2019-0338
[15] Lenné MG et al. The effects of cannabis and alcohol on simulated arterial driving: Influences of driving experience and task demand. Accid Anal Prev. 2010;42(3):859-866. doi:10.1016/j.aap.2009.04.021
[16] Hartman RL, Huestis MA. Cannabis effects on driving skills. Clin Chem. 2013;59(3):478-492. doi:10.1373/clinchem.2012.194381
[17] Hartman RL, Brown TL, Milavetz G, et al. Cannabis effects on driving lateral control with and without alcohol. Drug Alcohol Depend.
[18] ;154:25-37. doi:10.1016/j.drugalcdep.2015.06.015
[19] https://projectreporter.nih.gov/project_info_description.cfm?aid=9735170&icde=47797188

Dr. Volkow –

NIH Research into Medical Uses

NIH has supported research into the pharmacology of THC and other cannabinoids, and the National Academies report from 2017 found that orally administered THC is effective in treating some medical conditions.

- Do you think those studies are sufficient for patient use of those products? If not, what regulatory structure should be used to evaluate the safety and efficacy before they are prescribed?

Response:
While NIH supports research that generates evidence on the safety and efficacy of potential therapeutics, it is outside of NIH's purview to determine if there is sufficient evidence to support approval of such products for patient use. The U.S. Food and Drug Administration (FDA) is the Federal agency charged with determining whether medical products are safe and effective for their intended use, and the FDA has a rigorous evaluation process. To date, the FDA has not approved marijuana (the whole plant) for the treatment of any disease or condition. However, several synthetic or plant derived cannabinoid drugs have been approved. These include Marinol and Syndros for the treatment of anorexia associated with weight loss in AIDS patients and for nausea and vomiting associated with cancer treatment. Marinol and Syndros include the active ingredient dronabinol, a synthetic form of THC. The FDA also approved Cesamet, which contains the active ingredient nabilone, a synthetic chemical similar to THC. Cesamet is approved for nausea and vomiting related to cancer treatment. Epidiolex, which contains purified marijuana-derived cannabidiol, was approved for the treatment of seizures associated with Lennox-Gastaut and Dravet syndromes in patients two years of age and older.

- Do studies related to treating medical conditions typically utilize orally administered THC and cannabinoids?

Response:
Studies examining the therapeutic potential of cannabinoids use various routes of administration. Some studies use orally administered THC and/or cannabidiol, often as a capsule or a liquid extract, and others use vaporized or smoked forms. Observational studies examining the impact of marijuana use to self-treat health conditions include patients using marijuana in whatever form they choose. Most therapeutic studies (including those summarized in the NASEM report[20]) do not use marijuana plant material. Various factors make smoked marijuana less therapeutically promising than purified cannabinoid medications delivered through alternative routes of administration. These include the potential harmful effects on the lungs and heightened risk for addiction. In addition, the marijuana plant contain numerous poorly understood chemicals in

[20] The Health Effects of Cannabis and Cannabinoids: The Current State of Evidence and Recommendations for Research. Board on Population Health and Public Health Practice, Health and Medicine Division. The National Academies Press. 2017

addition to THC and CBD, and it is difficult to standardize dosages of a smoked plant with highly variable cannabinoid concentrations. Moreover, researchers who want to study the therapeutic use of marijuana plant material are required to obtain their product from the NIDA Drug Supply Program. This might be a disincentive for developing the plant as a medication insofar as it is not clear how developers would demonstrate equivalency between the marijuana available through NIDA that they would have to use in their clinical trials and the drug product that would ultimately be approved by the FDA for eventual marketing and sale.

- Are there any known medicinal uses for smoked marijuana?

Response:
There are currently no FDA-approved medicinal uses for smoked marijuana.

Senator Feinstein:

Questions for Nora Volkow, MD, Director of the National Institute on Drug Abuse (NIDA)

1. Using Marijuana to Treat Chronic Pain and Post Traumatic Stress Syndrome (PTSD)

A 2014 study published in the Journal of the American Medical Association found an association between lower opioid overdose death rates and marijuana use. This study was based on data from 1999 to 2010.

A subsequent study, published in the Proceedings of the National Academy of Sciences, which examined data from 1999 to 2017, found that states with medical marijuana laws actually saw a 23 percent increase in opioid overdose deaths.

a) What should we make of these studies, which seem to be in conflict?

Response:
The study published in 2014 in the *Journal of the American Medical Association (JAMA)*, which analyzed data through 2010, showed slower rates of increase in opioid analgesic overdose death rates in states with medical marijuana laws compared to states without such laws.[21] The subsequent study published in the *Proceedings of the National Academy of Sciences* reexamined this relationship using data through 2017. Similar to the previous study, it found that opioid overdose mortality rates between 1999-2010 in states allowing medical marijuana use were 21 percent lower than expected. However, when the analysis was extended through 2017, it was found that the trend reversed, such that states with medical marijuana laws experienced an overdose death rate 23

[21] Bachhuber MA, Saloner B, Cunningham CO, Barry CL. Medical Cannabis Laws and Opioid Analgesic Overdose Mortality in the United States, 1999-2010. JAMA Intern Med. 2014;174(10):1668–1673.

percent higher than expected.[22] This discrepancy suggests that overdose death rates are changing due to factors that weren't accounted for in the model, which could include a large range of influences from cultural shifts to state opioid policies to changes in the drug supply.

Many similar studies have assessed the impact of medical marijuana laws on opioid outcomes. Overall, results are inconsistent. There is some evidence to suggest that legalization of marijuana for recreational purposes and ready availability of marijuana dispensary products are associated with decreases in rates of opioid overdose.[23,24] There is also evidence that medical marijuana laws are associated with lower levels of opioid prescribing in Medicaid and Medicare Part D enrollees.[25,26] On the other hand, one study of a nationally representative sample found that medical marijuana law enactment was not associated with a reduction in nonmedical use of prescription opioids.[27] It should be emphasized that ecological studies that look at population measures of opioid outcomes cannot prove causation. More prospective studies controlling for important individual and state-level covariates are needed. It should also be emphasized that marijuana use carries risks, and the FDA has not approved marijuana or any cannabinoid drug for the treatment of pain, opioid misuse, or opioid use disorder.

b) Does medical marijuana have the potential to be an effective substitute for opioids in treating pain?

Response:
Preclinical and clinical research suggest that cannabinoids (chemicals found in marijuana) may have a role in treating pain, especially neuropathic pain; indeed, treatment of chronic pain is the most frequently cited reason for medical marijuana use.[28] In theory, marijuana could reduce or replace opioid use for pain, and this idea has significant anecdotal support. Survey data have shown that patients report substituting marijuana for opioids and benzodiazepines, and that patients replacing prescription opioids with marijuana have a preference for the pain relief to side-effect profile of marijuana.[29] However, a prospective study in Australia failed to confirm an opioid-sparing effect of marijuana over a four-year period.[30] Patients who used marijuana had more severe pain; continued to use opioids; had lower confidence in their ability to function while in pain; and had greater anxiety. It should be noted that this study was observational rather than a randomized clinical trial and is not conclusive.

---

[22] Shover CL, Davis CS, Gordon SC, Humphreys K. Association between medical cannabis laws and opioid overdose mortality has reversed over time. Proc Natl Acad Sci U S A. 2019 Jun 25;116(26):12624-12626.
[23] Livingston MD, Barnett TE, Delcher C, Wagenaar AC. Recreational Cannabis Legalization and Opioid-Related Deaths in Colorado, 2000-2015. Am J Public Health. 2017 Nov;107(11):1827-1829.
[24] Chihuri S, Li G. State marijuana laws and opioid overdose mortality. Inj Epidemiol. 2019 Sep 2;6:38.
[25] Wen H, Hockenberry JM. Association of Medical and Adult-Use Marijuana Laws With Opioid Prescribing for Medicaid Enrollees. JAMA Intern Med. 2018 May 1;178(5):673-679.
[26] Bradford AC, Bradford WD, Abraham A, Bagwell Adams G. Association Between US State Medical Cannabis Laws and Opioid Prescribing in the Medicare Part D Population. JAMA Intern Med. 2018 May 1;178(5):667-672..
[27] Segura LE, Mauro CM, Levy NS, et al. Association of US Medical Marijuana Laws With Nonmedical Prescription Opioid Use and Prescription Opioid Use Disorder. JAMA Netw Open. 2019;2(7):e197216.
[28] National Academies of Sciences, Engineering, and Medicine. 2017. The health effects of cannabis and cannabinoids: The current state of evidence and recommendations for research. Washington, DC: The National Academies Press.
[29] Khan SP, Pickens TA, Berlau DJ. Perspectives on cannabis as a substitute for opioid analgesics. Pain Manag. 2019 Mar 1;9(2):191-203.
[30] Campbell G, Hall WD, Peacock A, Lintzeris N, Bruno R, Larance B, Nielsen S, Cohen M, Chan G, Mattick RP, Blyth F, Shanahan M, Dobbins T, Farrell M, Degenhardt L. Effect of cannabis use in people with chronic non-cancer pain prescribed opioids: findings from a 4-year prospective cohort study. Lancet Public Health. 2018 Jul;3(7):e341-e350.

Along with ongoing preclinical work, two current NIDA-funded clinical trials are studying the safety and analgesic effects of combined treatment with cannabinoids and opioids.[31,32] A third NIDA-funded clinical trial is looking at this question prospectively to assess how medical marijuana use affects opioid analgesic use in HIV+ and HIV- adults with severe or chronic pain.[33] These studies will provide individual-level information on the opioid sparing potential of cannabinoids. There remains an urgent need for effective, non-opioid treatments for pain, including the treatment of low back pain, cancer and chemotherapy-induced pain, neuropathic pain, indigestion, and arthritis-induced pain.[34,35,36,37,38] This is an area of intense focus for NIH research.

The research regarding marijuana's effectiveness in treating PTSD appears to be limited.

a) Please explain what is currently known, particularly with respect to veterans, about the efficacy of using marijuana to treat PTSD.

Response:
NIMH is the lead Federal agency for research on mental disorders and supports a diverse research portfolio on post-traumatic stress disorder (PTSD) and related conditions. NIMH is supporting or conducting over 100 research projects relevant to posttraumatic psychopathology, including basic science research, translational and clinical research, and health care services research. NIMH-supported research involves participants across the lifespan and many different populations, including civilians, service members, and Veterans. Additionally, NIMH and other NIH Institutes and Centers, such as NIDA and the National Institute of Alcohol Abuse and Alcoholism (NIAAA), collaborate and coordinate with the Departments of Defense and Veterans Affairs in the area of service member and Veteran mental health research through the National Research Action Plan (NRAP).[39]

NIMH is invested in identifying and developing treatments for PTSD and related conditions. While there is not currently strong evidence to support the use of marijuana to treat PTSD, preliminary research is underway to learn whether short-term treatment with low doses of tetrahydrocannabinol (THC), the primary psychoactive ingredient in marijuana that affects the cannabinoid system in our brains, might help make current cognitive behavioral treatments more effective by priming certain brain circuits prior to therapy – making it easier to learn and remember not to fear trauma reminders.[40] Additionally, NIMH has participated in trans-NIH

31 https://clinicaltrials.gov/ct2/show/NCT03705559
32 https://clinicaltrials.gov/ct2/show/NCT03679949
33 https://clinicaltrials.gov/ct2/show/NCT03268551
34 https://clinicaltrials.gov/ct2/show/NCT02460692
35 https://projectreporter.nih.gov/project_info_description.cfm?aid=9608720&icde=47748806
36 https://projectreporter.nih.gov/project_info_description.cfm?aid=9614965&icde=47748701
37 https://projectreporter.nih.gov/project_info_description.cfm?aid=9796963&icde=47748842
38 https://projectreporter.nih.gov/project_info_description.cfm?aid=9895227&icde=47748866
39 https://obamawhitehouse.archives.gov/sites/default/files/uploads/nrap_for_eo_on_mental_health_august_2013.pdf
40 https://projectreporter.nih.gov/project_info_description.cfm?aid=9441033

meetings that included evaluation by experts into the neurological and psychiatric effects of marijuana, other cannabinoids, and the endocannabinoid system.[41]

2. Uniform Regulations

Thirty-three states and the District of Columbia have legalized marijuana in some form. Each state has its own laws and regulations.

The lack of uniformity across states, in terms of the testing, labeling, or packaging of marijuana products, the strength of products that may be sold, how they may be advertised, and how they may be accessed, could lead to consumer confusion. This may also produce unintended, acute public health effects, including increased emergency room visits.

In Colorado, for instance, there was a threefold increase in marijuana-related emergency room visits between 2012 and 2016.

a) Would uniform regulations across states be helpful to ensure consumer safety and reduce public health impacts, such as emergency room visits associated with marijuana use?

Response:
At present, there is insufficient data to determine which of the myriad state regulations would be most effective in reducing the adverse public health outcomes associated with marijuana use. This is an important area of scientific investigation, reflected by NIDA's support since 2011 for a robust portfolio of marijuana policy research. In 2017, recognizing the gaps in our understanding of how changing state marijuana laws affect public health, NIDA convened an expert working group to develop a marijuana policy research agenda. The working group report[42] included 28 recommendations for research in five broad areas, including research to: (1) develop standard measures of marijuana use; (2) better understand trends in use; (3) examine the health and social consequences of use, including motor vehicle accidents; (4) identify how product pricing, taxes, sales, promotion, and marketing affect use; and (5) develop prevention and treatment interventions that account for local variation in marijuana use and policies. NIDA is soliciting research applications on these and related marijuana policy issues[43] with the goal of supporting high quality science that can inform the development of evidence-based public health policies.

3. Barriers to Research

In your testimony, you noted that one of the difficulties associated with researching marijuana is that researchers are unable to legally access various strains of marijuana that are being used by individuals in states that have legalized its use. You further noted that the National Institute on

[41] https://www.drugabuse.gov/news-events/meetings-events/2016/03/marijuana-cannabinoids-neuroscience-research-summit
[42] National Institute on Drug Abuse. *Recommendation for NIDA's Cannabis Research Agenda: Report from the Cannabis Policy Research Workgroup. February 6, 2018.* https://www.drugabuse.gov/sites/default/files/nacda_cannabis_policy_research_workgroup_report_feb_2018.pdf
[43] https://grants.nih.gov/grants/guide/notice-files/NOT-DA-19-065.html

Drug Abuse has been working with the Drug Enforcement Administration to establish a mechanism through which researchers can legally access these strains in the future.

a) Can you please provide a status update on these ongoing conversations?

<u>Response:</u>
NIDA has not formally engaged the Drug Enforcement Agency (DEA) about permitting federally-funded researchers to access marijuana products on the market.

NIDA has been working with our interagency partners, including the White House Office of National Drug Control Policy (ONDCP), the FDA, and DEA, to identify opportunities for facilitating research with marijuana and other Schedule I substances, including opportunities to issue additional registrations for cultivating research marijuana. Presently, the University of Mississippi, which produces research marijuana through a contract with NIDA, is the only DEA registered marijuana manufacturer. It is not possible for the University to produce every marijuana product that is currently available in the various States. We were pleased that on August 26, 2019, the DEA signaled that it is moving forward with its review of additional grower applications[44] and that it would promulgate new regulations governing marijuana cultivation. NIDA looks forward to opportunities to provide input to the DEA as it develops a new regulatory framework that ensures an adequate and diverse supply of marijuana for research. NIDA would also remind researchers that the CSA permits researchers to import marijuana for research.

In collaboration with ONDCP, HHS, FDA, and DEA, NIDA has also been identifying ways to streamline the Schedule I research registration process.

b) In your view, is a legislative change required in order to enable researchers to legally access strains of marijuana that are being used in states that have legalized its use?

<u>Response:</u>
Under Federal law, researchers supported by NIDA and other Federal agencies are may not purchase marijuana available through state marijuana dispensaries, as marijuana is a Schedule I controlled substance under the CSA. Moreover, some universities have expressed reticence about allowing investigators to purchase dispensary products with non-Federal funds or do research with these products on university grounds for fear of violating Federal law. There is a significant gap in our understanding of their impact on health. The outbreak of e-cigarette or vaping product use associated lung injury (EVALI), which has been linked to informally-sourced THCcontaining vape products, underscores the critical importance of facilitating researcher access to different product sources.

---

[44] https://www.dea.gov/press-releases/2019/08/26/dea-announces-steps-necessary-improve-access-marijuana-research

c) *Would using marijuana in research that is obtained from states that have legalized its use present any challenges or safety concerns for research participants?*

Response

Marijuana available through state dispensaries is grown and processed under a variety of conditions and, like other botanical products, may include pesticides, pathogenic microbes, heavy metals, and other contaminants that could be harmful to humans. While most states with legal marijuana require product testing, there is no uniform testing standard. Likewise, product labeling varies, such that it may not be possible to determine the components of a marketed product, including the full range of cannabinoids present. Although the lack of testing and labeling standards presents challenges to conducting controlled research with these products, these challenges are surmountable. Before testing an unapproved drug or botanic product in humans, an investigator is required to submit to the FDA an investigational new drug (IND) application and to comply with FDA chemistry, manufacturing, and control requirements to ensure the proper identification, quality, purity, and strength of an investigational drug. We are aware of one study[45] for which the FDA approved an IND to conduct research with tablets containing THC and CBD derived from marijuana plants grown by a company that supplies Connecticut dispensaries. This study is not supported by the NIH, but it illustrates the feasibility of using products from suppliers of State dispensaries to develop research grade marijuana products that meet FDA's rigorous requirements. We anticipate that marijuana producers supplying dispensaries in other states would develop additional research-grade marijuana and marijuana-derived products if there was greater regulatory certainty about researchers' ability to use these products.

Senator Grassley

Dr. Volkow –

1. One of the biggest issues with marijuana is that people – particularly youth – think that since it's legalized in some states, it's therefore harmless. Marijuana and its derivatives have some medically recognized benefits, but like all drugs, it isn't without risk.

    a. How can we in the federal government make sure that the average American citizen understands the risks associated with marijuana use, particularly as it is simultaneously more normalized yet potent?

Response:

Research is at the heart of developing evidence-based public health information. The increasing potency of marijuana and the proliferation of new marijuana products and methods for consuming them raise new public health concerns. This is underscored by the outbreak of EVALI, which has been linked to THC-containing vape products. It is imperative that scientists

[45] https://reason.com/wp-content/uploads/2019/11/CTPharma-Yale-Study-news-release-11-8.pdf

have the opportunity to study marijuana products that the public is using so that we can identify and communicate any risks associated with them.

Effective communication is a critical component of NIDA's mission, and we are committed to serving as a trusted source of scientific information on drug use and addiction. NIDA strives to make addiction research accessible to people in the community by strategically leveraging social media, blogs, and the news media to promote new findings, inform the public about emerging drug trends, and educate the community on addiction science. NIDA engages adolescents, through our popular teen-oriented Drugs and Health Blog, our annual National Drug and Alcohol Facts Week events that engage participating schools across the country, and Drugs & Alcohol Chat Day, in which NIDA scientists answer questions from middle- and high-school students in an all-day, real-time virtual chat. Because it can be difficult to reach adolescents directly, it is important to engage people with influence over them, including parents, teachers, and the media. NIDA produces materials aimed at helping parents and teachers communicate with children and teens about drugs, such as web-based FAQs and our Family Checkup resource, which highlights parenting skills that are effective at preventing drug use among youth. Through our NIDAMED initiative, NIDA also develops educational resources and tools for healthcare providers across disciplines—not just those working in substance use—who are at the front lines of diagnosing, preventing, and treating substance misuse and addiction.

2. A number of studies state that the risk for psychotic disorders, such as schizophrenia, increases with the frequency of marijuana use, potency of the product, and as the age at first use decreases.
    a. What is it about marijuana that makes its users susceptible to psychotic disorders?

Response:

Research is needed to establish why individuals who use marijuana are at increased risk for psychotic disorders. The endocannabinoid system, through which marijuana exerts its effects, is thought to be involved. This system appears early in gestation and plays a critical role in brain development, especially in areas of the brain known to be involved in psychosis. One possible explanation for the link between marijuana use and psychosis is that marijuana use may lead to persistent disruptions in the endocannabinoid system, ultimately altering the developmental trajectory of circuits involved in psychosis. Importantly, a critical feature of mental illnesses, including psychotic disorders and substance use disorders, is the complicated interplay of biological and environmental factors that cause them and influence their progression. To the extent that marijuana contributes to the development of psychosis, it is likely a component cause, interacting with other known (e.g., family history) and, as of yet, unknown risk factors. Additional research is needed to identify these risk factors, determine their relative contribution to psychosis risk, and delineate the underlying mechanism by which they exert their effects.

Cornyn

Dr. Adams

Trends and Risks of High-Potency Marijuana

Your advisory raises awareness of the known and potential harms of marijuana use, especially for vulnerable populations like adolescents and pregnant women. Beyond the increased accessibility, you specifically note the increased potency of marijuana and wider variety of cannabis products being used as areas of significant public health concerns.

Could you expand on the trends you are seeing as in the onset of psychotic disorders and other mental health issues?

The scientific literature tells us that exposure to marijuana is associated with a range of psychosis outcomes from immediate, transient psychotic states that spontaneously resolve to delayed, persistent psychotic disorders such as schizophrenia (D'Souza et al, 2016). In an extensive review of the health effects of marijuana, the National Academies of Sciences, Engineering, and Medicine (NASEM) also found "...substantial evidence of a statistical association between cannabis use and the development of schizophrenia or other psychoses, with the highest risk among the most frequent users" (NASEM, 2017). The link between marijuana and psychosis has been found to be greater with earlier age of exposure to marijuana and genetic vulnerability.

Moreover, the findings of the 2018 National Survey on Drug Use and Health indicate an association between marijuana use and mental health concerns. In 2018, adults who had Any Mental Illness (AMI) or Serious Mental Illness (SMI) were more likely than those without any mental illness to be past-year users of marijuana (29.2 percent AMI and 38.9 percent SMI vs. 13.2 percent without mental illness)

- **Do cannabis concentrate and other high-THC products pose a greater public health risk than marijuana?**

  In addition to risks of dependence, addiction, psychosis, and harm to the developing brain, highly concentrated products raise the risks of harm from accidental ingestion, unintentional overdose, and repetitive cycles of nausea and vomiting known as cannabinoid hyperemesis syndrome.

Perceptions of Marijuana Risks and Consequences

The advisory also notes that perceptions of the safety and health risks of marijuana have change significantly over the past few years.

How has this change in perception impacted use by adolescents and pregnant women? Can you discuss the consequences of these changes?

As of yet, it is unclear what effects the changing perception of marijuana use among adolescents and pregnant women will have on public health. One concern is that a reduced perception of harm could increase the likelihood of experimentation, which could lead to harms to the developing brain. Additionally, marijuana use remains illegal for youth under Federal law and in all states; normalization of its use raises the potential for criminal consequences in this population. In addition to the health risks posed by marijuana use, sale or possession of marijuana remains illegal under Federal law notwithstanding some state laws to the contrary.

Feinstein

<u>Questions for Jerome Adams, MD, U.S. Surgeon General</u>

1. **Uniform Regulations**

Thirty-three states and the District of Columbia have legalized marijuana in some form. Each state has its own laws and regulations. The lack of uniformity across states, in terms of the testing, labeling, or packaging of marijuana products, the strength of products that may be sold, how they may be advertised, and how they may be accessed, could lead to consumer confusion. This may also produce unintended, acute public health effects, including increased emergency room visits.

In Colorado, for instance, there was a threefold increase in marijuana-related emergency room visits between 2012 and 2016.

a) ***Would uniform regulations across states be helpful to ensure consumer safety and reduce public health impacts, such as emergency room visits associated with marijuana use?***

Uniformity of ill-informed policy ensures safety for no one. A first step in ensuring consumer safety and reducing public health impacts is to disseminate scientifically sound information to the public and relevant stakeholders. The marijuana available today is much more potent than what was available in the past. The risks of physical dependence, addiction, and harm to the developing brain increase with frequent use, exposure to high concentrations of THC, and with younger age of initiation.

2. **Adolescent Marijuana Use and Risk-Perception**

According to the Youth Risk Behavior Study, in states that have legalized recreational marijuana, teen use dropped between 1993 and 2017: those who said they used marijuana in the previous 30 days dropped 8 percent, while those who used it 10 or more times fell by 9 percent. However, in your testimony before the Senate Caucus on International Narcotics Control you expressed concern that perceptions of risk related to marijuana use among youth has decreased.

a) ***Given that trends in reduced perceptions of harm may often indicate future increases in adolescent drug use, are you concerned that marijuana use among adolescents could increase, despite initial decreases in states that have legalized its use?***

Contemporaneous with widespread legalization, more high school students are reporting a decline in perceived harmfulness of marijuana. Despite an initial decrease in states that have legalized its use, there is still a large number of adolescents becoming new marijuana users. Each day 3,700 adolescents aged 12 to 17 become new marijuana users, and last year over 9 million 12-25 year olds reported marijuana use in the prior month. This lowered perceived harm must be considered a risk in the context of increased access, high potency, and the large variety of forms available. To our youth, marijuana is everywhere.

Importantly, nearly one in five people who begin marijuana use during adolescence become addicted. And the earlier and more often a person uses marijuana – especially at higher THC levels – the higher the risk of harmful consequences.

b) Given that marijuana seems to have more potential to harm the developing brain than the brain of an adult, should policies regarding marijuana use vary based on age? Is there any age at which marijuana use can be considered safe?

We know that the brain continues to develop through the mid-twenties and that these developing brains are more vulnerable to harm. But **we need to know much more.** We need to understand the mid- and long-term health consequences of prenatal and youth exposure to marijuana, as well as more about strategies to mitigate harms. Research is also needed to understand the impact of today's highly potent marijuana on chronic users of any age.

Cigarettes and alcohol are legal, but we know that doesn't mean they are safe. Based on the best scientific information we have right now, marijuana use poses particular dangers to youth, but there is no age at which marijuana use can be considered "safe."

Grassley

Surgeon General Adams

1. **One of the biggest issues with marijuana is that people – particularly youth – think that since it's legalized in some states, it's therefore harmless. Marijuana and its derivatives have some medically recognized benefits, but like all drugs, it isn't without risk.**
   a. **How can we in the federal government make sure that the average American citizen understands the risks associated with marijuana use, particularly as it is simultaneously more normalized yet potent?**

The Federal Government can produce and disseminate scientifically-sound information in formats that are easily consumable by the general public and targeted to specific stakeholders positioned to take action. Among the populations who need this information about the risks of marijuana use among youth and pregnant women are parents and parents-to-be, educators, healthcare and public health professionals, and policy makers at local, state, and national levels. The President donated his quarterly salary to support a digital ad campaign focused on parents of adolescents and on pregnant women. These ads are available for widespread use.

2. **A number of studies state that the risk for psychotic disorders, such as schizophrenia, increases with the frequency of marijuana use, potency of the product, and as the age at first use decreases.**
   a. **What is it about marijuana that makes its users susceptible to psychotic disorders?**

Multiple studies have shown that the risk for psychotic disorders like schizophrenia rises with higher concentrations of THC, daily use, and earlier age of initiation. This association needs to be more deeply researched, including genetic and other susceptibilities.

5/21/20

Please note that my responses are shown in blue. If you have any questions I would be happy to discuss by phone (858-657-5733) or email (rfitzgerald@ucsd.edu). Thanks for your leadership in addressing these important issues.

Best regards,

Rob Fitzgerald, PhD
Professor of Pathology
UC San Diego Health

Cornyn

Fitzgerald

Impaired Driving
Dr. Fitzgerald, it has been noted that there is no scientific basis for the adoption of THC per se laws for driving. You have also mentioned the difficulties of using blood tests to establish a threshold for impairment.

- Can you discuss some approaches that states have taken to try to address impaired driving given these limitations?

Response: Several states have enacted per se legislation. Generally these states have implemented per se concentrations between 1 and 5 ng/mL of THC. At this time, there is no data to support this practice. Most states depend on officer observations, standard field sobriety tests, drug recognition expert (DRE) findings and results of blood testing to determine impairment. There are on-going studies to further evaluate these processes in relation to cannabis-related driving impairment. The combination of officer observations with toxicology lab findings is the most objective and scientific approach we have to date.

- What steps can be taken at the federal level to provide a stronger foundation for developing these policies?

Response: The following steps would be helpful:
1. Support efforts to train more police officers in the Advanced Roadside Impairment Driving Enforcement program (ARIDE). ARIDE is a NHTSA developed program that bridges training between standardized field sobriety tests and DRE exams.
2. Support efforts to train additional DREs.
3. Support forensic laboratories to enable them to acquire instrumentation required for these types of toxicology analyses.
4. Provide research funding focused on driving under the influence of cannabis and cannabis combined with alcohol. An important focus of such research should include the development of new behavioral and toxicological methods for identifying impairment and/or time since substance use. The federal government should partner with states like California, which have already begun funding these types of projects, in order to leverage federal investment.
5. Support legislation that would standardize reporting of driving under the influence of drugs, so we can get a better understanding of the national importance of this problem.

Gruber

Mental Illness and Tie to Higher THC Content

Dr. Gruber, you've noted how THC levels are rising in recreational marijuana products, CBD has declined to nearly untraceable levels, and that CBD has been shown to mitigate some of the negative effects of THC including adverse psychological symptoms.

- Do you believe that increased use of this higher-potency marijuana could increase the risks of developing mental health issues? Would that risk change depending on the age and frequency of the user?

- How impactful is the age of use to the short- and long-term risks of recreational marijuana use?

Risks for Drug Interactions

Studies have shown that cannabinoids, including CBD, can inhibit the liver's enzyme system, increasing both plasma levels and toxicity of other drugs, and potentially causing interactions with other drugs.

- Have there been sufficient studies into this risk? To what extent are we aware of adverse drug reactions between cannabinoids and prescription drugs?

Issues with Standardization in Research

Your testimony also notes that there is no consensus regarding the definition of chronic, regular, or heavy use versus casual or light use, and how that contributes to mixed findings across studies. It also notes that there isn't much standardization of measurements of marijuana.

- Have studies found a difference in outcomes based on the type of marijuana product used? For example, a study that calculates an estimate of grams of marijuana used by the subjects regardless of the product or model of use?

- What are some of the consequences of this lack of standardization?

Hennessy

Mental Illness Findings In NASEM Study

Dr. Hennessy, the National Academies report found substantial evidence of a statistical association between cannabis use and the development of schizophrenia or other psychoses. The highest risk was among the most frequent users.

- What factors contribute to this higher risk, and is it related to the higher potency of marijuana?
- Is there any evidence that using concentrates could negatively impact users who have existing mental health issues?

Feinstein

Questions for Dr. Robert Fitzgerald, Clinical Pathologist, University of California, San Diego

1. Marijuana Impaired Driving

It is my understanding that marijuana impairment is difficult to detect in roadside tests, and that each state has a different standard of impairment, if it has any standard at all.

a) Based on your research, what are the biggest challenges in determining whether a driver is impaired by marijuana?

Response: Let me first say that it's not quite accurate to say that each state has a different standard of impairment. While that is true when it comes to per se laws, many states strive to follow the guidelines established by the International Association of Chiefs of Police criteria regarding field sobriety tests and the determination of impairment, thus aiming to have some consistency in officer determinations.

The biggest challenges to determining if a driver is impaired by marijuana are:

1. There is no correlation between THC concentration in blood and effect on driving (unlike alcohol where there is a reasonably good relationship between blood alcohol concentration and severity of driving impairment).
2. We have not developed an objective measure of THC impairment. The degree to which the field sobriety tests, which were developed to detect alcohol related impairment, accurately identify THC-related impairment is still a subject of research. Coming back to my response to Senator Cornyn, research aimed at the development of roadside test protocols that are specific to identifying cannabis associated driving impairment would help advance the field.

b) As you noted in your testimony, blood alcohol concentration is a clear indicator of alcohol-induced impairment. Is there, or will there soon be, any similar standard that can be applied to marijuana? You noted that oral fluids may be able to be used to determine marijuana impairment. Are there any drawbacks to using this testing method?

Response: Currently there are no analogous measures of THC that are similar to a blood alcohol for driving impairment. It is possible that oral fluid and/or breath testing for THC (or a metabolite) could be developed that would indicate recent use, but I'm not convinced that they would necessarily indicate impairment. Being able to demonstrate recent use is a necessary step that could be combined with officer observations of impairment to identify people who are under the influence of marijuana. Drawbacks to oral fluid and breath testing is that results will probably vary depending on the route of administration (Smoked/vaped vs Oral).

c) Are drug recognition experts adequately trained to determine whether a driver is impaired by marijuana?

Response: DREs undergo extensive training in the identification of presence of various drug classes, and their impairing effects. Due to some of the challenges in conducting research with cannabis (classified as a Schedule I drug), there are have only been limited studies examining the relationship between field sobriety and DRE evaluations and cannabis-related driving impairment. More research is needed to demonstrate how good drug recognition experts are. To date they have not been tested in large samples using a blinded randomized placebo controlled manner. We are working with the California Highway Patrol to conduct these kinds of studies. Results of this work would have implications for highway safety across the nation and it would be appropriate for the federal government to provide funds to match state investments.

2. Public Health Perspective

During the hearing, it was made clear that marijuana has the potential to cause both harms and benefits.

a) *With this in mind, from a public health perspective, what are the biggest challenges related to marijuana, where are the most significant research gaps, and what should policymakers be focusing on moving forward?*

Response: The biggest challenge currently facing understanding effects of marijuana on human health is the inability of research institutions like the University of California to study the products that our population is exposed to. Because of federal scheduling of marijuana (schedule 1) we cannot investigate the concentrated forms of marijuana that the general public has access to, and thus have no mechanism to understand the health and public safety implications of these substances.

Policy makers should work on creating an exemption that allows established research institutions to perform studies using the products our population is exposed to. One of the primary strengths of the United States is our research engine. We need to unleash the power of our scientific enterprise to better understand both the beneficial and harmful effects of marijuana on human health. Our research universities, including in California, are reluctant to expand clinical research on cannabis because of concern that they might violate Federal law, and that the institutions and investigators may be subject to prosecution, or have their Federal awards withdrawn. Thus, creating exemptions, so that institutions can study and administer products that are legal in a State would be an important step. Related to this, the current single source of marijuana for medical research is the Federal Government itself (grown at the University of Mississippi). Expanding the supply base is important. Again, I would recommend that the federal government partner with states that have robust medicinal cannabis research enterprises to support studies on products that residents of those states have access to. Another important way to facilitate research on marijuana and health is to reschedule marijuana to reflect the emerging science. Based on the data, the most appropriate is Schedule 3.

<u>Questions for Dr. Staci Gruber, Associate Professor of Psychiatry, Harvard Medical School</u>

1. Comparing Medical and Recreational Use

There doesn't seem to be a great deal of information available about the differences between the use of marijuana for medical versus recreational purposes. Given that much of your research has involved subjects who use medical marijuana, can you comment on the following:

a) *Have you found that there is a difference in the types, quantity, and concentration of marijuana products used by medical marijuana patients compared to recreational patients?*

b) *Should these differences be taken into consideration when developing policies to address marijuana?*

c) *Given the lack of research and information on appropriate dosing, etc., how do medical marijuana users know what products are effective for their particular condition, and is there any reason to be concerned about adverse impacts on the body?*

2. Marijuana Strains

It is my understanding that different strains of marijuana contain different chemical profiles. Depending on the specific strain, the marijuana could produce more positive than negative effects.

a) *Can you speak to the differences in strains that contain high levels of cannabidiol compared to tetrahydrocannabinol, and vice-versa, and how these strains might have different effects on the body?*

b) *Should different strains of marijuana be regulated differently?*

3. <u>Veterans</u>

You noted during your testimony that ongoing research, through the MIND study, is being conducted with respect to veterans' use of marijuana products to treat a variety of conditions, including post-traumatic stress disorder, insomnia, and chronic pain. It is my understanding that you have already conducted two studies related to veterans and that you are currently enrolling participants in the third study.

a) *Please discuss your findings from the first two studies that have been conducted.*

b) *Does marijuana use to treat veterans, particularly as it relates to Post Traumatic Stress Disorder (PTSD), seem to be effective? Is there any concern that marijuana use could exacerbate problems associated with PTSD?*

3. Public Health Perspective

During the hearing, it was made clear that marijuana has the potential to cause both harms and benefits.

a) *With this in mind, from a public health perspective, what are the biggest challenges related to marijuana, where are the most significant research gaps, and what should policymakers be focusing on moving forward?*

<u>Questions for Sean Hennessy, PharmD ,PhD, University of Pennsylvania School of Medicine</u>

1. Evidence Regarding Use of Marijuana for Medical Purposes

You were a member of the committee of the National Academies of Sciences, Engineering, and Medicine that produced the 2017 report titled "The Health Effects of Marijuana and Cannabinoids."

Based on your work on this report:

a) *Does enough information exists to conclude what the proper dosage and delivery mechanisms for medical marijuana patients should be?*

b) *Does enough information exist to determine how marijuana might interact with other medications?*

2. Public Health Perspective

During the hearing, it was made clear that marijuana has the potential to cause both harms and benefits.

a) With this in mind, from a public health perspective, what are the biggest challenges related to marijuana, where are the most significant research gaps, and what should policymakers be focusing on moving forward?

Questions for Dr. Madeline Meier, Assistant Professor of Psychology, Arizona State University

1. Research on Marijuana Use and IQ levels

In 2012, you authored a longitudinal study, which found that early persistent use of marijuana by adolescents could result in the loss of up to eight IQ points, which are not recoverable, even after a person stops using. It is my understanding that these findings held true, even when controlling for socio-economic status.

However, subsequent longitudinal studies involving twins, published in the Proceedings of the National Academy of Sciences, found that there was no predictable difference in the twins' IQ when one used marijuana in adolescence and the other did not.

a) Can you speak to the differences in these two studies and discuss whether we should be concerned about the loss of IQ among adolescents when they are early, persistent users of marijuana?

As a follow up, it is my understanding that you recently authored a study, which found that adolescent marijuana use is not associated with changes in the adult brain structure.

b) How, if at all, are the findings in this study related to the findings of your previous longitudinal study on IQ?

2. Marijuana Strains

It is my understanding that different strains of marijuana contain different chemical profiles. Depending on the specific strain, the marijuana could produce more positive than negative effects.

a) Can you speak to the differences in strains that contain high levels of cannabidiol compared to tetrahydrocannabinol, and vice-versa, and how these strains might have different effects on the body?

b) *Should different strains of marijuana be regulated differently?*

3. Public Health Perspective

In your testimony before the Senate Caucus on International Narcotics Control, you spoke about the facts, research and conclusions at which you have arrived with your research and work regarding marijuana use. As discussed during the hearing, these facts, the research already conducted and potential future research hold the answer to policy-making regarding marijuana.

a) From a public health perspective, what are the biggest challenges related to marijuana, where are the most significant research gaps, and what should policymakers be focusing on moving forward?

Grassley

Dr. Robert Fitzgerald

1. An obstacle with drugged driving is measuring impairment. You stated in your testimony that "officer observations combined with results of toxicology testing" can be used to measure impairment.
   a. Would this assessment replace or supplement measuring THC levels in a sample? Why or why not?

Response: Since there is no correlation between concentrations of THC in blood with impairment it is essential that toxicology testing of biological specimens is combined with officer observations. Both the officer observations and the analysis of THC (and/or metabolites) in biological specimens are essential components of keeping our roads safe with respect to drugged driving. Officers can document impairment and toxicology testing can help identify the cause.

2. Drug Recognition Experts, or DREs, are the gold standard in recognizing and identifying signs of impairment. A DRE, however, is a person with his or her own subjective points of view and experiences.
   a. How can we ensure consistency in assessment and due process protections?

Response: Currently the combination of a DRE's findings and toxicology testing is the best way to provide objective data for identifying driving impairment. This is an imperfect system and we need to continue to investigate other methods for objectively identifying impairment.

Dr. Sean Hennessy

1. You stated in your written testimony that there is "substantial evidence" of an association between cannabis use and the development of schizophrenia or other psychoses. However, you also qualify this by stating, "there is reason to question the directionality of this association."
   a. Please expand on the risks of marijuana use and why its users are particularly susceptible to psychoses, and why there is a question as to the directionally of this association.

Senate Follow-Up Questions

Mental Illness and Tie to Higher THC Content

Dr. Gruber, you've noted how THC levels are rising in recreational marijuana products, CBD has declined to nearly untraceable levels, and that CBD has been shown to mitigate some of the negative effects of THC including adverse psychological symptoms.

- Do you believe that increased use of this higher-potency marijuana could increase the risks of developing mental health issues? Would that risk change depending on the age and frequency of the user?
    - *While there are no direct studies that objectively quantify real-world use of high potency products and mental health outcomes, it is likely that higher potency products could exacerbate existing or prodromal symptoms of psychotic disorders given studies which cite a dose-response relationship, such that increased potency is associated with an increased risk for psychotic symptoms. Importantly, however, in the majority of these naturalistic studies, the actual potency of cannabis products has not been directly assessed. Similarly, a number of acute administration studies show increased "psychotic-like" behaviors (i.e., feelings of paranoia) following exposure to higher potency products. However, the effects reported in these studies are only observed during acute intoxication in a laboratory setting and can therefore considered transient. Individuals who are potentially vulnerable to developing a psychotic disorder (i.e., those with a genetic predisposition/family history of psychosis) may be at increased risk the earlier they initiate cannabis use, and the more frequently and heavily they use cannabis. Importantly though, a number of additional factors are likely to moderate outcomes. Overall, although a body of research provides important evidence suggesting that higher potency products may increase the risk for psychosis or psychotic-like behaviors, studies that directly assess and quantify the potency of the products patients are actually using are needed to elucidate the specific relationship between marijuana potency and mental health outcomes; this is best done in studies of those with and without genetic liability.*

- How impactful is the age of use to the short- and long-term risks of recreational marijuana use?
    - *In general, most agree that earlier, heavier and more frequent exposure to marijuana is related to an increased likelihood of negative consequences, particularly in terms of cognition, given that adolescents and emerging adults are still in the midst of critical brain maturation processes, which leaves them vulnerable to outside influences such as injury, illness, or drugs, including (but not limited to) marijuana.*

Risks for Drug Interactions

Studies have shown that cannabinoids, including CBD, can inhibit the liver's enzyme system, increasing both plasma levels and toxicity of other drugs, and potentially causing interactions with other drugs.

- Have there been sufficient studies into this risk? To what extent are we aware of adverse drug reactions between cannabinoids and prescription drugs?
    - *Although this research is vital to determine the safety of cannabinoid-based products, empirical data is generally lacking in this area. To date, a handful of studies have identified enzymes that are strong inducers/inhibitors of the Cytochrome P450 enzyme system, which has implications for the efficacy and safety of certain conventional medications that patients may be taking concurrently with cannabinoid-based products.*

Issues with Standardization in Research

Your testimony also notes that there is no consensus regarding the definition of chronic, regular, or heavy use versus casual or light use, and how that contributes to mixed findings across studies. It also notes that there isn't much standardization of measurements of marijuana.

- Have studies found a difference in outcomes based on the type of marijuana product used? For example, a study that calculates an estimate of grams of marijuana used by the subjects regardless of the product or model of use?
  - *Historically, must studies examining the impact of marijuana use have quantified use by collecting data on number of episodes of use per week, number of "joints" or "marijuana cigarettes" smoked, or grams of marijuana used. When studies use these types of calculations, these measurements do not reflect the specific amount of each individual cannabinoid, or other components contained in cannabis plants, that a person is exposed to. Although it is more difficult to measure exposure to the compounds within a plant (samples must be sent to a laboratory for analyses, which can be logistically difficult due to Schedule I restrictions, as well as cost prohibitive), this type of data will ultimately help elucidate the unique effects of individual cannabinoids as well as other constituents and compounds found within cannabis plants. It is likely that some compounds may confer negative outcomes (e.g., THC), while other compounds such as cannabidiol and potentially certain terpenoids, may be neuroprotective. In addition, it is also possible that potential contaminants, including heavy metals, pesticides, and yeast/mold could contribute to negative outcomes.*
  - *To date, no studies have directly compared specified preset/predetermined or quantifiable amounts between product types (e.g., matched amount of specific cannabinoids within flower vs edibles vs oils). More research is needed to more fully understand how specific modes of use/routes of administration moderate the effects of cannabinoids as well as the effects of other compounds found within the cannabis plant.*

- What are some of the consequences of this lack of standardization?
  - *Due to the lack of standardization, it is difficult to answer questions regarding safe limits of cannabis use. While many studies have reported decrements among heavy, recreational cannabis users, studies often define "chronic," "heavy," or "frequent" differently. For example, these criteria are often based on descriptions/definitions from within the literature but are often somewhat arbitrary numbers that can reflect different time frames (i.e., lifetime vs monthly vs weekly use), different amounts of cannabis used (i.e., a particular amount of grams of cannabis, or a particular number of use episodes). In addition, there is no standard 'serving size' or dose of THC, CBD, or any other cannabinoids although some states, including Colorado, consider a 'standard dose' of edibles as 10 mg. This aspect of the lack of standardization makes it difficult to directly compare product types.*

Questions for Dr. Staci Gruber, Associate Professor of Psychiatry, Harvard Medical School

1. Comparing Medical and Recreational Use

There doesn't seem to be a great deal of information available about the differences between the use of marijuana for medical versus recreational purposes. Given that much of your research has involved subjects who use medical marijuana, can you comment on the following:

a) Have you found that there is a difference in the types, quantity, and concentration of marijuana products used by medical marijuana patients compared to recreational patients?

   a. *Although products sold to recreational users and medical marijuana patients can be the same, recreational users primarily seek products with considerable amounts of THC, as they desire the "high" or mood altering, often euphoric or mellowing, effects of cannabis. In contrast, medical marijuana patients typically initiate use with the primary goal of symptom alleviation, and often times look to actively avoid feelings of intoxication. As such, MC patients frequently seek products with rich and varied cannabinoid profiles (e.g., high-CBD products). In fact, preliminary data from my lab's longitudinal, observational study suggests that on average, medical marijuana patients have higher exposure to CBD relative to THC. Products high in CBD and other cannabinoids in addition to THC have the potential to confer a variety of benefits. A number of studies have indicated that THC appears to serve as an effective analgesic, antiemetic, and appetite stimulant.*

b) Should these differences be taken into consideration when developing policies to address marijuana?

   a. *It is important to recognize that cannabis is a complex plant. As such, cannabinoid formulations will likely exert unique effects depending on which cannabinoids are contained within a product, as well as which other constituents (e.g., terpenoids, flavonoids,) are present. The impact of cannabis products are not only related to the presence of these individual compounds, but also depend on the* <u>*amount*</u> *of each of these constituents in a given product, their interaction with other compounds, and an individual's unique response to product administration. Therefore, research examining the actual products patients are using will help determine safety, efficacy, and side effect profiles; data from these investigations, which must employ empirically sound, controlled models (whether preclinical or clinical), should be used to help guide public policies.*

c) Given the lack of research and information on appropriate dosing, etc., how do medical marijuana users know what products are effective for their particular condition, and is there any reason to be concerned about adverse impacts on the body?

   a. *Currently, there is a lack of research on appropriate dosing of medical cannabis products, which is at least in part due to the fact that researchers cannot study commercially available cannabis-based products in research participants using clinical trial models. Moreover, as the cannabis plant contains over 100 phytocannabinoids and over 400 chemical compounds, each of which may have an impact, it is currently difficult for researchers, clinicians, and consumers to know what specific products might be most effective for a particular condition. While research remains in its infancy, some studies have suggested that individual cannabinoids demonstrate unique therapeutic properties, such as the anti-anxiety and anti-inflammatory effects of CBD, or the analgesic and anti-emetic effects of THC. More research is needed to clarify the impact of these primary cannabinoids as well as many of the other cannabinoids and compounds within the plant. When using any cannabinoid-based product, particularly those containing THC, it is recommended to 'start low and go slow," meaning that medical marijuana patients should start with low doses of a product and wait to determine if a larger dose is needed. It is also important for patients who are taking other conventional medications to be aware of potential interactions between cannabinoids and their medications. For example, CBD has been shown to impact the Cytochrome P450 enzyme system, which means that CBD may strengthen or weaken the effects of many conventional medications.*

b. *In terms of side effects, potential negative effects of THC have been well-documented and include the potential of increasing heart rate, inducing psychomimetic effects like hallucinations/paranoia/anxiety, and decreasing cognitive performance. Some preliminary evidence also suggests that CBD may cause drowsiness, and for some, high doses of purified CBD products may also have gastrointestinal side effects.*

2. Marijuana Strains

It is my understanding that different strains of marijuana contain different chemical profiles. Depending on the specific strain, the marijuana could produce more positive than negative effects.

a) Can you speak to the differences in strains that contain high levels of cannabidiol compared to tetrahydrocannabinol, and vice-versa, and how these strains might have different effects on the body?

   a. *Strains, also known as cultivars, are each unique and vary with regard to concentrations of the primary constituents (THC and CBD), and with regard to other cannabinoids and compounds, including terpenoids and flavonoids, which are thought to exert their own biobehavioral effects. More research is needed to understand the effects of individual strains, but given that THC is the primary intoxicating constituent of cannabis and is often associated with negative effects at high doses (e.g., cognitive decrements, increased heart rate, paranoia, anxiety), those using high THC strains are potentially more likely to experience adverse effects related to cannabis use. High CBD strains are typically considered to have therapeutic effects, such as anti-anxiety, anti-inflammatory, and anti-epileptic properties, but a number of factors, including the amount of THC and other cannabinoids that are also present in the product, will influence the effects of a particular strain.*

b) Should different strains of marijuana be regulated differently?

   a. Given the potential negative impact of higher THC product, particularly on our most vulnerable consumers (i.e., youth), many have considered requiring a higher tax or age restrictions for products containing THC levels about a certain level. Conversely, some may consider requiring a threshold for minimum levels of CBD, which may have the ability to mitigate the effects of THC and/or confer neuroprotective properties.

3. <u>Veterans</u>

You noted during your testimony that ongoing research, through the MIND study, is being conducted with respect to veterans' use of marijuana products to treat a variety of conditions, including post-traumatic stress disorder, insomnia, and chronic pain. It is my understanding that you have already conducted two studies related to veterans and that you are currently enrolling participants in the third study.

a) Please discuss your findings from the first two studies that have been conducted.
   a. *While we have a number of ongoing studies focused on assessing the impact of cannabis and cannabinoid-based products in veterans, thus far, none have been completed to date; all are currently ongoing and remain in the data collection phase.*

b) Does marijuana use to treat veterans, particularly as it relates to Post Traumatic Stress Disorder (PTSD), seem to be effective? Is there any concern that marijuana use could exacerbate problems associated with PTSD?
   a. *According to available literature, evidence is mixed; there have been concerns that cannabis could exacerbate existing symptoms of PTSD, but other reports indicate that cannabis products could confer benefits. For example, small studies suggest that THC or synthetic, non-plant derived THC (e.g., nabilone) could enhance sleep quality in those with PTSD; however, the positive effects of THC for PTSD symptoms do not appear to address many of the other symptoms associated with PTSD. Studies of CBD or CBD-containing products have found evidence suggesting amelioration of symptoms such as nightmares and anxiety, and reported that CBD could be beneficial in fear extinction processes. These seemingly mixed findings are likely due to the fact that cannabis itself is a heterogeneous plant containing hundreds of cannabinoids, terpenoids, and flavonoids. Given that studies of veterans are often observational or survey-based studies, the products used by veterans in each of these studies is often not directly assessed or profiled and can vary greatly. Clinical trials assessing products specifically formulated to target symptoms of PTSD and reduce potential negative side effects (e.g., anxiety, paranoia) are needed.*

4. Public Health Perspective

During the hearing, it was made clear that marijuana has the potential to cause both harms and benefits.

a) With this in mind, from a public health perspective, what are the biggest challenges related to marijuana, where are the most significant research gaps, and what should policymakers be focusing on moving forward?
   a. *Currently, the legal status of cannabis contributes to a number of complexities and difficulties when conceptualizing cannabis-based research studies. In the future, reconciling federal and state law will help facilitate researchers' abilities to conduct empirically sound research. In addition, allowing researchers to study real-world products that are available to patients and that are actually being used will provide critical data regarding the benefits and harms associated with specific cannabinoid formulations. Future research focused on safety and efficacy of unique formulations of cannabinoids for specific medical/psychiatric conditions and symptoms is clearly needed. Research directly examining the impact of high potency products and novel, marijuana concentrates products (which contain extremely high levels of THC) are also needed. Further, given that older adults represent the fastest growing population of cannabis consumers, researchers focused on the impact of cannabis in this population is critical. Preclinical data suggests that older adults may experience unique outcomes given a number of important factors in this population; adults have slower metabolisms, high rates of comorbid conditions and conventional medication use, and often experience age-related cognitive decline as well as age-related changes in the endocannabinoid system.*

Response to Questions Submitted by Members of the
Senate Caucus on International Narcotics Control
submitted by Sean Hennessy
University of Pennsylvania
27 May 2020

Senator Cornyn

Mental Illness Findings In NASEM Study

Dr. Hennessy, the National Academies report found substantial evidence of a statistical association between cannabis use and the development of schizophrenia or other psychoses. The highest risk was among the most frequent users.

- What factors contribute to this higher risk, and is it related to the higher potency of marijuana?
Response: Numerous factors are believed to affect one's risk of developing schizophrenia or other psychotic disorders. A 2016 meta-analysis (that is, a study of studies) conducted by Marconi and colleagues[1] examined the relationship between a person's level of cannabis use and their risk of developing schizophrenia and other psychotic disorders. That meta-analysis examined studies, published through 2013, that classified participants' self-reported cannabis use into at least three different categories—non-use plus at least two other levels. Those studies did not ask participants about the potency of the cannabis that they used, nor did they directly measure potency. Thus, the studies that found that a higher level of cannabis use is associated with a higher risk of psychosis did not include information on the potency of the cannabis.

- Your testimony also notes that there is reason to question the directionality of the statistical association. Could you share those reasons?
Response: The study committee of the National Academies of Science, Engineering and Medicine (NASEM) noted that there are at least three potential explanations for the observed associations between use of cannabis and the development of psychotic disorders: 1) cannabis use may contribute to the development of psychotic disorders; 2) psychotic disorders or their precursors may contribute to cannabis use; or 3) the same factors (e.g., genetic vulnerability, environment) may contribute to both cannabis use and to the development of psychotic disorders. A dose-response relationship between cannabis use and psychotic disorders may be present under any of these three explanations. Further, none of these explanations excludes the others—they could all be working in concert. Given that schizophrenia and other psychotic disorders may develop slowly over many years, it can be difficult to know even from longitudinal studies that measure drug use before schizophrenia was diagnosed, whether cannabis use actually preceded the emergence of early symptoms of schizophrenia in any given person. Therefore, as noted in the report (e.g., Box 12-1 on page 296), making conclusions about the direction of causation underlying such associations is challenging.

The report found moderate evidence of increased symptoms of mania, hypomania in individuals diagnosed with bipolar disorder and regular cannabis use.

---

[1] Marconi, A., Di Forti, M., Lewis, C. M., Murray, R. M., & Vassos, E. (2016). Meta-analysis of the association between the level of cannabis use and risk of psychosis. Schizophrenia bulletin, 42(5), 1262-1269.

- Were the users taking orally administered THC, cannabis-derived products, or smoking marijuana?

Response: The studies that examined symptoms of mania and hypomania in persons with bipolar disorder looked at smoked cannabis.

- Is this evidence significant enough to advise patients with bipolar disorder to not utilize medicinal marijuana?

Response: Decisions regarding whether or not to use medical cannabis involve weighing the potential benefits and harms in the specific person in whom use is being considered. The NASEM study committee did not assess the balance of potential benefits and harms of medical cannabis in either the general population or in specific subgroups, such as persons with bipolar disorder.

Evaluation of Medical Claims

The National Academies report did find conclusive evidence that orally administered THC is effective in treating some medical conditions, and that the clinical trials were utilized to gain FDA approval of the first drug comprised of an active ingredient derived from marijuana to treat rare, severe forms of epilepsy. It is my sense that any medical claims related to marijuana and cannabis derived products should receive the same through review that this drug received before being made available.

 Do you agree with that?

Response: The NASEM report did not articulate any findings or conclusions regarding the level of review or evidence that should be required from a regulatory perspective to either support medical claims for cannabis or cannabis-derived products, or to support the availability of cannabis or cannabis-derived products for medical use. Given the unique history and cultural context of cannabis in the US, the issues concerning its regulation are complex. Personally, I have not engaged in sufficient consideration or discussion of these issues to have formed well-founded views on this question.

Senator Feinstein

1. Evidence Regarding Use of Marijuana for Medical Purposes

You were a member of the committee of the National Academies of Sciences, Engineering, and Medicine that produced the 2017 report titled "The Health Effects of Marijuana and Cannabinoids."

Based on your work on this report:

a) Does enough information exists to conclude what the proper dosage and delivery mechanisms for medical marijuana patients should be?

Response: No. Even for the few FDA-unapproved uses for which there is at least moderate evidence for the effectiveness of cannabis or cannabis-derived products, there is very little evidence about the comparative effects of different doses or of different mechanisms of delivery. This represents a significant knowledge gap concerning therapeutic uses of cannabis and cannabis-derived products.

b) Does enough information exist to determine how marijuana might interact with other medications?

Response: No. Although the 2017 NASEM report did not specifically address the question of drugdrug interactions, there are a number of mechanisms by which THC, CBD, and other constituents of cannabis and cannabis-derived products might be expected to interact with prescription drugs.[2] However, very little research has been performed to evaluate such interactions, including their health effects in real-world patient populations.

2. Public Health Perspective

During the hearing, it was made clear that marijuana has the potential to cause both harms and benefits.

a) With this in mind, from a public health perspective, what are the biggest challenges related to marijuana, where are the most significant research gaps, and what should policymakers be focusing on moving forward?

Response: The 2017 NASEM report examined the available evidence concerning the benefits and harms of cannabis and cannabis-derived products. A common theme of our findings was that the available evidence was sparse and of uneven quality. To support and improve the cannabis research agenda, the NASEM study committee made recommendations to address research gaps, improve research quality, improve surveillance capacity, and address research barriers.

To specifically address your question, the study committee recommended that public agencies, philanthropic and professional organizations, private companies, and clinical and public health research groups provide funding and support for a national cannabis research agenda that addresses key evidence gaps. Prioritized research objectives should include, but need not be limited to:

Clinical and Observational Research

- Examine the health effects of cannabis use in at-risk or under-researched populations, such as children and youths and older populations, pregnant and breastfeeding women, and heavy cannabis users.
- Investigate the pharmacokinetic and pharmacodynamic properties of cannabis, modes of delivery, different concentrations, in various populations, including the dose–response relationships of cannabis and THC or other cannabinoids.
- Determine the harms and benefits associated with understudied cannabis products, such as edibles, concentrates, and topicals.
- Conduct well-controlled trials on the potential harmful and beneficial health effects of using different forms of cannabis, such as inhaled (smoked or vaporized) whole cannabis plant and oral cannabis.
- Characterize the health effects of cannabis on unstudied and understudied health endpoints, such as epilepsy in pediatric populations; symptoms of posttraumatic stress disorder; childhood and adult cancers; cannabis-related overdoses and poisonings; and other highpriority health endpoints.

Health Policy and Health Economics Research

- Identify models, including existing state cannabis policy models, for sustainable funding of national, state, and local public health surveillance systems.

---

[2] Foster, B. C., Abramovici, H., & Harris, C. S. (2019). Cannabis and cannabinoids: Kinetics and interactions. American Journal of Medicine, 132(11), 1266-1270.

- Investigate the economic impact of recreational and medical cannabis use on national and state public health and health care systems, health insurance providers, and patients.

Public Health and Public Safety Research

- Identify gaps in the cannabis-related knowledge and skills of health care and public health professionals, and assess the need for, and performance of, continuing education programs that address these gaps.
- Characterize public safety concerns related to recreational cannabis use and evaluate existing quality assurance, safety, and packaging standards for recreational cannabis products.

In addition, to ensure that sufficient data are available to inform research on the short- and longterm health effects of cannabis use (both harmful and beneficial effects), the committee recommended that the Centers for Disease Control and Prevention, the Substance Abuse and Mental Health Services Administration, the Association of State and Territorial Health Officials, the National Association of County and City Health Officials, the Association of Public Health Laboratories, and state and local public health departments fund and support improvements to federal public health surveillance systems and state-based public health surveillance efforts.

Senator Grassley

1. You stated in your written testimony that there is "substantial evidence" of an association between cannabis use and the development of schizophrenia or other psychoses. However, you also qualify this by stating, "there is reason to question the directionality of this association."

   a. Please expand on the risks of marijuana use and why its users are particularly susceptible to psychoses, and why there is a question as to the directionally of this association. Response: The NASEM report did indeed note that there is substantial evidence of a statistical association between cannabis use and the development of schizophrenia and other psychotic disorders (Conclusion 12-1; page 295). The committee noted that at least three potential mechanisms may explain these associations: 1) cannabis use may contribute to the development of psychotic disorders; 2) psychotic disorders or their precursors may contribute to cannabis use; or 3) the same factors (e.g., genetic vulnerability, environment) may contribute to both cannabis use and the development of psychotic disorders. None of these explanations excludes the others— they could all be working in concert. Given that schizophrenia and other psychotic disorders can develop slowly over many years, it can be difficult to know even from longitudinal studies that measured cannabis use before schizophrenia was diagnosed whether cannabis use actually preceded the emergence of early symptoms of schizophrenia in any given person. Therefore, as noted in the report (e.g., Box 12-1 on page 296), making conclusions about the direction of causation underlying such associations is challenging.

Senate Caucus on International Narcotics Control Hearing, Marijuana and Public Health, October 23, 2019, Written Statement from: Robert L. Fitzgerald, PhD., Professor of Pathology, University of California-San Diego

Introduction

Senators Cornyn and Feinstein, and Members of the Caucus it is a pleasure to be here today to discuss issues related to the use of marijuana and driving. As a way of a brief introduction, my first job out of graduate school was as a forensic toxicologist in Virginia helping to determine the cause and manner of death in Medical Examiner cases. At the Medical Examiner's office, I saw the devastating effects of driving under the influence on a routine basis. I also had the opportunity to work with State and Local police along with prosecution and defense attorneys to present scientific data in courts of law. Currently I am clinical toxicologist at UC San Diego where my research focuses on developing analytical methods to measure concentrations of THC and metabolites following recent marijuana exposure. I am part of a large team of investigators at the UCSD Center for Medical Cannabis Research (CMCR) focused on understanding both beneficial and detrimental effects of cannabis on human health. We recently completed enrolling subjects in one of the largest studies to date looking at the effect of smoked marijuana on driving performance and are in the initial stages of analyzing data.

The relationship between marijuana use and driving impairment is complex because of the unique pharmacokinetic and pharmacodynamic properties of delta-9-tetrahydrocannabinol (THC). With ethanol there is a clear relationship between amount of alcohol consumed, blood concentrations, and effects on driving performance. With marijuana these types of relationship are much more complex. The relationship between blood THC concentrations and crash risk has not been established, but there is a clear understanding that THC impairs driving performance. The question that remains is how to best identify drivers who are impaired by marijuana. There are no perfect solutions and legislative directives must balance keeping our roadways safe with due process.

Problems with determining the relationship between concentrations of THC and impairment is that levels of THC in blood vary widely depending on the route of administration, the time of sampling after dosing and the characteristics of the individual using marijuana. Generally, smoked marijuana causes effects that start shortly after inhalation and last about 3 hours, while subjects who eat marijuana start feeling effects about an hour later and can have effects up to 8 hours. Unlike alcohol which is cleared with 24 hours of drinking, THC and several metabolites accumulate in the body with repeated dosing so frequent users have baseline concentrations that exceed the per se limits currently used in some states for driving under the influence. After smoking, THC concentrations in blood change rapidly and our studies have documented the poor relationship between blood concentrations of THC and measures of impairment. Studies like this led the National Safety Council to put out a position statement in 2017 that reads:

"It is further concluded that due to rapid changes in blood THC concentrations over time, there is no minimum safe threshold blood concentration below which a driver can be considered to have been unaffected while driving following recent marijuana use. Consequently, there is no scientific basis for the adoption of THC per se laws for driving." This statement was also supported by the International Association of Police Chiefs. Despite these position statements, 18 States currently have some form of per se statutes.

How do we keep our roads safe? In California prosecution of driving under the influence of drugs is currently based on officer observations combined with results of toxicology testing. This practice will likely continue for the foreseeable future.

Since there is no reasonable expectation that THC or a metabolite of THC will be useful for per se impairment an alternative would be to develop methods to identify "recent use" biomarkers. The biological specimens that could be used to determine if a driver has recently used marijuana are blood, breath, and oral fluid. The primary advantages of breath and oral fluid over blood is that they can be collected at the roadside at the time of a traffic stop as opposed to blood which typically takes about 90 minutes to collect. This is an important consideration because unlike ethanol, concentrations of THC can fall by more than 90% in this short timeframe. There are a variety of ongoing efforts to identify markers of recent use.

In respect of my time limit I would like to close my initial statement by mentioning two items that this caucus needs to be aware of so they can help shape appropriate regulations.

1) Due to federal restrictions, investigators cannot study the cannabis products our population is exposed to. This is a critically important public health issue that needs to be changed.
2) Currently there is no standardized data collection for driving under the influence of drugs. Without good data it is difficult to develop good policy.

I hope my testimony was helpful and look forward to answering any questions members of the caucus may have.

Testimony of Dr. Staci Gruber, before the Senate Caucus on International Narcotics Control, "Marijuana and America's Health: Questions and Issues for Policy Makers," October 23, 2019

The term "marijuana" typically describes *all* constituents derived from the plant *Cannabis Sativa L*, which contains more than 100 phytocannabinoids that interact with the body's natural endocannabinoid system (ECS). Delta-9-tetrahydrocannabinol (THC), the primary psychoactive constituent of MJ, is mainly responsible for the subjective "high" felt by recreational MJ users who often seek strains and products with high concentrations of THC. Given that the ECS affects growth, differentiation, positioning, and connectivity among neurons, exposure to exogenous cannabinoids such as THC may disrupt neural development, especially during adolescence.

However, preliminary evidence also suggests that MJ and its constituents likely hold extraordinary potential for the treatment of a number of medical conditions[1]. Cannabidiol (CBD), the primary non-intoxicating constituent of the plant, has become well-known for its role in treating intractable pediatric-onset seizure disorders[2], and has demonstrated promise in treating other medical conditions including pain and multiple sclerosis[3], as well as psychiatric conditions including anxiety[4] and psychosis[5,6]. CBD has been shown to mitigate some of the negative effects of THC, including adverse

---

[1] Whiting PF, Wolff RF, Deshpande S, et al. Cannabinoids for Medical Use: A Systematic Review and Meta-analysis. *JAMA*. 2015;313(24):2456-2473.

[2] Devinsky O, Marsh E, Friedman D, et al. Cannabidiol in patients with treatment-resistant epilepsy: an open-label interventional trial. *Lancet Neurol.* 2016;15(3):270-278.

[3] Giacoppo S, Soundara Rajan T, Galuppo M, et al. Purified Cannabidiol, the main non-psychotropic component of Cannabis sativa, alone, counteracts neuronal apoptosis in experimental multiple sclerosis. *Eur Rev Med Pharmacol Sci.* 2015;19(24):4906-4919.

[4] Blessing EM, Steenkamp MM, Manzanares J, Marmar CR. Cannabidiol as a Potential Treatment for Anxiety Disorders. *Neurotherapeutics.* 2015;12(4):825-836.

[5] Leweke FM, Piomelli D, Pahlisch F, et al. Cannabidiol enhances anandamide signaling and alleviates psychotic symptoms of schizophrenia. *Transl Psychiatry.* 2012;2:e94.

[6] Zuardi AW, Crippa JA, Hallak JE, et al. Cannabidiol for the treatment of psychosis in Parkinson's disease. *J Psychopharmacol.* 2009;23(8):979-983.

psychological symptoms[7] and structural alterations in the brain[8,9]. It is of note that while THC levels are rising in *recreational* MJ products, CBD levels have declined to nearly undetectable levels[10].

Despite a body of evidence demonstrating structural and functional brain alterations among MJ users, more than 24 million Americans report past month MJ use[11]. Current deliberations over the legalization of MJ often highlight the potential benefits of medical marijuana (MMJ), and with the majority of states legalizing MMJ, it is not surprising that perceived risk related to MJ use is at an all-time low. In fact, recent US national survey data indicate that more high school seniors use MJ daily (5.9%) than smoke cigarettes (4.2%), more than 37% of seniors reported past-year MJ use, and only 29% of all seniors surveyed thought regular MJ use was harmful[12]. Further, almost 9% of the national population aged 12 or older currently use MJ[11], which is potentially concerning given critical neurodevelopmental changes that take place throughout adolescence. During adolescence, a period often marked by increased risk-taking behaviors including experimentation with substance use, brain regions, particularly those associated with executive functioning (e.g., problem solving, planning, inhibition), undergo processes that refine and strengthen neural networks, which continue until at least the mid-20s[13,14]. Throughout emerging adulthood, white matter volume and integrity also increase, which are associated with improvements in neural

---

[7] Morgan CJ, Gardener C, Schafer G, et al. Sub-chronic impact of cannabinoids in street cannabis on cognition, psychotic-like symptoms and psychological well-being. *Psychol Med.* 2012;42(2):391-400.

[8] Lorenzetti V, Solowij N, Yucel M. The Role of Cannabinoids in Neuroanatomic Alterations in Cannabis Users. *BiolPsychiatry.* 2016;79(7):e17-31.

[9] Yucel M, Lorenzetti V, Suo C, et al. Hippocampal harms, protection and recovery following regular cannabis use. *Transl Psychiatry.* 2016;6:e710.

[10] Chandra S, Radwan MM, Majumdar CG, Church JC, Freeman TP, ElSohly MA. New trends in cannabis potency in USA and Europe during the last decade (2008-2017). *Eur Arch Psychiatry Clin Neurosci.* 2019;269(1):5-15.

[11] *Key substance use and mental health indicators in the United States: Results from the 2016 National Survey on Drug Use and Health* Rockville, MD: Substance Abuse and Mental Health Services Administration;2017. HHS Publication No. SMA 17-5044, NSDUH Series H-52.

[12] National Adolescent Drug Trends in 2017: Findings Released. [press release]. Ann Arbor, MI: Monitoring the Future, December 14, 2017 2017.

[13] Gogtay N, Nugent TF, 3rd, Herman DH, et al. Dynamic mapping of normal human hippocampal development.*Hippocampus.* 2006;16(8):664-672.

[14] Houston SM, Herting MM, Sowell ER. The neurobiology of childhood structural brain development: conception through adulthood. *Curr Top Behav Neurosci.* 2014;16:3-17.

conductivity[15,16]. As adolescence is marked by ongoing neuromaturational processes and given increasing evidence that the adolescent brain is more vulnerable to the effects of drugs than the adult brain, *those at the greatest risk for adverse consequences represent a vast and vulnerable population of MJ consumers, a combination that poses serious public health concerns.*

To date, the majority of data regarding the impact of MJ is derived from studies of individuals with chronic, heavy recreational use; given public health concerns regarding adolescent use, many studies have specifically examined adolescent users or those with adolescent onset of MJ use. These studies have yielded a large body of research documenting the neurocognitive impact of recreational MJ use on the brain using both neuropsychological assessment and neuroimaging techniques, which have helped to clarify the underlying structural and functional alterations associated with recreational MJ use. Given heterogeneity across study findings, potential moderating variables must be taken into account given overall implications for public policy and considerations for continued research efforts.

Neurocognitive Impact of Recreational MJ Use

Cognition

Numerous studies have documented the effects of MJ across a wide range of cognitive domains[17],[18,19,20].

With regard to studies of memory function, several reviews indicate that recreational MJ use appears to impact a number of individual aspects of

---

[15] Giedd JN, Blumenthal J, Jeffries NO, et al. Brain development during childhood and adolescence: a longitudinal MRI study. *Nat Neurosci.* 1999;2(10):861-863.

[16] Jernigan TL, Gamst AC. Changes in volume with age--consistency and interpretation of observed effects. *NeurobiolAging.* 2005;26(9):1271-1274; discussion 1275-1278.

[17] Crane NA, Schuster RM, Fusar-Poli P, Gonzalez R. Effects of cannabis on neurocognitive functioning: recent advances, neurodevelopmental influences, and sex differences. *Neuropsychol Rev.* 2013;23(2):117-137.

[18] Ganzer F, Broning S, Kraft S, Sack PM, Thomasius R. Weighing the Evidence: A Systematic Review on Long-Term Neurocognitive Effects of Cannabis Use in Abstinent Adolescents and Adults. *Neuropsychol Rev.* 2016;26(2):186-222.

[19] Gruber SA, Sagar KA. Marijuana on the Mind? The Impact of Marijuana on Cognition, Brain Structure, and Brain Function, and Related Public Policy Implications. *Policy Insights from the Behavioral and Brain Sciences.* 2017;4(1):104-111.

[20] Lisdahl KM, Wright NE, Kirchner-Medina C, Maple KE, Shollenbarger S. Considering Cannabis: The Effects of Regular Cannabis Use on Neurocognition in Adolescents and Young Adults. *Curr Addict Rep.* 2014;1(2):144-156.

memory[18,21,22]; however, findings are most robust for measures of verbal learning, where decrements have been observed in terms of encoding, recall, and recognition[22].

Despite strong evidence for verbal memory impairment among recreational MJ consumers, findings from other areas of memory function, namely associative and visuospatial memory, are less clear[21,23,24]. Studies of executive function which examine response inhibition, planning, and decision-making, generally report decrements in MJ users[25,26,27,28,29,30,31,32]. Further, several investigations also report that poorer executive function is a

---

[21] Broyd SJ, van Hell HH, Beale C, Yucel M, Solowij N. Acute and Chronic Effects of Cannabinoids on Human Cognition-A Systematic Review. *Biol Psychiatry.* 2016;79(7):557-567.

[22] Solowij N, Battisti R. The chronic effects of cannabis on memory in humans: a review. *Curr Drug Abuse Rev.* 2008;1(1):81-98.

[23] Hermann D, Sartorius A, Welzel H, et al. Dorsolateral prefrontal cortex N-acetylaspartate/total creatine (NAA/tCr) loss in male recreational cannabis users. *Biol Psychiatry.* 2007;61(11):1281-1289.

[24] Sneider JT, Gruber SA, Rogowska J, Silveri MM, Yurgelun-Todd DA. A preliminary study of functional brain activation among marijuana users during performance of a virtual water maze task. *J Addict.* 2013;2013:461029.

[25] Becker MP, Collins PF, Luciana M. Neurocognition in college-aged daily marijuana users. *J Clin Exp Neuropsychol.* 2014;36(4):379-398.

[26] Dougherty DM, Mathias CW, Dawes MA, et al. Impulsivity, attention, memory, and decision-making among adolescent marijuana users. *Psychopharmacology (Berl).* 2013;226(2):307-319.

[27] Fontes MA, Bolla KI, Cunha PJ, et al. Cannabis use before age 15 and subsequent executive functioning. *Br J Psychiatry.* 2011;198(6):442-447.

[28] Hanson KL, Thayer RE, Tapert SF. Adolescent marijuana users have elevated risk-taking on the balloon analog risk task. *J Psychopharmacol.* 2014;28(11):1080-1087.

[29] Jacobus J, Bava S, Cohen-Zion M, Mahmood O, Tapert SF. Functional consequences of marijuana use in adolescents. *Pharmacol Biochem Behav.* 2009;92(4):559-565.

[30] Sagar KA, Dahlgren MK, Gonenc A, Racine MT, Dreman MW, Gruber SA. The impact of initiation: Early onset marijuana smokers demonstrate altered Stroop performance and brain activation. *Dev Cogn Neurosci.* 2015;16:84-92.

[31] Solowij N, Jones KA, Rozman ME, et al. Reflection impulsivity in adolescent cannabis users: a comparison with alcohol-using and non-substance-using adolescents. *Psychopharmacology (Berl).* 2012;219(2):575-586.

[32] Winward JL, Hanson KL, Tapert SF, Brown SA. Heavy alcohol use, marijuana use, and concomitant use by adolescents are associated with unique and shared cognitive decrements. *J Int Neuropsychol Soc.* 2014;20(8):784-795.

predictor of MJ use[33,34] and MJ-related problems[35]. Although only a small number of studies have examined processing speed, most have observed deficits in MJ users[36,37,38] relative to non-users. Findings with regard to overall intelligence are largely inconsistent. While some studies have reported lower IQ among recreational MJ users relative to non-users[37,39], more recent longitudinal studies with larger sample sizes challenge these findings. In one investigation of twins discordant for MJ use, MJ users demonstrated lower IQ relative to non-users, but MJ-using twins failed to show significantly greater IQ decline relative to their abstinent siblings, suggesting that the observed decline in IQ might be attributable to familial factors, rather than a direct result of MJ use[40]. Similarly, a second large-scale, longitudinal study[41] did not find IQ differences between MJ users and controls after adjusting for confounding variables.

Brain Function

Neuroimaging techniques have facilitated researchers' ability to clarify the underlying neural substrates associated with cognitive decrements in MJ users. Using a variety of paradigms, researchers have studied functional correlates across cognitive domains. While the direction and magnitude of findings are often variable, overall, MJ use is typically associated with altered patterns of neural activation across multiple brain regions. For example, during measures

---

[33] Dahlgren MK, Sagar KA, Racine MT, Dreman MW, Gruber SA. Marijuana Use Predicts Cognitive Performance on tasks of Executive Function. *Journal of studies on alcohol and drugs.* 2016;77:298-208.

[34] Squeglia LM, Jacobus J, Nguyen-Louie TT, Tapert SF. Inhibition during early adolescence predicts alcohol and marijuana use by late adolescence. *Neuropsychology.* 2014;28(5):782-790.

[35] Day AM, Metrik J, Spillane NS, Kahler CW. Working memory and impulsivity predict marijuana-related problems among frequent users. *Drug Alcohol Depend.* 2013;131(1-2):171-174.

[36] Auer R, Vittinghoff E, Yaffe K, et al. Association Between Lifetime Marijuana Use and Cognitive Function in Middle Age: The Coronary Artery Risk Development in Young Adults (CARDIA) Study. *JAMA Intern Med.* 2016;176(3):352-361.

[37] Fried PA, Watkinson B, Gray R. Neurocognitive consequences of marihuana--a comparison with pre-drug performance. *Neurotoxicol Teratol.* 2005;27(2):231-239.

[38] Thames AD, Arbid N, Sayegh P. Cannabis use and neurocognitive functioning in a non-clinical sample of users. *Addict Behav.* 2014;39(5):994-999.

[39] Meier MH, Caspi A, Ambler A, et al. Persistent cannabis users show neuropsychological decline from childhood to midlife. *Proc Natl Acad Sci U S A.* 2012;109(40):E2657-2664.

[40] Jackson NJ, Isen JD, Khoddam R, et al. Impact of adolescent marijuana use on intelligence: Results from two longitudinal twin studies. *Proc Natl Acad Sci U S A.* 2016;113(5):E500-508.

[41] Mokrysz C, Landy R, Gage SH, Munafo MR, Roiser JP, Curran HV. Are IQ and educational outcomes in teenagers related to their cannabis use? A prospective cohort study. *J Psychopharmacol.* 2016;30(2):159-168.

of executive function, a number of studies have reported altered activation in the frontal cortex[30,42,43,44]. Although many have examined verbal memory using traditional neuropsychological measures, the majority of fMRI studies have utilized spatial working memory tasks. Interestingly, MJ users generally demonstrate similar behavioral performance compared to non-users on these paradigms, yet neural alterations have been observed across studies[24,45,46,47,48], suggesting that less efficient neural strategies may be used by MJ users in order to achieve the same level of performance as non-users. Other aspects of cognition proposed to be associated with drug use, including associative memory, error monitoring, and reward processing have also been examined using fMRI methods in recreational MJ users. Overall, functional correlates of each of these processes appear to be altered in MJ users relative to non-MJ users[49].

Brain Structure

Brain imaging techniques have also afforded researchers the opportunity to examine the impact of MJ use on brain structure, including measures of both grey and white matter. Studies assessing the structural impact of MJ use often report bidirectional findings, which are typically related to the brain region

---

[42] Gruber SA, Yurgelun-Todd DA. Neuroimaging of marijuana smokers during inhibitory processing: a pilot investigation. *Brain Res Cogn Brain Res.* 2005;23(1):107-118.

[43] Hatchard T, Fried PA, Hogan MJ, Cameron I, Smith AM. Marijuana Use Impacts Cognitive Interference: An fMRI Investigation in Young Adults Performing the Counting Stroop Task. *Journal of Addiction Research & Therapy.* 2014;05(04).

[44] Kober H, DeVito EE, DeLeone CM, Carroll KM, Potenza MN. Cannabis abstinence during treatment and one-year follow-up: relationship to neural activity in men. *Neuropsychopharmacology.* 2014;39(10):2288-2298.

[45] Padula CB, Schweinsburg AD, Tapert SF. Spatial Working Memory Performance and fMRI Activation Interactions in Abstinent Adolescent Marijuana Users. *Psychol Addict Behav.* 2007;21(4):478-487.

[46] Schweinsburg AD, Nagel BJ, Schweinsburg BC, Park A, Theilmann RJ, Tapert SF. Abstinent adolescent marijuana users show altered fMRI response during spatial working memory. *Psychiatry Res.* 2008;163(1):40-51.

[47] Smith AM, Longo CA, Fried PA, Hogan MJ, Cameron I. Effects of marijuana on visuospatial working memory: an fMRI study in young adults. *Psychopharmacology (Berl).* 2010;210(3):429-438.

[48] Kanayama G, Rogowska J, Pope HG, Gruber SA, Yurgelun-Todd DA. Spatial working memory in heavy cannabis users: a functional magnetic resonance imaging study. *Psychopharmacology (Berl).* 2004;176(3-4):239-247.

[49] Sagar KA, Gruber SA. Interactions between recreational cannabis use and cognitive function: lessons from functional magnetic resonance imaging. *Ann N Y Acad Sci.* 2018.

under examination[50]. Interestingly, however, alterations are most often observed in areas with high densities of CB1 receptors[8] and may also be influenced by age of onset and increased MJ use[51]. A recent review reported that while larger cerebellar and striatal volumes have been observed in MJ users, regular MJ users often exhibit reductions in grey matter volume in several other regions, particularly in the hippocampus[8]. Importantly, studies have found that structural alterations in a number of brain regions appear to be related to increased executive dysfunction[52,53,54,55] and poorer verbal memory[56].

White matter, critical for efficient communication between brain regions, has also been assessed among MJ-using populations. In general, reduced white matter fiber tract integrity, measured using diffusion tensor imaging (DTI) techniques, has been observed in several prefrontal, limbic, parietal and cerebellar tracts in adolescent and emerging adult MJ users[57,58,59,60]. A relationship between earlier age of onset of MJ use and lower white matter integrity has also been reported[57-60]. Interestingly, these alterations have also

---

[50] Batalla A, Bhattacharyya S, Yucel M, et al. Structural and functional imaging studies in chronic cannabis users: a systematic review of adolescent and adult findings. *PLoS One.* 2013;8(2):e55821.

[51] Filbey FM, McQueeny T, DeWitt SJ, Mishra V. Preliminary findings demonstrating latent effects of early adolescent marijuana use onset on cortical architecture. *Dev Cogn Neurosci.* 2015;16:16-22.

[52] Churchwell JC, Lopez-Larson M, Yurgelun-Todd DA. Altered frontal cortical volume and decision making in adolescent cannabis users. *Front Psychol.* 2010;1:225.

[53] Medina KL, McQueeny T, Nagel BJ, Hanson KL, Yang TT, Tapert SF. Prefrontal cortex morphometry in abstinent adolescent marijuana users: subtle gender effects. *Addict Biol.* 2009;14(4):457-468.

[54] Medina KL, Nagel BJ, Tapert SF. Abnormal cerebellar morphometry in abstinent adolescent marijuana users. *PsychiatryRes.* 2010;182(2):152-159.

[55] Price JS, McQueeny T, Shollenbarger S, Browning EL, Wieser J, Lisdahl KM. Effects of marijuana use on prefrontal and parietal volumes and cognition in emerging adults. *Psychopharmacology (Berl).* 2015;232(16):2939-2950.

[56] Ashtari M, Avants B, Cyckowski L, et al. Medial temporal structures and memory functions in adolescents with heavy cannabis use. *J Psychiatr Res.* 2011;45(8):1055-1066.

[57] Clark DB, Chung T, Thatcher DL, Pajtek S, Long EC. Psychological dysregulation, white matter disorganization and substance use disorders in adolescence. *Addiction.* 2012;107(1):206-214.

[58] Epstein KA, Kumra S. White matter fractional anisotropy over two time points in early onset schizophrenia and adolescent cannabis use disorder: A naturalistic diffusion tensor imaging study. *Psychiatry Res.* 2015;232(1):34-41.

[59] Gruber SA, Dahlgren MK, Sagar KA, Gonenc A, Lukas SE. Worth the wait: effects of age of onset of marijuana use on white matter and impulsivity. *Psychopharmacology (Berl).* 2014;231(8):1455-1465.

[60] Gruber SA, Silveri MM, Dahlgren MK, Yurgelun-Todd D. Why so impulsive? White matter alterations are associated with impulsivity in chronic marijuana smokers. *Exp Clin Psychopharmacol.* 2011;19(3):231-242.

been correlated with impulsivity[59,60] and appear to be a risk factor for poorer executive function and for cannabis use disorders, specifically in adolescent users[57].

Variables Moderating the Impact of MJ Use on the Brain

Age of Onset of MJ use

As noted, overall, investigations have revealed functional and structural alterations associated with MJ use, but a number of studies have also reported that decrements observed in adults tend to be more significant, or persist for longer periods in those who began using MJ during adolescence[29,61]. This is not surprising given the fact that the brain is neurodevelopmentally vulnerable during adolescence and sensitive to exposure to drugs, alcohol, illness, and injury. Additionally, some investigations have noted that earlier age of MJ onset appears to be inextricably linked to higher frequency of use and amount of MJ used[30], suggesting that increased MJ use may be a trait characteristic specific to early onset users. As such, individuals with earlier MJ onset may have an "additive vulnerability," marked by a brain that is susceptible to the impact of MJ coupled with an increased likelihood to engage in higher levels of MJ use, relative to those with later MJ onset. Age of MJ onset is therefore an important variable to include in research endeavors as individuals who begin using MJ during adolescence are characterized by relatively "immature" brains and a tendency to use MJ more regularly, potentially posing a greater risk for cognitive decrements. Further, as differences between MJ users and non-users are often attributable to those with early versus late MJ onset[27,62,63,64], collecting data regarding onset of MJ use is likely to help reduce heterogeneity of study findings in future investigations.

---

[61] Schneider M. Puberty as a highly vulnerable developmental period for the consequences of cannabis exposure. *AddictBiol.* 2008;13(2):253-263.

[62] Ehrenreich H, Rinn T, Kunert HJ, et al. Specific attentional dysfunction in adults following early start of cannabis use. *Psychopharmacology.* 1999;142:295-301.

[63] Gruber SA, Sagar KA, Dahlgren MK, Racine M, Lukas SE. Age of onset of marijuana use and executive function. *Psychol Addict Behav.* 2012;26(3):496-506.

[64] Pope HG, Gruber AJ, Hudson JI, Cohane G, Huestis MA, Yurgelun-Todd D. Early-onset cannabis use and cognitive deficits: what is the nature of the association? *Drug and Alcohol Dependence.* 2003;69(3):303-310.

Exposure to MJ: Frequency, Magnitude, Potency & Novel Modes of Use

Increased frequency and magnitude of MJ use have been shown to be predictive of poorer cognitive performance[30,33]. To date, most studies regarding MJ use have examined the impact of heavy, chronic recreational MJ use. Accordingly, conclusions regarding the effects of MJ use on the brain are generally reflective of chronic, heavy use and may not necessarily be generalizable to light or more casual MJ users. However, it is important to recognize that there is no consensus regarding the definition or criteria required for "chronic," "regular," or "heavy" use versus "casual" or "light use." Discrepancies among what constitutes heavy relative to light MJ use has likely contributed to mixed findings across studies. Further, although most studies base assessments of MJ use on current number of days of MJ use or number of episodes of use per week, some investigators utilize estimates based on longer periods of time, such as lifetime smoking episodes. Each of these definitions account for frequency of use, but none specifically account for magnitude or amount of cannabis consumed, which can be difficult to assess especially across multiple products types. Unlike alcohol or other drugs, there is no standardized measure of MJ, which stems from a variety of difficulties in calculating exposure to MJ. For example, some derive the magnitude of MJ consumed by calculating the total number of joints smoked or "puffs" taken, while others calculate an estimate of actual grams of MJ used, which is becoming increasingly difficult with the advent of novel products and varied modes of use. Even if individuals can quantify the number of grams of MJ used, it does not account for other factors that influence overall exposure.

Individuals often use MJ products of various strengths, or potencies. Over the last several decades, the potency of recreational MJ, measured as THC concentration, has increased exponentially. Analyses of recreational MJ products revealed that between 1995 and 2017 levels of THC more than quadrupled, increasing from 4% to 17%[10]. In addition, highly potent products termed "concentrates" have also had a surge in popularity in recent years, raising additional concerns about the impact of recreational MJ use on the brain. These products are made by extracting THC from MJ flower to yield products with extremely high levels of THC that can exceed 80%[65]. Concentrated products, including "dabs" (the colloquial name for concentrated oil created by extracting THC from flower-based MJ products),

[65] Stogner JM, Miller BL. Assessing the Dangers of "Dabbing": Mere Marijuana or Harmful New Trend? *Pediatrics.* 2015;136(1):1-3.

shatter, wax, budder, and others all have significantly higher potency relative to conventional flower products[66]. Although no studies thus far have directly examined the impact of concentrates on the brain, survey studies have associated the use of concentrates with negative physiological consequences,[67] stronger intoxicating effects[68], and higher levels of physical dependence[69] and self-reported depression and anxiety[70]. In addition, one study assessing the relationship between brain structure and potency of MJ flower products (classified as either "high" or "low" potency by self-report) noted alterations in corpus callosum white matter microstructure in high-potency MJ users compared to low-potency users and controls[71]. Findings suggest that use of high potency MJ products, including concentrates, may impart negative consequences on the brain. This raises concern that adverse consequences associated with MJ use may be more significant now than in the past, particularly among young users.

Length of Abstinence

Throughout the literature, studies have employed a range of abstinence periods, generally ranging from 12 hours to one month, in order to examine the residual effects of MJ use. Length of abstinence may also influence study findings, as studies have shown changes in cognition over the course of abstinence periods. While some have reported recovery of function after one to three months of MJ abstinence,[37,72] others have shown that decrements are sustained over time[18]. Additional research is needed in this area, particularly studies examining the impact of *extended* abstinence periods.

---

[66] Mehmedic Z, Chandra S, Slade D, et al. Potency trends of Delta9-THC and other cannabinoids in confiscated cannabis preparations from 1993 to 2008. *J Forensic Sci.* 2010;55(5):1209-1217.

[67] Cavazos-Rehg PA, Sowles SJ, Krauss MJ, Agbonavbare V, Grucza R, Bierut L. A content analysis of tweets about high-potency marijuana. *Drug Alcohol Depend.* 2016;166:100-108.

[68] Loflin M, Earleywine M. A new method of cannabis ingestion: the dangers of dabs? *Addict Behav.* 2014;39(10):1430-1433.

[69] Meier MH. Associations between butane hash oil use and cannabis-related problems. *Drug Alcohol Depend.* 2017;179:25-31.

[70] Chan GCK, Hall W, Freeman TP, Ferris J, Kelly AB, Winstock A. User characteristics and effect profile of Butane Hash Oil: An extremely high-potency cannabis concentrate. *Drug Alcohol Depend.* 2017;178:32-38.

[71] Rigucci S, Marques TR, Di Forti M, et al. Effect of high-potency cannabis on corpus callosum microstructure. *Psychol Med.* 2016;46(4):841-854.

[72] Pope HG, Gruber AJ, Yurgelun-Todd D. Residual Neuropsychologic Effects of MJ. *Curr Psychiatry Rep.* 2001;3(6):507-512.

Chronologic Age: The Impact of MJ Use in Older Adults

Historically, increasing rates of MJ use have been noted among adolescents and young adults, which raised public health concerns given their neurodevelopmental vulnerability, driving research efforts to focus on youth and young adult populations. Recently, however, with expanded legalization across the US for both medical and recreational use, rates of use are now climbing fastest among older adults. According to data from the National Survey of Drug Use and Health (NSDUH), from 2002-2014, the proportion of adults aged 55 to 64 who reported MJ use in the past year increased by 455% from 1.1% to 6.1%; among those 65 and older, this proportion also increased dramatically, rising from 0.3% to 1.3%[73]. In comparison, rates among 18- to 25-year-olds rose only 13% in the same period, while rates among 12-17 year-olds actually *decreased* 10%. Despite the prevalence of MJ use among older adults, consequences of use are relatively unknown in this population, although preclinical evidence suggests that THC may impact older individuals differently. One preclinical study reported a *reversal* of age-related cognitive decline in mature and old mice treated with low doses of THC, while the same exposure resulted in cognitive decrements among young mice[74]. It is of note, however, that older adults may also have specific vulnerabilities with regard to MJ use. As overall metabolism slows with age, MJ may take longer to "clear the body," increasing the likelihood of experiencing higher levels of intoxication or an adverse event. Further, cannabinoids, including CBD, can inhibit the liver's cytochrome P450 enzyme system, increasing both plasma levels and toxicity of other drugs and potentially causing drug-drug interactions[75]. This is important, as approximately one-third of all prescription drugs in the US are used by older adults[76]. Additional studies aimed at identifying the specific impact of MJ use in older adults are clearly warranted, especially given the shifting landscape of legal recreational and medical use in a growing number of states.

---

[73] Azofeifa A, Mattson ME, Schauer G, McAfee T, Grant A, Lyerla R. National Estimates of Marijuana Use and Related Indicators - National Survey on Drug Use and Health, United States, 2002-2014. In. Vol 65: MMWR Surveill Summ; 2016:1-25.

[74] Bilkei-Gorzo A, Albayram O, Draffehn A, et al. A chronic low dose of Delta(9)-tetrahydrocannabinol (THC) restores cognitive function in old mice. *Nat Med.* 2017;23(6):782-787.

[75] Zendulka O, Dovrtelova G, Noskova K, et al. Cannabinoids and Cytochrome P450 Interactions. *Curr Drug Metab.* 2016;17(3):206-226.

[76] *NIDA Community Drug Alert Bulletin: Prescription Drugs.* Washington, DC: U.S. : National Institute on Drug Abuse;2005.

Can the Effects of Recreational MJ Use Be Generalized to Medical MJ Use?

Historically, THC, the primary intoxicating constituent of MJ, has been the most commonly studied cannabinoid. Recreational users typically seek products high in THC, given their goal to "alter their current state of being" or "get high." In contrast, MMJ patients are typically *not* interested in getting high, but instead seek symptom relief. Accordingly, MMJ patients are inclined to use products with varied cannabinoid constituent profiles, which often include those with high levels of CBD and other non-intoxicating cannabinoids, as well as THC. While CBD has been shown to mitigate some of the negative effects related to THC[9] and has been hypothesized to have tremendous therapeutic potential for a variety of conditions and indications[1], studies investigating the properties of additional cannabinoids, including cannabigerol (CBG), cannabichromene (CBC), and cannabinol (CBN), also cite positive effects, such as anti-inflammatory and neurogenic effects[77,78,79,80.] In addition to the unique effects of each individual cannabinoid, many posit the existence of an "entourage effect," which describes the synergistic action that occurs in the presence of multiple cannabinoids and terpenoids[81]. Terpenoids, the essential oils responsible for the flavor and fragrance components of cannabis, also exert their own biobehavioral health effects. This potential entourage effect may help explain why products from whole-plant extractions appear to be more efficacious than isolated cannabinoid compounds[82,83].

---

[77] Borrelli F, Fasolino I, Romano B, et al. Beneficial effect of the non-psychotropic plant cannabinoid cannabigerol on experimental inflammatory bowel disease. *Biochem Pharmacol.* 2013;85(9):1306-1316.

[78] Izzo AA, Borrelli F, Capasso R, Di Marzo V, Mechoulam R. Non-psychotropic plant cannabinoids: new therapeutic opportunities from an ancient herb. *Trends Pharmacol Sci.* 2009;30(10):515-527.

[79] Shinjyo N, Di Marzo V. The effect of cannabichromene on adult neural stem/progenitor cells. *Neurochem Int.* 2013;63(5):432-437.

[80] Valdeolivas S, Navarrete C, Cantarero I, Bellido ML, Munoz E, Sagredo O. Neuroprotective properties of cannabigerol in Huntington's disease: studies in R6/2 mice and 3-nitropropionate-lesioned mice. *Neurotherapeutics.* 2015;12(1):185-199.

[81] Russo EB. Taming THC: potential cannabis synergy and phytocannabinoid-terpenoid entourage effects. *Br J Pharmacol.* 2011;163(7):1344-1364.

[82] Gallily R, Yekhtin Z, Hanuš LO. Overcoming the Bell-Shaped Dose-Response of Cannabidiol by Using <i>Cannabis</i> Extract Enriched in Cannabidiol. *Pharmacology & Pharmacy.* 2015;06(02):75-85.

[83] Pamplona FA, da Silva LR, Coan AC. Potential Clinical Benefits of CBD-Rich Cannabis Extracts Over Purified CBD in Treatment-Resistant Epilepsy: Observational Data Meta-analysis. *Front Neurol.* 2018;9:759.

Although additional research is needed to fully understand the effects of individual cannabinoids as well as interactions between cannabinoids, terpenoids, flavonoids and other compounds present in the plant, differences between recreational and medical users' goals of use and choice of products raise the question as to whether the documented effects of recreational MJ use can be generalized to MMJ use. Despite the literature on recreational MJ use, few studies thus far have specifically examined the impact of MMJ on the brain, which may differ from recreational use given a number of factors, including but not limited to goal of use, product choice, and age of the consumer. Recent work from the first longitudinal, observational study of MMJ patients suggests that following three months of MMJ treatment, patients exhibit improvements in mood, quality of life, and sleep disturbance as well as *improved* cognitive performance on measures of executive function relative to baseline[84,85]. Additionally, in the first study to use neuroimaging techniques to examine functional correlates of MMJ use, three months of MMJ treatment was related to an apparent normalization of brain activation during the completion of the Multi-Source Interference Test (MSIT), a robust measure of cognitive control[84]. These improvements, which are in stark contrast to previous findings in recreational MJ users, particularly those with adolescent onset, may be related to potentially protective factors such as the presence of CBD and other therapeutic cannabinoids in MMJ patients' products or are perhaps attributable to the fact that most MMJ patients are adults and beyond the period of neurodevelopmental vulnerability when they initiate use. Further, these MMJ patients reported significant symptom alleviation and a notable decrease in the use of conventional medication (including opioids) following three months of MMJ treatment; these factors may also contribute to the cognitive improvements observed in this population. Additional research is needed to fully explore mechanisms of action among medical MJ patients in order to identify specific factors which moderate the adverse effects of MJ primarily observed in young, recreational users.

---

[84] Gruber SA, Sagar KA, Dahlgren MK, et al. The Grass Might Be Greener: Medical Marijuana Patients Exhibit Altered Brain Activity and Improved Executive Function after 3 Months of Treatment. *Frontiers in Pharmacology*. 2018;8.

[85] Gruber SA, Sagar KA, Dahlgren MK, Racine MT, Smith RT, Lukas SE. Splendor in the Grass? A Pilot Study Assessing the Impact of Medical Marijuana on Executive Function. *Front Pharmacol.* 2016;7:355.

Marijuana and Public Policy

The rapid pace of legalization efforts has caused policy to outpace science, and while additional research is needed, it is imperative to use scientific evidence to guide policy decisions. Studies of recreational MJ use report decrements in cognitive performance and alterations in brain structure and function, and most agree that individuals who begin to use MJ in adolescence or those with earlier onset of use are more likely to demonstrate neurobiologic alterations relative to those who initiate use later in life.

This finding is consistent with work demonstrating that the adolescent brain is not fully mature during adolescence and thus more vulnerable to the effects of drugs and alcohol than adults. It is critical for policymakers to carefully consider age-related guidelines to help prevent or reduce adolescent exposure. In addition, advertising of MJ products should not target youth, and safe guidelines for packaging of MJ products should be established to prevent accidental ingestion by children.

Policymakers are encouraged to engage in dialogue regarding safe limits of MJ use. In addition to frequency and magnitude of MJ used, safe limits of MJ use should consider potency of MJ products used and novel modes of administration, specifically those designed to deliver large doses of THC very quickly. Some have considered increased tax rates for higher potency products or limiting the total amount of THC within products available to specific consumer populations (e.g., young adults). Given that a number of cannabinoid constituents have potentially beneficial and neuroprotective effects, it is also important to determine whether implementing minimums for certain constituents, such as CBD, could help to mitigate some of the adverse effects related to THC. In light of data demonstrating a significant increase in THC and decline in CBD within recreational products, reversing this trend could prove to be helpful.

Barriers to Cannabis Research

In order to fully understand the potential benefit and possible risks associated with cannabis use, researchers *should be able to study actual cannabis products currently available to consumers* for both recreational and medical use. However, despite a growing need for information to help inform public policy and safe use guidelines, a number of barriers currently hinder research efforts. First, the Schedule I status of MJ poses significant challenges.

Currently, cannabis and all cannabinoids derived from plants containing >.3% THC by weight, fall under Schedule I of the CSA, the most restrictive category, despite the fact that numerous constituents, particularly CBD, are non-intoxicating and have been deemed "safe" by a number of sources[86,87]. While MJ may be legal in a particular state for medical and/or recreational/adult purposes, MJ remains illegal at the Federal level making it difficult for scientists to gain access to appropriate products for investigation. The Schedule I status of MJ can also lead to delays in conducting research, as multiple approvals are required, including applying for and receiving a Schedule I license, and a number of other safeguards must be in place to prevent potential diversion, such as storage, security, and surveillance considerations.

Current regulations stipulate that all cannabis to be used in clinical trials must be obtained from a single Federal source, currently the National Institute on Drug Abuse (NIDA). Although the DEA announced in 2016 that it would accept applications for non-NIDA entities to become registered to manufacture MJ and related products to supply researchers in the US, NIDA currently remains the only source of cannabis material for researchers. Over the last several years, NIDA's Drug Supply Program (DSP) has exponentially expanded the number of conventional MJ flower products (and one high CBD extract) available to researchers, which vary in constituent composition (low, medium, high THC, CBD, etc.) and potency.

However, investigations using only products from NIDA's drug supply may suffer from a lack of ecological or external validity, as potency and constituent profiles and ratios may not be consistent with consumers' products. Further, the majority of products available through the DSP are in conventional flower form, and do not reflect the wide range and types of products/modes that MJ consumers and patients often use.

Mechanisms allowing cannabis growers, providers or dispensaries to have their products tested, vetted, and ultimately made available to researchers for use in clinical research studies are a potential step in facilitating the assessment of actual MJ products used by consumers, including concentrate products, edibles, topicals, and tinctures, as well as products supplied by medical and recreational dispensaries.

---

[86] Iffland K, Grotenhermen F. An Update on Safety and Side Effects of Cannabidiol: A Review of Clinical Data and Relevant Animal Studies. *Cannabis Cannabinoid Res.* 2017;2(1):139-154.

[87] Volkow ND. Researching Marijuana for Therapeutic Purposes: The Potential Promise of Cannabidiol (CBD). In:2015, July 20.

Conclusion

Decades of research have focused on the impact of recreational MJ use, documenting cognitive decrements and structural and functional brain alterations in chronic, heavy users. These changes are most evident among adolescent users or those with early onset of MJ use, as adolescence represents a critical period of neurodevelopment, making youth more vulnerable to exogenous influences, including MJ. Accordingly, frequency and magnitude of use, product choice, potency, mode of use, and age of the consumer are all likely to influence the effects of MJ on the brain. It is important, however, to recognize that cannabis is a diverse and complex plant comprised of hundreds of constituents, many of which are likely to exhibit unique effects when studied alone as well as in the presence of other cannabinoids, terpenoids, flavonoids, and other compounds. Despite the range of effects conferred by individual constituents, many of which are non-intoxicating and have no diversion potential, cannabis and cannabinoids extracted from plants with >0.3%THC by weight is currently treated as a single entity and classified as a Schedule I substance, the most restrictive drug class, significantly hindering research efforts. While the impact of recreational MJ use among adolescents and early onset users is often the focus of research investigations, resulting in a body of literature, the impact of medical MJ use is vastly understudied. Investigations are needed to clarify the impact of MMJ on the brain and health-related outcomes (e.g., changes in conventional medication use, impact on pain, sleep, quality of life, mental health conditions, etc.), both short- and long-term consequences of high potency products and novel modes of use, effects of recreational and medical MJ use in older adults, and the efficacy and safety of existing products as well as those in development, ideally using clinical trial models. As the nation has warmed toward both medical and adult recreational MJ, the need for empirically sound data is critical to help patients and consumers make informed decisions about their use.

Testimony by Sean Hennessy, before the Senate Caucus on International Narcotics Control, October 23, 2019

Good afternoon. My name is Sean Hennessy and I am a pharmacist-epidemiologist and faculty member at the University of Pennsylvania. I was a member of the 16-person committee that wrote the report entitled *The Health*

Effects of Cannabis and Cannabinoids[88] that the National Academies of Science, Engineering and Medicine released in January 2017.

More than 150 years ago, the National Academy of Sciences was created through a congressional charter signed by Abraham Lincoln to serve as an independent, authoritative body outside the government that could advise the nation on matters pertaining to science and technology. It later expanded to include engineering and medicine. Every year, approximately 6,000 National Academies members and volunteers serve pro bono on consensus study committees or convening activities. The National Academies' consensus study process is considered the gold standard of independent, nonpartisan, evidence-based advice.

Our committee conducted a comprehensive review and synthesis of the existing evidence regarding the potential health effects—both therapeutic and harmful—of cannabis and cannabis-derived products. Our 487-page report lists nearly 100 different conclusions about these effects. It also lists four recommendations to address research gaps, improve research quality, improve surveillance capacity, and address research barriers. I'd like to briefly summarize what our committee found and recommended. I have attached a copy of the report's highlights for your reference.

For each potentially therapeutic or harmful health effect that we examined, our committee classified the evidence as either *conclusive*, *substantial*, *moderate*, *limited*, or as *no or insufficient evidence*.

Potential Therapeutic Effects

We found *conclusive evidence* that orally administered tetrahydrocannabinol (THC) is effective in treating chemotherapy-induced nausea and vomiting. Synthetic THC (dronabinol) and a synthetic analogue of THC (nabilone) are both FDA-approved for this use.

We found *substantial evidence* that some cannabis products are effective for the treatment of chronic pain in adults. Of the trials examined, 13 studied a product called *nabiximols* (an oral-mucosal cannabis extract containing equal amounts of THC and CBD), 7 studied cannabis flower that was either

---

[88] National Academies of Sciences, Engineering, and Medicine. 2017. The health effects of cannabis and cannabinoids: The current state of evidence and recommendations for research. Washington, DC: The National Academies Press. doi:10.17226/24625.

smoked or vaped, 5 studied orally administered synthetic THC, and 3 studied THC oramucosal spray.

We found *substantial evidence* that orally administered cannabinoids (nabiximols and nabilone) can improve patient-reported symptoms of muscle spasticity in persons with multiple sclerosis.

We found *moderate evidence* that cannabis-derived products, primarily nabiximols, can improve short- term sleep in persons with sleep disturbance associated with obstructive sleep apnea, fibromyalgia, chronic pain, and multiple sclerosis.

We found only *limited evidence* that cannabis and oral cannabinoids can increase appetite and reduce weight loss associated with HIV/AIDS; that that oral cannabinoids can improve clinician-measured muscle spasticity in persons with multiple sclerosis; that oral THC can improve symptoms of Tourette syndrome; that oral CBD can improve anxiety symptoms in individuals with social anxiety disorders; and that nabilone can improve symptoms of posttraumatic stress disorder.

There were many conditions for which we found *no or insufficient evidence* that cannabis or cannabis- derived products were effective, including cancers, irritable bowel syndrome, and Parkinson disease.

After we issued our report, the results of clinical trials were made available that served as the basis for the approval by the US Food and Drug Administration of concentrated CBD oil (Epidiolex®) for use as part of a multi-drug treatment for two rare and severe forms of epilepsy.[89] For reasons of transparency, I note that I served as a consultant for Greenwich Biosciences, Inc. in 2018 and received consulting fees that were less than the $5000 threshold for a "significant financial interest" set by the US Department of Health and Human Services.

Potential Harmful Health Effects

We found *substantial evidence* of a statistical association between recent cannabis use and an increased risk of motor vehicle crashes.

We found *substantial evidence* of a statistical association between maternal cannabis smoking and lower birth weight of the offspring.

---

[89] https://www.fda.gov/news-events/press-announcements/fda-approves-first-drug-compri-sed-active-ingredient-derived-marijuana-treat-rare-severe-forms, accessed 16 October 2019.

We found *substantial evidence* of a statistical association between long-term cannabis smoking and worse respiratory symptoms including cough, increased sputum production, wheeze, and more frequent chronic bronchitis episodes.

We found *substantial evidence* that initiating cannabis use at an earlier age is a risk factor for the development of problem cannabis use.

We found *substantial evidence* of a statistical association between cannabis use and the development of schizophrenia or other psychoses, with the highest risk among the most frequent users. However, there is reason to question about the directionality of this association.

We found *moderate evidence* of a statistical association between acute cannabis use and impairment in learning, memory, and attention.

We found *moderate evidence* of a statistical association between regular cannabis use and increased symptoms of mania and hypomania in individuals diagnosed with bipolar disorders.

We found *moderate evidence* of a statistical association between cannabis use and a small increased risk for the development of depressive disorders.

We found *moderate evidence* of a statistical association between cannabis use and increased incidence of suicidal ideation, suicide attempts, and completed suicide.

We found *moderate evidence* of a statistical association between regular cannabis use and increased incidence of social anxiety disorder.

We found *moderate evidence* that during adolescence the frequency of cannabis use, oppositional behaviors, a younger age of first alcohol use, nicotine use, parental substance use, poor school performance, antisocial behaviors, and childhood sexual abuse are risk factors for the development of problem cannabis use.

We found *moderate evidence* of a statistical association between cannabis use and the development of substance dependence and/or a substance abuse disorder for substances, including alcohol, tobacco, and other illicit drugs.

We found *moderate evidence* of a statistical association between cannabis use and an increased risk of overdose injuries among pediatric populations in U.S. states where cannabis is legal according to state law.

Barriers to Research on the Effects of Cannabis and Cannabis-derived Products

Our committee identified four challenges to conducting research on the health effects of cannabis:

1) There are specific regulatory barriers, including the classification of cannabis as a Schedule I substance, that impede the advancement of cannabis and cannabinoid research.
2) It is often difficult for researchers to gain access to the quantity, quality, and type of cannabis product necessary to address specific research questions on the health effects of cannabis use.
3) A diverse network of funders is needed to support cannabis and cannabinoid research that explores the beneficial and harmful health effects of cannabis use.
4) To develop conclusive evidence for the effects of cannabis use on short- and long-term health outcomes, improvements and standardization in research methods are needed.

Recommendations

Our committee made the following four recommendations:

1) To develop a comprehensive evidence base on the short- and long-term health effects of cannabis use (both beneficial and harmful effects), public agencies, philanthropic and professional organizations, private companies, and clinical and public health research groups should provide funding and support for a national cannabis research agenda that addresses key gaps in the evidence base.
2) To promote the development of conclusive evidence on the short- and long-term health effects of cannabis use (both beneficial and harmful effects), agencies of the U.S. Department of Health and Human Services should jointly fund a workshop to develop a set of research standards and benchmarks to guide and ensure the production of high-quality cannabis research.
3) To ensure that sufficient data are available to inform research on the short- and long-term health effects of cannabis use, the federal, state,

and local health authorities should fund and support improvements to federal public health surveillance systems and state-based public health surveillance efforts.

4) The Centers for Disease Control and Prevention, National Institutes of Health, U.S. Food and Drug Administration, industry groups, and nongovernmental organizations should fund the convening of a committee of experts tasked to produce an objective and evidence-based report that fully characterizes the impacts of regulatory barriers to cannabis research and that proposes strategies for supporting development of the resources and infrastructure necessary to conduct a comprehensive cannabis research agenda.

Thank you for your attention and the opportunity to discuss these issues. I look forward to answering your questions.

The Health Effects of Cannabis and Cannabinoids

The Current State of Evidence and Recommendations for Research

Recent years have seen a rapid rise in the medical and recreational use of cannabis: a broad term that can be used to describe the various products and chemical compounds (e.g., marijuana, cannabinoids) derived from different species of the cannabis plant. Despite increased cannabis use and a changing state-level policy landscape, conclusive evidence regarding the short- and long-term health effects—both harms and benefits—of cannabis use remains elusive.

A lack of definitive evidence has resulted in insufficient information on the health implications of cannabis use, causing a significant public health concern for vulnerable populations such as adolescents, pregnant women, and others. Unlike with substances such as alcohol or tobacco, no accepted standards exist to help guide individuals as they make choices regarding if, when, where, and how to use cannabis safely and, in regard to therapeutic uses, effectively.

With support from a host of federal, state, philanthropic and nongovernmental organizations, the National Academies of Sciences, Engineering, and Medicine convened an ad hoc, expert committee to develop a comprehensive, in-depth review of the most recent evidence regarding health effects of using cannabis and cannabis-derived products. In the resulting report, *The Health Effects of Cannabis and Cannabinoids: The Current State of Evidence and Recommendations for Research,* the committee presents nearly 100 research conclusions. The committee also formulated recommendations to expand and improve the quality of cannabis research efforts, enhance data collection efforts to support the advancement of research, and address the current barriers to cannabis research.

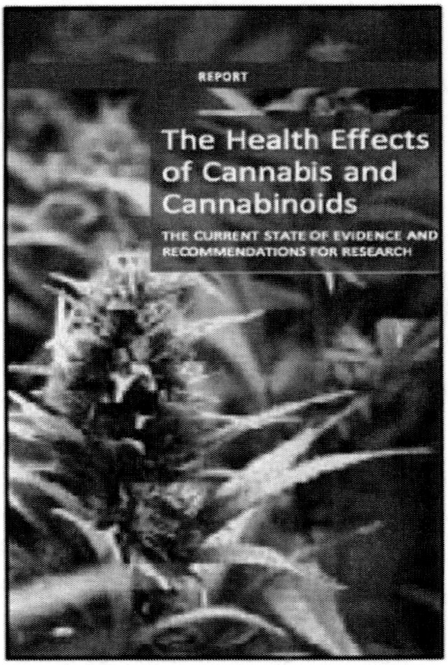

Despite increased cannabis use and a changing state-level policy landscape, conclusive evidence regarding the short- and long-term health effects— both harms and benefits— of cannabis use remains elusive.

The Study Process

The committee conducted an extensive search of literature databases to identify relevant articles published since the 1999 release of the National Academies report *Marijuana and Medicine: Assessing the Science Base.* As a result of their search efforts, the committee considered more than 10,000 scientific abstracts for their relevance to the report. Given the large scientific literature on cannabis, the breadth of the statement of task, and other constraints of the study, the committee gave primacy to recently published systematic reviews and high-quality primary research for 11 groups of health topics and concerns, including therapeutic effects for a variety of diseases and conditions; cancer incidence; respiratory disease; prenatal, perinatal, and neonatal outcomes; psychosocial and mental health concerns, and others.

The committee was charged to conduct a comprehensive, in-depth review of health topics with the greatest public health impact rather than to conduct multiple systematic reviews, which would have required a lengthy and robust series of processes. The committee did, however, adopt key features of that process: a comprehensive literature search, assessments by more than one person of the quality of the literature and the conclusions, pre-specification of the questions of interest before conclusions were formulated, standard language to allow for comparisons between conclusions, and declarations of conflict of interest via the National Academies conflict-of-interest policies.

Because of the practical steps taken to narrow a very large literature to one that was manageable within the timeframe available to the committee, there is a possibility that some literature was missed. Furthermore, some research may not be reflected in this report if it did not directly address the health endpoint research questions that were prioritized by the committee.

The Committee's Conclusions

The committee arrived at nearly 100 different research conclusions related to cannabis or cannabinoid use and health, organizing these into 5 categories: conclusive, substantial, moderate, limited, and no/insufficient evidence.

For a definition of these levels of evidence and a full listing of the conclusions, please see the "Committee's Conclusions" document by visiting the report's website at nationalacademies.org/CannabisHealthEffects.

The Committee's Recommendations

Based on their research conclusions, the committee members formulated four recommendations that outline priorities to inform a research agenda. The recommendations prioritize research approaches and objectives to:

- address current research gaps, highlighting the need for a national cannabis research agenda that includes clinical and observational research, health policy and health economics research, and public health and public safety research;
- identify actionable strategies to improve research quality and promote the development of research standards and benchmarks;
- highlight the potential for improvements in data collection efforts and the enhancement of surveillance capacity; and
- propose strategies for addressing the current barriers to the advancement of the cannabis research agenda.

The full text of the committee's recommendations appears on the pages that follow.

Conclusion

This is a pivotal time in the world of cannabis policy and research. Shifting public sentiment, conflicting and impeded scientific research, and legislative battles have fueled the debate about what, if any, harms or benefits can be attributed to the use of cannabis or its derivatives. This report provides a broad set of evidence-based research conclusions on the health effects of cannabis and cannabinoids and puts forth recommendations to help advance the research field and better inform public health decisions.

To read the full report, please visit nationalacademies.org/CannabisHealthEffects.

Recommendations

Recommendation 1: To develop a comprehensive evidence base on the short- and long-term health effects of cannabis use (both beneficial and harmful effects), public agencies, philanthropic and professional organizations, private companies, and clinical and public health research groups should provide funding and support for a national cannabis research agenda that addresses key gaps in the evidence base. Prioritized research streams and objectives should include, but need not be limited to:

Clinical and Observational Research

- Examine the health effects of cannabis use in at-risk or under-researched populations, such as children and youth (often described as less than 18 years of age) and older populations (generally over 50 years of age), pregnant and breastfeeding women, and heavy cannabis users.
- Investigate the pharmacokinetic and pharmacodynamic properties of cannabis, modes of delivery, different concentrations, in various populations, including the dose–response relationships of cannabis and THC or other cannabinoids.
- Determine the benefits and harms associated with understudied cannabis products, such as edibles, concentrates, and topicals.
- Conduct well-controlled trials on the potential beneficial and harmful health effects of using different forms of cannabis, such as inhaled (smoked or vaporized) whole cannabis plant and oral cannabis.
- Characterize the health effects of cannabis on unstudied and understudied health endpoints, such as epilepsy in pediatric populations; symptoms of posttraumatic stress disorder; childhood and adult cancers; cannabis-related overdoses and poisonings; and other high-priority health endpoints.

Health Policy and Health Economics Research

- Identify models, including existing state cannabis policy models, for sustainable funding of national, state, and local public health surveillance systems.
- Investigate the economic impact of recreational and medical cannabis use on national and state public health and health care systems, health insurance providers, and patients.

Public Health and Public Safety Research

- Identify gaps in the cannabis-related knowledge and skills of health care and public health professionals, and assess the need for, and performance of, continuing education programs that address these gaps.
- Characterize public safety concerns related to recreational cannabis use and evaluate existing quality assurance, safety, and packaging standards for recreational cannabis products.

Recommendation 2: To promote the development of conclusive evidence on the short- and long-term health effects of cannabis use (both beneficial and harmful effects), agencies of the United States Department of Health and Human Services, including the National Institutes of Health and the Centers for Disease Control and Prevention should jointly fund a workshop to develop a set of research standards and benchmarks to guide and ensure the production of high-quality cannabis research. Workshop objectives should include, but need not be limited to:

- The development of a minimum dataset for observational and clinical studies, standards for research methods and design, and guidelines for data collection methods.
- Adaptation of existing research-reporting standards to the needs of cannabis research.
- The development of uniform terminology for clinical and epidemiological cannabis research.
- The development of standardized and evidence-based question banks for clinical research and public health surveillance tools.

Recommendation 3: To ensure that sufficient data are available to inform research on the short- and long-term health effects of cannabis use, (both beneficial and harmful effects), the Centers for Disease Control and Prevention, the Substance Abuse and Mental Health Services Administration, the Association of State and Territorial Health Officials, National Association of County and City Health Officials, the Association *of Public Health Laboratories, and state and local public health departments should fund and support improvements to federal public health surveillance systems and state-based public health surveillance efforts. Potential efforts should include, but need not be limited to:*

- The development of question banks on the beneficial and harmful health effects of therapeutic and recreational cannabis use and their incorporation into major public health surveys, including: the National Health and Nutrition Examination Survey, National Health Interview Survey, Behavioral Risk Factor Surveillance System, National Survey on Drug Use and Health, Youth Risk Behavior Surveillance System, National Vital Statistics System, Medical Expenditure Panel Survey, and the National Survey of Family Growth.

- Determining the capacity to collect and reliably interpret data from diagnostic classification codes in administrative data (e.g., International Classification of Diseases-10)
- The establishment and utilization of state-based testing facilities to analyze the chemical composition of cannabis and products containing cannabis, cannabinoids, or THC.
- The development of novel diagnostic technologies that allow for rapid, accurate, and noninvasive assessment of cannabis exposure and impairment.
- Strategies for surveillance of harmful effects of cannabis for therapeutic use.

Recommendation 4: The Centers for Disease Control and Prevention, National Institutes of Health, Food and Drug Administration, industry groups, and nongovernmental organizations should fund the convening of a committee of experts tasked to produce an objective and evidence-based report that fully characterizes the impacts of regulatory barriers to cannabis research and that proposes strategies for supporting development of the resources and infrastructure necessary to conduct a comprehensive cannabis research agenda. Committee objectives should include, but need not be limited to:

- Proposing strategies for expanding access to research-grade marijuana, through the creation and approval of new facilities for growing and storing cannabis.
- Identifying nontraditional funding sources and mechanisms to support a comprehensive national cannabis research agenda.
- Investigating strategies for improving the quality, diversity, and external validity of research-grade cannabis products.

Committee on the Health Effects of Marijuana

Marie McCormick (Chair),
Harvard T.H. Chan School of Public Health

Donald I. Abrams
Zuckerberg San Francisco General Hospital

Margarita Alegría
Massachusetts General Hospital

William Checkley
Johns Hopkins University

R. Lorraine Collins
State University of New York at Buffalo

Ziva Cooper
Columbia University Medical Center

Adre J. Du Plessis
Children's National Health System

Sarah Feldstein Ewing
Oregon Health & Science University

Sean Hennessy
University of Pennsylvania

Kent Hutchison
University of Colorado Boulder

Norbert E. Kaminski
Michigan State University

Sachin Patel
Vanderbilt University Medical Center

Daniele Piomelli
University of California, Irvine

Stephen Sidney
Kaiser Permanente Northern California

Robert B. Wallace
University of Iowa College of Public Health

John Williams
Duke University Medical Center

Study Sponsors

Alaska Mental Health Trust Authority
Arizona Department of Health Services
California Department of Public Health
CDC Foundation
Centers for Disease Control and Prevention
Food and Drug Administration Mat-Su Health Foundation
National Cancer Institute— National Institutes of Health
National Highway Traffic Safety Administration
National Institute on Drug Abuse—National Institutes of Health
Oregon Health Authority
Robert W. Woodruff Foundation
The ColoradoHealth Foundation
Truth Initiative
Washington State Department of Health

Study Staff

Leigh Miles Jackson
Study Director

Jennifer Cohen
Program Officer

Kelsey Geiser
Research Associate *(from July 2016)*

R. Brian Woodbury
Research Associate

Sara Tharakan
Research Associate *(until July 2016)*

Hope Hare
Administrative Assistant

Matthew Masiello
Research Assistant *(from June 2016)*

Marjorie Pichon
Senior Program Assistant *(from August 2016)*

Kathleen Stratton
Scholar

Brownsyne Tucker-Edmonds
Norman F. Grant/American Board of Obstetrics and Gynecology Fellow

Rose Marie Martinez
Senior Board Director, Board on Population Health and Public Health Practice

* * *

Good afternoon, Mr. Chairman and members of the Caucus. Thank you for inviting me to contribute my knowledge about adolescent vulnerability to cannabis effects on cognitive functioning.

Summary

What We Know:

1) Cannabis use is associated with cognitive deficits that persist beyond the period of acute intoxication
2) Cannabis-related cognitive deficits are subtle
3) More frequent, persistent, and earlier-onset cannabis use is associated with larger cognitive deficits

What We Still Need to Know:

1) What are the mechanisms underlying cannabis-related cognitive deficits?

2) What are the parameters of cannabis use that determine the magnitude and persistence of cognitive deficits (quantity, frequency, age-of-onset, duration, THC content)?
3) Does cognitive functioning recover with abstinence?
4) Are there individual differences in susceptibility to cannabis-related cognitive deficits?

Cannabis Effects on Cognitive Function

Cannabis intoxication results in temporary cognitive impairment,[90,91,92] but it is less clear if cannabis use results in enduring cognitive impairment – impairment that persists beyond the period of acute intoxication. Studies comparing heavy cannabis users with nonusers have collectively shown that heavy cannabis users, even when not intoxicated by cannabis, perform worse on cognitive tests, including tests of learning and memory, attention, and other executive functions.[93,94,95] The magnitude of cognitive deficits in these heavy cannabis users is small,[4-6] though some evidence suggests that cognitive deficits might be larger among more frequent, chronic, and earlier-onset

---

[90] Crean RD, Crane NA, Mason BJ. An evidence-based review of acute and long-term effects of cannabis use on executive cognitive functions. *J Addict Med.* 2011;5(1):1-8.

[91] Crane NA, Schuster RM, Fusar-Poli P, Gonzalez R. Effects of cannabis on neurocognitive functioning: Recent advances, neurodevelopmental influences, and sex differences. *Neuropsychol Rev.* 2013;23(2):117-137.

[92] Solowij N, Pesa N. Cannabis and cognition: short and long-term effects. *Marijuana and Madness.* 2012;2:91-102.

[93] Grant I, Gonzalez R, Carey CL, Natarajan L, Wolfson T. Non-acute (residual) neurocognitive effects of cannabis use: A meta-analytic study. *J Int Neuropsych Soc.* 2003;9(5):679-689.

[94] Schreiner AM, Dunn ME. Residual effects of cannabis use on neurocognitive performance after prolonged abstinence: A meta-analysis. *Exp Clin Psychopharm.* 2012;20(5):420-429.

[95] Scott JC, Slomiak ST, Jones JD, Rosen AF, Moore TM, Gur RC. Association of cannabis with cognitive functioning in adolescents and young adults: A systematic review and meta-analysis. *JAMA Psychiatry.* 2018;75(6):585-595.

cannabis users.[3,96,97,98,99,100,101] Some evidence suggests that cognitive deficits might resolve with prolonged abstinence.[5,6,102]

The extant evidence base draws largely on studies that compared heavy cannabis users with nonusers on cognitive test performance, and these studies have two commonly cited limitations. First, the studies lack information on initial cognitive functioning before the onset of cannabis use. Therefore, the studies do not address the possibility that cognitive differences between cannabis users and comparison individuals represent pre-existing rather than cannabis-induced deficits. Second, the studies rely on cannabis users' retrospective reports of their frequency, quantity, age-of-onset, and duration of cannabis use, with reports often obtained years after initiation of heavy use. Therefore, retrospective reports of cannabis use might not be accurate.

To redress these limitations, prospective longitudinal studies are needed. Prospective longitudinal studies assess cognitive functioning in youth before the initiation of cannabis use, obtain prospective information about cannabis use as the sample is followed over a number of years, and then reassess cognitive functioning again, after some individuals in the sample have developed a persistent pattern of cannabis use. The most comprehensive prospective longitudinal study of cannabis use and cognitive functioning was published by our group in 2012 (Meier et al., 2012).[103] Our study found that persistent cannabis use was associated with IQ decline from childhood to adulthood, and IQ decline was concentrated in adolescent-onset persistent cannabis users. Here I (1) describe our 2012 study and explain the findings, (2) address questions about whether cannabis-associated IQ decline could be

---

[96] Solowij N, Jones KA, Rozman ME, et al. Verbal learning and memory in adolescent cannabis users, alcohol users and non-users. *Psychopharmacology.* 2011;216(1):131-144.

[97] Ehrenreich H, Rinn T, Kunert HJ, et al. Specific attentional dysfunction in adults following early start of cannabis use. *Psychopharmacology.* 1999;142(3):295-301.

[98] Pope HG, Gruber AJ, Hudson JI, Cohane G, Huestis MA, Yurgelun-Todd D. Early-onset cannabis use and cognitive deficits: What is the nature of the association? *Drug Alcohol Depen.* 2003;69(3):303-310.

[99] Fontes MA, Bolla KI, Cunha PJ, et al. Cannabis use before age 15 and subsequent executive functioning. *Brit J Psychiat.* 2011;198(6):442-447.

[100] Hall W, Lynskey M. Long-term marijuana use and cognitive impairment in middle age. *JAMA Internal Medicine.* 2016;176(3):362-363.

[101] Auer R, Vittinghoff E, Yaffe K, et al. Association between lifetime marijuana use and cognitive function in middle age: the Coronary Artery Risk Development in Young Adults (CARDIA) study. *JAMA Internal Medicine.* 2016;176(3):352-361.

[102] Jacobus J, F Tapert S. Effects of cannabis on the adolescent brain. *Current Pharmaceutical Design.* 2014;20(13):2186-2193.

[103] Meier MH, Caspi A, Ambler A, et al. Persistent cannabis users show neuropsychological decline from childhood to midlife. *Proc Natl Acad Sci U S A.* 2012;109(40):E2657-E2664.

accounted for by factors such as low socioeconomic status and poor childhood self-regulation, and (3) explain why the study is unique and why we need more studies like it.

Cannabis and IQ (Discussion of Meier et al., 2012)

The Findings

We studied the association between persistent cannabis use and IQ decline and asked whether IQ decline was concentrated among adolescent-onset cannabis users. Findings come from the Dunedin Multidisciplinary Health and Development Study. The Study has followed a group of 1,037 children, who were born in 1972-73 in Dunedin, New Zealand, from birth to age 38 years, with 96% of the sample taking part at age 38. IQ was tested at age 13, before cannabis use, and again at age 38, after some study members had used cannabis for years.

We found that:

1) Persistent cannabis use was associated with IQ decline from childhood to adulthood, and IQ decline was concentrated among adolescent-onset persistent cannabis users. For example, individuals who began using cannabis in adolescence (before age 18) and used it for years thereafter showed an average 8-point IQ decline from childhood to adulthood (circled in red in the figure). Individuals who used cannabis short-term in adolescence showed only weak evidence of IQ decline (3-point IQ decline; circled in black dashes in the figure). Individuals who began using cannabis in adulthood (after age 18) did not show IQ decline (gray bars), even when they used persistently.
   In the figure below, 1 diagnosis = the study member met criteria for cannabis dependence at only one of the five assessment phases (ages 18, 21, 26, 32, 38); 2 diagnoses = the study member met criteria for cannabis dependence at two of the five assessment phases.; 3+ diagnoses = the study member met criteria for cannabis dependence at three or more of the five assessment phases. More diagnoses = greater persistence.
2) Quitting or reducing cannabis use did not appear to fully restore intellectual functioning among adolescent-onset former persistent cannabis users.

3) IQ decline could not be explained by alcohol or other drug use or by reduced years of education among persistent cannabis users.
4) IQ decline could also not be explained by low childhood socioeconomic status or poor childhood self-regulation.[104]
5) Third-party informants (e.g., friends, relatives) reported noticing more attention and memory problems in everyday life among persistent cannabis users (e.g, losing focus when they should be paying attention, forgetting to do errands, return calls, pay bills).

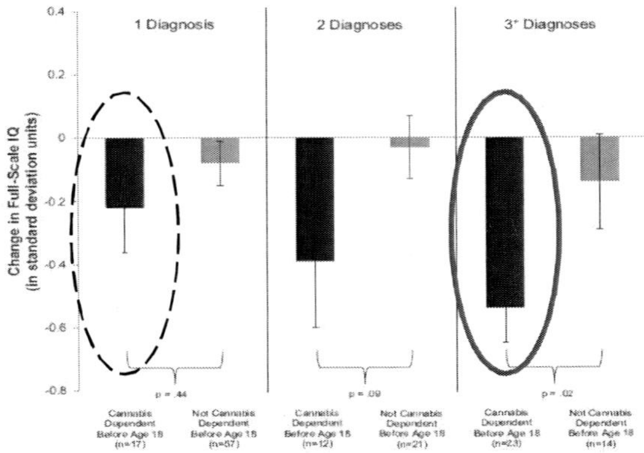

Adolescent vulnerability. Shown is change in full-scale IQ (in SD units) from childhood to adulthood among study members with 1, 2, or 3+ diagnoses of cannabis dependence as a function of age of onset of cannabis dependence. Individuals with adolescent-onset cannabis dependence (black bars) experienced greater IQ decline than individuals with adult-onset cannabis dependence (gray bars). IQ decline of approximately −0.55 SD units among individuals with adolescent-onset cannabis dependence in the 3+ group represents a decline of 8 IQ points. Error bars = SEs.

Why Are These Findings Important?

The importance of "before and after" IQ testing. Previous studies have suggested that adolescents may be particularly vulnerable to the effects of cannabis on cognitive functioning.[8-10,105,106,107] However, until our study, research had not been able to rule out the possibility that poorer cognitive test performance among adolescent-onset cannabis users predates cannabis use initiation. We showed that regardless of their initial (pre-cannabis) test

[104] Moffitt TE, Meier MH, Caspi A, Poulton R. Reply to Rogeberg and Daly: No evidence that socioeconomic status or personality differences confound the association between cannabis use and IQ decline. *Proc Natl Acad Sci U S A.* 2013;110(11):E980-E982.

[105] Gruber SA, Sagar KA, Dahlgren MK, Racine M, Lukas SE. Age of onset of marijuana use and executive function. *Psychology of Addictive Behaviors.* 2012;26(3):496.

[106] Lisdahl KM, Shollenbarger S, Sagar KA, Gruber SA. The Neurocognitive impact of alcohol and marijuana use on the developing adolescent and young adult brain. *Brief Interventions for Adolescent Alcohol and Substance Abuse.* 2018:50.

[107] Lubman DI, Cheetham A, Yücel M. Cannabis and adolescent brain development. *Pharmacol Therapeut.* 2015;148:1-16.

performance, adolescent-onset persistent cannabis users performed worse than non-users and adult-onset cannabis users on cognitive tests in adulthood.

What Is the Size of the IQ Decline?

The extent of IQ decline among adolescent-onset persistent cannabis users (8 IQ points) is non-trivial. For example, an average person has an IQ of 100, placing them in the 50th percentile for intelligence compared to their same-age peers. If this average person loses 8 IQ points, they drop from the 50th to the 29th percentile for intelligence.

Why Is an 8-Point Decline in IQ Significant?

Research has shown that IQ is a strong predictor of a person's access to a college education, their lifelong total income, their access to a good job, their performance on the job, and even early death.[108,109] Individuals who lose 8 points may be disadvantaged, relative to their same-age peers, in many important aspects of life. In fact, the adolescent-onset persistent cannabis users from the Dunedin Study experienced downward social mobility. That is, they ended up in occupations that were less prestigious, less skilled, and less well paid than their parents' occupation.[110]

How Many People Does This Affect?

Only approximately 2% of the 1,037 individuals born in one year in Dunedin became adolescent-onset persistent cannabis users. Thus, any effect of cannabis on IQ is confined to a relatively small segment of the population. Nonetheless, findings are concerning given that fewer adolescents today believe that regular cannabis use presents a serious health risk.[111]

---

[108] Batty GD, Deary IJ, Gottfredson LS. Premorbid (early life) IQ and later mortality risk: Systematic review. *Annals of epidemiology*. 2007;17(4):278-288.

[109] Gottfredson LS. Social consequences of group differences in cogntive ability. Newark, DE: University of Delaware; 2004.

[110] Cerdá M, Moffitt TE, Meier MH, et al. Persistent cannabis dependence and alcohol dependence represent risks for midlife economic and social problems: A longitudinal cohort study. *Clinical Psychological Science*. 2016;4:1028-1046.

[111] Johnston LD, Miech, R.A., O'Malley, P.M., Bachman, J.G., Schulenberg, J.E., Patrick, M.E. Monitoring the Future national survey results on drug use, 1975-2018: Overview, key findings on adolescent drug use. Ann Arbor: Institute for Social Research, The University of Michigan; 2019.

What Should We Do?

We should direct efforts toward delaying the onset of cannabis use in young people and encourage cessation, particularly for cannabis users who began using in adolescence.

What Additional Research Is Needed?

Additional research is needed to answer the following questions:

1. *What are the mechanisms underlying cannabis-related IQ decline?*

One hypothesis is that cannabis use causes brain changes that result in IQ decline. Further, adolescents might be particularly vulnerable to the effects of cannabis because cannabis use might disrupt critical neuromaturational processes (e.g., synaptic pruning [culling of weak/unused synapses, which might result in more efficient information processing] and white matter development [which is important for efficient brain signaling]) that occur during adolescence.[13,18] Our 2012 study on cannabis and IQ lacked brain imaging data, and so we could not test this hypothesis. Findings from extant brain imaging studies of cannabis users and comparison individuals have been somewhat inconsistent,[23] but functional imaging studies have found evidence of altered brain activity in cannabis users in at least some brain regions,[112,113] and structural imaging studies have consistently found that cannabis users have lower hippocampal volume.[23,114,115] The consistent finding of lower hippocampal volume among cannabis users is interesting because the hippocampus has a high density of cannabinoid receptors and is involved in learning and memory. Nonetheless, most brain imaging studies lack data from before cannabis initiation, leaving open the possibility that differences between cannabis users and non-users in terms of brain structure or function reflect pre-existing differences. Overall, there is a clear need for large-scale

---

[112] Batalla A, Bhattacharyya S, Yucel M, et al. Structural and functional imaging studies in chronic cannabis users: A systematic review of adolescent and adult findings. *Plos One.* 2013;8(2).

[113] Yanes JA, Riedel MC, Ray KL, et al. Neuroimaging meta-analysis of cannabis use studies reveals convergent functional alterations in brain regions supporting cognitive control and reward processing. *J Psychopharmacol.* 2018;32(3):283-295.

[114] Lorenzetti V, Solowij N, Yucel M. The role of cannabinoids in neuroanatomic alterations in cannabis users. *Biol Psychiatry.* 2016;79(7):E17-E31.

[115] Lorenzetti V, Chye Y, Silva P, Solowij N, Roberts CA. Does regular cannabis use affect neuroanatomy? An updated systematic review and meta-analysis of structural neuroimaging studies. *European Archives of Psychiatry and Clinical Neuroscience.* 2019;269(1):59-71.

longitudinal studies to follow youth from before to well after cannabis initiation and to combine cognitive testing with brain imaging. The Adolescent Brain and Cognitive Development Study (ABCD Study) was launched, in part, to meet this need.

Although adolescence is receiving attention as a developmental period of heightened vulnerability to cannabis effects, there are likely other sensitive periods in development. For example, cannabis exposure during prenatal development is receiving increased attention, and evidence suggests that the children of mothers who used cannabis during pregnancy show poorer cognitive functioning.[116] Another example is that cannabis use in older adulthood might be associated with serious cognitive consequences. With continued follow-up of the Dunedin Study cohort, who are now age 45, our team can answer new questions about cannabis effects on the aging brain.

2. *What are the parameters of cannabis use that determine the magnitude and persistence of cognitive deficits?*

Additional work is needed to identify the frequency, quantity, age-of-onset, and duration of cannabis use that is sufficient to produce cognitive deficits. Findings from our 2012 study on cannabis use and IQ suggest that cannabis use that begins before age 18 and continues for many years is associated with IQ decline from childhood to adulthood, but short-term cannabis use in adolescence might not be associated with IQ decline (see above Figure). Several recent longitudinal studies,[117,118,119] including a study from our group using data from a different cohort,[120] found little evidence of cannabis-related IQ decline in adolescence. Importantly, these studies do not conflict with our 2012 study. Rather, the studies collectively suggest that short-term cannabis use in adolescence might not be associated with IQ

---

[116] Huizink AC, Mulder EJ. Maternal smoking, drinking or cannabis use during pregnancy and neurobehavioral and cognitive functioning in human offspring. *Neuroscience & Biobehavioral Reviews.* 2006;30(1):24-41.

[117] Jackson NJ, Isen JD, Khoddam R, et al. Impact of adolescent marijuana use on intelligence: Results from two longitudinal twin studies. *Proc Natl Acad Sci U S A.* 2016;113(5):E500-E508.

[118] Mokrysz C, Landy R, Gage S, Munafò M, Roiser J, Curran H. Are IQ and educational outcomes in teenagers related to their cannabis use? A prospective cohort study. *J Psychopharmacol.* 2016:0269881115622241.

[119] Boccio CM, Beaver KM. Examining the influence of adolescent marijuana use on adult intelligence: Further evidence in the causation versus spuriousness debate. *Drug Alcohol Depen.* 2017.

[120] Meier MH, Caspi A, Danese A, et al. Associations between adolescent cannabis use and neuropsychological decline: a longitudinal co-twin control study. *Addiction.* 2018;113(2):257-265.

decline, but long-term cannabis use from adolescence onward might. A caveat is that the adolescents in these recent longitudinal studies had relatively low levels of cannabis use. For example, adolescents were classified as cannabis users if they had ever used cannabis or if they had used cannabis 50+ times. It is possible that cannabis-related IQ decline in adolescence might only become apparent after heavier use. Consistent with this, an earlier longitudinal study of youth followed to adolescence found evidence of IQ deficits among heavy adolescent cannabis users (>5 joints per week) but not lighter uses.[121]

One parameter of cannabis use that has received almost no research attention is cannabis potency, which refers to the THC content of cannabis. (THC is the main psychoactive constituent of cannabis.) In our 2012 study on cannabis and IQ, the cannabis users had access to low-potency cannabis – 3.5% THC.[122] Today's teenagers have access to cannabis with much higher potency. For example, the average THC content of confiscated marijuana (flower) in the US was 12% in 2014,[123] and the average THC content of marijuana sold in US dispensaries is now ~20%.[124,125] In addition, work from my group showed that nearly 1 in 4 adolescents have used cannabis concentrates,[126] which are cannabis plant extracts with unprecedentedly high THC content.[127,128] Cannabis concentrates have estimated average THC content of ~40-70%,[38] but THC content of concentrates can exceed 80%. Because THC has been shown to have dose effects on drug reinforcement (e.g., liking of the drug), cognitive impairment, and psychotic-like

---

[121] Fried PA, Watkinson B, Gray R. Neurocognitive consequences of marihuana - a comparison with pre-drug performance. *Neurotoxicol Teratol.* 2005;27(2):231-239.

[122] Poulsen H, Sutherland G. The potency of cannabis in New Zealand from 1976 to 1996. *Science & Justice: Journal of the Forensic Science Society.* 2000;40(3):171-176.

[123] ElSohly MA, Mehmedic Z, Foster S, Gon C, Chandra S, Church JC. Changes in cannabis potency over the last two decades (1995-2014): Analysis of current data in the United States. *Biol Psychiatry.* 2016;79:613-619.

[124] Vergara D, Bidwell LC, Gaudino R, et al. Compromised external validity: Federally produced cannabis does not reflect legal markets. *Sci Rep-Uk.* 2017;7:46528.

[125] Smart R, Caulkins JP, Kilmer B, Davenport S, Midgette G. Variation in cannabis potency and prices in a newly-legal market: Evidence from 30 million cannabis sales in Washington State. *Addiction.* 2017.

[126] Meier MH, Docherty M, Leischow SJ, Grimm KJ, Pardini D. Cannabis concentrate use in adolescents. *Pediatrics.* 2019;144(3):e20190338.

[127] Raber JC, Elzinga S, Kaplan C. Understanding dabs: Contamination concerns of cannabis concentrates and cannabinoid transfer during the act of dabbing. *J Toxicol Sci.* 2015;40(6):797-803.

[128] Carlini BH, Garrett SB, Harwick RM. Beyond joints and brownies: Marijuana concentrates in the legal landscape of WA State. *International Journal of Drug Policy.* 2017;42:26-29.

experiences,[129,130,131,132] there is speculation that use of cannabis with higher THC content might increase risk for addiction, cognitive deficits, psychosis, and other adverse consequences.[41,133,134,135,136,137,138] However, an alternative hypothesis is that higher THC cannabis might not pose greater risks, because cannabis users might titrate their use (use less cannabis when THC content is high). My recent work showed that cannabis users who used concentrates had higher rates of physiological dependence (symptoms of addiction) on cannabis than cannabis users who did not use concentrates.[139] However, additional research on this topic is needed. Moreover, research is needed to ascertain if cannabidiol (CBD), another constituent of cannabis, might attenuate the negative effects of THC.[140,141]

To summarize, research is needed to understand how cannabis frequency, quantity, duration, age-of-onset, and potency impact cognitive functioning. To do this work, cannabis researchers must work together to develop standardized measures of each of these cannabis parameters.

---

[129] Curran HV, Freeman TP, Mokrysz C, Lewis DA, Morgan CJ, Parsons LH. Keep off the grass? Cannabis, cognition and addiction. *Nature Reviews Neuroscience.* 2016;17(5):293-306.

[130] Freeman TP, van der Pol P, Kuijpers W, et al. Changes in cannabis potency and first-time admissions to drug treatment: a 16-year study in the Netherlands. *Psychol Med.* 2018:1-7.

[131] D'Souza DC, Perry E, MacDougall L, et al. The psychotomimetic effects of intravenous delta-9-tetrahydrocannabinol in healthy individuals: implications for psychosis. *Neuropsychopharmacology.* 2004;29(8):1558-1572.

[132] Chait LD, Burke KA. Preference for high-versus low-potency marijuana. *Pharmacol Biochem Behav.* 1994;49(3):643-647.

[133] Smith N. High potency cannabis: The forgotten variable. *Addiction.* 2005;100(10):1558-1560.

[134] Freeman T, Winstock A. Examining the profile of high-potency cannabis and its association with severity of cannabis dependence. *Psychol Med.* 2015;45(15):3181-3189.

[135] Murray RM, Quigley H, Quattrone D, Englund A, Di Forti M. Traditional marijuana, high-potency cannabis and synthetic cannabinoids: Increasing risk for psychosis. *World Psychiatry: Official Journal of the World Psychiatric Association.* 2016;15(3):195-204.

[136] Di Forti M, Marconi A, Carra E, et al. Proportion of patients in south London with first-episode psychosis attributable to use of high potency cannabis: a case-control study. *Lancet Psychiat.* 2015;2(3):233-238.

[137] Loflin M, Earleywine M. A new method of cannabis ingestion: the dangers of dabs? *Addict Behav.* 2014;39(10):1430-1433.

[138] Rigucci S, Marques T, Di Forti M, et al. Effect of high-potency cannabis on corpus callosum microstructure. *Psychol Med.* 2016;46(4):841-854.

[139] Meier MH. Associations between butane hash oil use and cannabis-related problems. *Drug Alcohol Depen.* 2017;179:25-31.

[140] Morgan CJ, Schafer G, Freeman TP, Curran HV. Impact of cannabidiol on the acute memory and psychotomimetic effects of smoked cannabis: naturalistic study. *The British Journal of Psychiatry.* 2010;197(4):285-290.

[141] Englund A, Morrison PD, Nottage J, et al. Cannabidiol inhibits THC-elicited paranoid symptoms and hippocampal-dependent memory impairment. *J Psychopharmacol.* 2013;27(1):19-27.

3. *Does cognitive functioning recover with abstinence?*

In our 2012 study, we found that adolescent-onset persistent cannabis users performed worse in adulthood than in childhood even after they had quit or reduced their use in the year leading up to cognitive testing in adulthood. This suggests that quitting or reducing use might not fully restore functioning among adolescent-onset persistent cannabis users, but longer-term follow-up is needed. In general, the evidence on recovery with abstinence is mixed. Some studies have found evidence of cognitive deficits among cannabis users who were abstinent for approximately a month or more.[142,143,144,145] Yet, studies that compared heavy cannabis users with comparison individuals have collectively found little evidence of cognitive deficits among longer-term abstinent cannabis users.[5,6] Carefully designed studies are needed to understand the extent and time course of recovery associated with quitting cannabis, and to understand if recovery depends on age-of-onset of use, duration of use, or other cannabis use parameters.

4. *Are there individual differences in susceptibility to cannabis-related cognitive deficits?*

   One intriguing possibility is that some individuals are less likely than others to experience negative effects of cannabis. Research is needed to identify these individuals and to isolate the factors that offer them protection. For example, evidence suggests that some people might be genetically less susceptible than others to experiencing cannabis-related cognitive deficits.[146,147] This could have significant implicants for prevention. Relatedly, research is needed on sex differences in

---

[142] Hanson KL, Winward JL, Schweinsburg AD, Medina KL, Brown SA, Tapert SF. Longitudinal study of cognition among adolescent marijuana users over three weeks of abstinence. *Addict Behav.* 2010;35(11):970-976.

[143] Medina KL, Hanson KL, Schweinsburg AD, Cohen-Zion M, Nagel BJ, Tapert SF. Neuropsychological functioning in adolescent marijuana users: Subtle deficits detectable after a month of abstinence. *J Int Neuropsych Soc.* 2007;13(5):807-820.

[144] Schwartz RH, Gruenewald PJ, Klitzner M, Fedio P. Short-term-memory impairment in cannabis-dependent adolescents. *Am J Dis Child.* 1989;143(10):1214-1219.

[145] Bolla KI, Brown K, Eldreth D, Tate K, Cadet JL. Dose-related neurocognitive effects of marijuana use. *Neurology.* 2002;59(9):1337-1343.

[146] Verdejo-García A, Fagundo AB, Cuenca A, et al. COMT val158met and 5-HTTLPR genetic polymorphisms moderate executive control in cannabis users. *Neuropsychopharmacology.* 2013;38(8):1598.

[147] Tunbridge EM, Dunn G, Murray RM, et al. Genetic moderation of the effects of cannabis: catechol-O-methyltransferase (COMT) affects the impact of Δ9-tetrahydrocannabinol (THC) on working memory performance but not on the occurrence of psychotic experiences. *J Psychopharmacol.* 2015;29(11):1146-1151.

vulnerability to cannabis effects on cognitive function.[40] For example, one recent study found that an earlier age of onset of cannabis use was associated with poorer memory in women but not men.[148]

Appendix

Supporting Details for Meier et al., 2012

How we measured cannabis use. We measured cannabis use in two ways: cannabis dependence and regular cannabis use. Persistence of cannabis dependence was defined as the total number of study waves out of five (ages 18, 21, 26, 32, and 38) at which a study member met DSM criteria for cannabis dependence. Study members were grouped according to their number of dependence diagnoses: (a) those who never used cannabis at any study wave and thus could not have become dependent; (b) those who used cannabis at least once at one or more study waves but never diagnosed; (c) those who diagnosed at one wave; (d) those who diagnosed at two waves; and (e) those who diagnosed at three or more waves.

Cannabis dependence is a substance use disorder as defined in the Diagnostic and Statistical Manual of the American Psychiatric Association (known as DSM-IV). The purpose of the DSM-IV diagnosis is to predict a patient's future prognosis, and to identify which patients are most in need of treatment. A diagnosis of cannabis dependence generally reflects an individual's continued use of cannabis despite experiencing significant health, social, and/or legal problems related to cannabis use.

Persistence of regular cannabis use. Because some people use cannabis on a regular basis but never develop problems, we also examined IQ decline as a function of persistent regular cannabis use. This was defined as the total number of study waves out of five at which a study member reported using cannabis four or more days per week (the majority of days in a week). Study members were grouped as those who: (a) never used cannabis; (b) used but never regularly; (c) used regularly at one wave; (d) used regularly at two waves; and (e) used regularly at three or more waves.

---

[148] Crane NA, Schuster RM, Mermelstein RJ, Gonzalez R. Neuropsychological sex differences associated with age of initiated use among young adult cannabis users. *J Clin Exp Neuropsyc.* 2015(ahead-of-print):1-13.

Results were similar for persistent cannabis dependence and persistent regular cannabis use.

How we defined adolescent-onset cannabis use. We defined adolescent-onset cannabis in two ways: 1) cannabis dependence before age 18 or 2) weekly cannabis use before age 18. Results were similar across both definitions.

How we measured IQ. We assessed intelligence in childhood (ages 7, 9, 11, and 13) and again in adulthood at age 38 using standard tests for the field.

How we measured everyday life cognitive functioning. Study members nominated people "who knew them well." These informants were mailed questionnaires and asked to complete a checklist, including whether the study member had problems with their attention (e.g., "can't concentrate, mind wanders) and memory (e.g., forgets to do errands, return calls, pay bills) over the past year at age 38.

Written Testimony of VADM Jerome M. Adams, M.D., M.P.H., U.S. Surgeon General and Nora D. Volkow, M.D., Director, National Institute on Drug Abuse, Caucus on International Narcotics Control, October 23, 2019

Chairman Cornyn, Co-Chairwoman Feinstein and members of the Caucus on International Narcotics Control, we appreciate the opportunity to share the content of the recent Surgeon General's Advisory on Marijuana Use and the Developing Brain with you, and to join national experts to discuss this complex issue that demands our attention and action. Recent increases in access to marijuana and in its potency, along with misperceptions of its safety, endanger our most precious resource, our nation's youth.

Background

Marijuana, or cannabis, is the most commonly used illicit drug in the United States. In 2018, 43.5 million people reported using marijuana in the past year [1]. Marijuana acts by binding to cannabinoid receptors in the brain to produce a variety of effects, including euphoria, intoxication, and memory and motor impairments. These cannabinoid receptors are part of an extensive endocannabinoid system that regulates a wide range of functions, including brain development.

The endocannabinoid system appears relatively early during fetal development. As the fetal brain grows, this system influences how brain cells develop and connect with one another, and it plays a major role in the formation of brain circuits including those important for decision making, mood, and responding to stress [2]. Not surprisingly, animal studies have shown that in utero exposure to marijuana can interfere with the proper development and regulation of brain circuitry. Moreover, the endocannabinoid system is a critical regulator of the neuronal hardwiring that translates experience throughout the teen years and young adulthood into mature brain architecture. This helps explain why the developing brain is particularly vulnerable to chronic exposure to delta-9-tetrahydrocannabinol (THC), the component of marijuana responsible for euphoria, intoxication, and addiction.

Marijuana and its related products are widely available in multiple forms, with varying concentrations of constituent chemicals, the most salient of which are known collectively as "cannabinoids" [3]. In addition to varying levels of THC, marijuana also contains cannabidiol (CBD). While pure CBD is not intoxicating and does not lead to addiction, its long-term effects are largely unknown. In addition to THC and CBD, the marijuana plant also contains hundreds of other cannabinoid and non-cannabinoid components, many of which have not been studied extensively.

Marijuana has changed over time; the marijuana available today is much more potent than what was available in the past. The THC concentration in commonly cultivated marijuana plants increased three-fold between 1995 and 2014 (4 percent and 12 percent, respectively) [4], and marijuana available in dispensaries in some states has average concentrations of THC between 17.7 percent and 23.2 percent [5]. Concentrated products, commonly known as dabs or waxes, are widely available to recreational users today and may contain between 23.7 percent and 75.9 percent THC [6].

The risks of physical dependence, addiction, and other negative consequences increase with frequent use, exposure to high concentrations of THC [7] and with younger age of initiation. Higher doses of THC are more likely to produce anxiety, agitation, paranoia, and psychosis [8]. Use of edible marijuana can increase the risk of unintentional overdose due to its lengthy absorption time and delayed effect, often prompting the user to take a second dose. Edibles, which may have the appearance of desserts or snacks, are also increasingly a cause of accidental ingestion by children [9] and adolescents [10]. In addition, chronic users of marijuana with a high THC content are at risk for developing a condition known as cannabinoid hyperemesis syndrome, which is marked by severe cycles of nausea and vomiting [11]. The increase in the THC content of marijuana, combined with the growing availability of loosely regulated cannabis products, has led to a worrisome upward trend in the rate of calls to poison control centers and emergency department visits over the past decade.

Surgeon General's Advisory on Marijuana Use and the Developing Brain

On August 29, 2019, the Surgeon General's Advisory on Marijuana Use and the Developing Brain was issued to emphasize the importance of protecting our Nation from the health risks of marijuana use in adolescence and during pregnancy. This advisory is intended to raise awareness of the known and potential harms that the increasing availability of highly-potent marijuana in multiple, concentrated forms poses to the developing brain of youth and young adults who consume it. These harms can be long-lasting and costly to individuals and to our society, impacting mental health and educational achievement and raising the risks of addiction and other psychiatric disorders. In addition to the health risks posed by marijuana use, the sale or possession of marijuana remains illegal under federal law, notwithstanding some state laws to the contrary.

Marijuana Use during Pregnancy

Pregnant women use marijuana more than any other illicit drug. In a national survey, marijuana use in the past month among pregnant women doubled (3.4 percent to 7 percent) between 2002 and 2017 [12], although this trend may be starting to reverse based on the most recent data reported in the National Survey on Drug Use and Health. In a study conducted in a large health system in California, marijuana use rose by 69 percent (4.2 percent to 7.1 percent) between 2009 and 2016 among pregnant women, with the highest rates of use occurring among pregnant women under the age of 25. These researchers found that 22 percent of pregnant girls under the age of 18 and 19 percent of pregnant women ages 18-24 used marijuana in 2016 [13]. Alarmingly, many retail dispensaries recommended marijuana to pregnant women for morning sickness [14].

Since the THC in marijuana crosses the placenta, it may disrupt the important role the endocannabinoid system plays in fetal brain development and in maintaining a healthy pregnancy [2]. Moreover, the placenta itself has cannabinoid receptors, which might contribute to restricted fetal growth with cannabis use during pregnancy [15, 34]. Indeed, studies have shown that marijuana use in pregnancy is associated with adverse outcomes, including lower birth weight and [16] and preterm delivery [35]. For example, The Colorado Pregnancy Risk Assessment Monitoring System reported that maternal marijuana use was associated with a 50 percent increased risk of low birth weight regardless of maternal age, race, ethnicity, education, and tobacco use [16].

The American College of Obstetricians and Gynecologists holds that "[w]omen who are pregnant or contemplating pregnancy should be encouraged to discontinue marijuana use. Women reporting marijuana use should be counseled about concerns regarding potential adverse health consequences of continued use during pregnancy" [17]. In a 2018 clinical guidance statement, the American Academy of Pediatrics recommended that health professionals "…advise all adolescents and young women that if they become pregnant, marijuana should not be used during pregnancy" [18].

While cannabis use *during* pregnancy is associated with increased risk of adverse birth outcomes, later effects on the child due to exposure to THC through breastmilk are still unclear. This is in part due to challenges disentangling the long-term effects associated with marijuana exposure *in utero* versus during nursing. Although additional research is needed in this area, there is ample reason for caution, as THC has been detected in breastmilk for up to six days after the last recorded use [19, 20, 21]. Additionally, marijuana smoke contains many of the same harmful components as tobacco smoke [22]; no one should smoke marijuana or tobacco around a baby.

Marijuana Use during Adolescence

Each day in 2018, 3700 adolescents aged 12 to 17 became new users of marijuana [1]. Although marijuana use declined among 8th graders and remains unchanged among 10th and 12th graders compared to five years ago, high school students' perception of the harm from regular marijuana use has been steadily declining over the last decade [24]. In 2018, only about a third (34.9 percent) of adolescents aged 12 to 17 perceived great risk from weekly marijuana use [1]. During this same period, a number of states legalized adult and/or so-called medicinal use of marijuana, though it remains illegal under federal law. Importantly, medical marijuana laws may allow for use at a younger age than adult recreational laws. The legalization movement may be impacting youth perception of harm from marijuana.

The human brain continues to develop from before birth into the mid-20s and is vulnerable to the effects of addictive substances [25, 26]. Frequent marijuana use during adolescence is associated with structural and functional changes in areas of the brain involved in attention, memory, decision-making, and motivation, and in deficits in attention and memory [27]. Marijuana can also impair learning in adolescents. Chronic use is linked to declines in IQ and school performance, which may jeopardize professional and social achievements, and life satisfaction [28]. Regular use of marijuana in adolescence is linked to increased rates of school absence and drop-out, as well as suicide attempts [29].

Marijuana use is also linked to both overall risk for and early onset of psychotic disorders, such as schizophrenia. The risk for psychotic disorders increases with frequency of use, potency of the marijuana product, and younger age of initiation [30]. Adolescent marijuana use is also associated with other substance use [31, 32]. In 2017, teens 12-17 reporting frequent use of marijuana showed a 130 percent greater likelihood of misusing opioids [23]. 2018 data from 8th, 10th, and 12th graders show that a third reported lifetime cannabis use and almost a quarter reported lifetime use of concentrated products. Adolescents using concentrates show higher rates of other substance use and risk factors for substance use-related problems [33]. Marijuana's increasingly widespread availability in multiple and highly potent forms, coupled with a false and dangerous perception of safety among youth, merits a nationwide call to action.

Research Supported by the National Institutes of Health's (NIH) National Institute on Drug Abuse (NIDA)

NIH supports a broad range of research aimed at understanding the public health effects of marijuana use at all stages of life. NIDA's portfolio includes research on the pharmacology of THC and other cannabinoids in the marijuana plant; the molecular mechanisms underlying the effect of marijuana use on the brain, including its development; epidemiologic studies to elucidate the prevalence and patterns of marijuana use; research to understand the brain changes associated with cannabis addiction and other adverse effects such as amotivation, an unwillingness to participate in normal social situations; research on the potentially beneficial effects of marijuana and its constituent compounds; applied research aimed at preventing and treating cannabis misuse and addiction; as well as research aimed at understanding how marijuana policies affect public health.

There is still much we do not know about the impact of marijuana exposure during the vulnerable periods of adolescence and pregnancy; therefore, these remain key areas of focus for NIDA. Two current studies with great potential to advance knowledge in these areas are the Adolescent Brain Cognitive Development (ABCD) study and the HEALthy Brain and Child Development (HBCD) study. ABCD, the largest long-term study of brain development and child health in the United States, is expected to yield an unprecedented amount of information about normal brain development and how it is affected by substance use—including use of marijuana—and other childhood experiences. The ABCD study has recruited over 11,000 children ages 9-10 and is following them into early adulthood. By integrating structural and functional brain imaging with genetic and biological markers, along with psychological, behavioral, and other health assessments, ABCD will increase our understanding of the many factors that can enhance or disrupt a young person's life trajectory. Complementing ABCD is the HBCD Study, which is currently in its planning phase. HBCD would establish a large cohort of pregnant women and assess maternal and child outcomes over the course of at least 10 years. In parallel to the ABCD study, findings from this cohort will help researchers understand both normal childhood brain development as well as the long-term impact of prenatal and postnatal drug and environmental exposures.

Key Messages and Critical Actions

No amount of marijuana use during pregnancy or during youth when the brain is under development is known to be safe. Until and unless more is known about the long-term impact, the safest choice for pregnant women and youth is not to use marijuana. Although women generally tend to limit drug use during pregnancy, education efforts on marijuana's adverse effects during pregnancy should be expanded and improved. Pregnant women and youth--and those who love them--need the facts and resources to support healthy decisions. It is critical to educate women and youth, as well as family members, school officials, state and local leaders, and health professionals, about the risks of marijuana.

Science-based messaging campaigns and targeted prevention programming are urgently needed to ensure that risks are clearly communicated and amplified by local, state, and national organizations. Clinicians can help by asking about marijuana use, and by informing pregnant women, new mothers, young people, and those vulnerable to psychotic disorders of the risks associated with marijuana use. Clinicians can also prescribe safe, effective, and FDA-approved treatments for nausea, depression, and pain during pregnancy.

What we know now about the impact of marijuana exposure during adolescence, as well as during prenatal development is enough to warrant concern and action. Still, further research is needed to understand the full effects of marijuana exposure on biological, cognitive, and social development, especially the mid- and long-term consequences of prenatal and youth exposures. The wide and ever-increasing array of cannabis products used both recreationally and for therapeutic purposes also raise significant public health concerns, particularly when used by young people and pregnant women. Additional research aimed at evaluating the health effects of these products is critical.

Thank you for the opportunity to share this summary of the current trends in marijuana use among youth and pregnant women; the state of the evidence regarding the harms to developing brains; and the steps we can take together to understand more about and to mitigate those harms in order to protect our youth, the future of our nation. I am happy to answer any questions you may have.

References

[1] Substance Abuse and Mental Health Services Administration. (2019). *Key substance use and mental health indicators in the United States: Results from the 2018 National Surveyon Drug Use and Health* (HHS Publication No. PEP19-5068, NSDUH Series H-54). Rockville, MD: Center for Behavioral Health Statistics and Quality, Substance Abuse and Mental Health Services Administration. Retrieved from https://www.samhsa.gov/data/.

[2] Brents L. K. (2016). Marijuana, the Endocannabinoid System and the Female Reproductive System. *The Yale journal of biology and medicine*, 89(2), 175–191.

[3] National Center for Chronic Disease Prevention and Health Promotions, Centers for Disease Control and Prevention. *Marijuana and Public Health: How is*

marijuana used? https://www.cdc.gov/marijuana/faqs/how-is-marijuana-used.html.

[4] Elsohly, M. A., Mehmedic, Z., Foster, S. (2016). Changes in Cannabis Potency Over the Last 2 Decades (1995-2014): Analysis of Current Data in the United States. *Biological Psychiatry,* 79(7), 613-619. doi:10.1016/j.biopsych.2016.01.004.

[5] Jikomes, N., & Zoorob, M. (2018). The Cannabinoid Content of Legal Cannabis in Washington State Varies Systematically Across Testing Facilities and Popular Consumer Products. *Scientific reports,* 8(1), 4519. doi:10.1038/s41598-018-22755-2.

[6] Alzghari, S. K., Fung, V., Rickner, S. S., Chacko, L., & Fleming, S. W. (2017). To Dab or Not to Dab: Rising Concerns Regarding the Toxicity of Cannabis Concentrates. *Cureus,* 9(9), e1676. doi:10.7759/cureus.1676.

[7] Freeman, T. P., & Winstock, A. R. (2015). Examining the profile of high-potency cannabis and its association with severity of cannabis dependence. Psychological medicine, 45(15), 3181– 3189. doi:10.1017/S0033291715001178.

[8] Volkow N. D., Baler R. D., Compton W. M., Weiss S. R. B. Adverse Health Effects of Marijuana Use. *N Engl J Med.* 2014 June 5; 370(23): 2219–2227. doi:10.1056/NEJMra1402309.

[9] Richards, J. R., Smith N. E., Moulin, A. K. Unintentional Cannabis Ingestion in Children: A Systematic Review. *J Pediatr* 2017; 190:142-52.

[10] Cao, D., Sahaphume, S., Bronstein, A. C., Hoyte, C.O., Characterization of edible marijuana product exposures reported to the United States poison centers. *Clinical Toxicology,* 54:9, 840-846, DOI: 10.1080/15563650.2016.1209761.

[11] Galli, J. A., Sawaya, R. A., Friedenberg, F. K. Cannabinoid Hyperemesis Syndrome. *Curr Drug Abuse Rev.* 2011 Dec; 4(4): 241–249.

[12] Volkow N. D., Han B., Compton W. M., McCance-Katz E. F. Self-reported Medical and Non-medical Cannabis Use Among Pregnant Women in the United States. *JAMA.* 2019 doi:10.1001/jama.2019.7982.

[13] Young-Wolff K. C., Tucker L., Alexeeff S., et al. Trends in Self-reported and Biochemically Tested Marijuana Use Among Pregnant Females in California From 2009-2016. *JAMA.* 2017;318(24):2490–2491. doi:10.1001/jama.2017.17225.

[14] Dickson, B. (2018). Recommendations From Cannabis Dispensaries About First-Trimester Cannabis Use. *Obstetrics & Gynecology.* 2018; 0029-7844. doi:10.1097/AOG.0000000000002619.

[15] National Academies of Sciences, Engineering, and Medicine. 2017. The health effects of cannabis and cannabinoids: Current state of evidence and recommendations for research. Washington, DC: The National Academies Press.

[16] Crume et al.: Cannabis use during the perinatal period in a state with legalized recreational and medical marijuana: the association between maternal characteristics, breastfeeding patterns, and neonatal outcomes. *J Pediatr.* 2018;197:90-96.

[17] American College of Obstetricians and Gynecologists: Marijuana use during pregnancy and lactation. Committee Opinion No. 722. *Obstet Gynecol.* 2017;130(4):e205-e209.

[18] Ryan et al: Marijuana use during pregnancy and breastfeeding: implications for neonatal and childhood outcomes. *Pediatrics.* 2018; 142(3):,e20181889.

[19] Bertrand, K. A., Hanan, N. J., Honerkamp-Smith, G., Best, B. M., & Chambers, C. D. (2018). Marijuana Use by Breastfeeding Mothers and Cannabinoid Concentrations in Breast Milk. *Pediatrics,* 142(3). doi:10.1542/peds.2018-1076.

[20] Metz T. D., Stickrath E. H.: Marijuana use in pregnancy and lactation: a review of the evidence. *Am J Obstet Gynecol.* 2015;213(6):761-778.

[21] Effects while pregnant or breastfeeding. (2017, March 02). Retrieved from https://www.colorado.gov/pacific/marijuana/effects-while-pregnant-or-breastfeeding.

[22] Moir, D., et al., A comparison of mainstream and sidestream marijuana and tobacco cigarette smoke produced under two machine smoking conditions. *Chem Res Toxicol* 21: 494-502. (2008).

[23] Substance Abuse and Mental Health Services Administration. (2018). Key Substance Use and Mental Health Indicators in the United States: Results from the 2017 National Survey on Drug Use and Health (HHS Publication No. SMA 18-5068, NSDUH Series H-53). Rockville, MD: Center for Behavioral Health Statistics and Quality, Substance Abuse and Mental Health Services Administration.

[24] Johnston, L. D., Miech, R. A., O'Malley, P. M., Bachman, J. G., Schulenberg, J. E., & Patrick, M. E. (2019). *Monitoring the Future national survey results on drug use, 1975-2018: Overview, key findings on adolescent drug use.* Ann Arbor: Institute for Social Research, The University of Michigan, 119 pp.

[25] Pujol, J., Vendrell, P., Junqué, C., Martí-Vilalta, J. L., & Capdevila, A. (1993). When does human brain development end? Evidence of corpus callosum growth up to adulthood. *Annals of Neurology,* 34(1), 71-75. doi:10.1002/ana.410340113.

[26] Levine, A., Clemenza, K., Rynn, M., & Lieberman, J. (2017). Evidence for the Risks and Consequences of Adolescent Cannabis Exposure. *Journal of the American Academy of Child & Adolescent Psychiatry,* 56(3), 214-225. doi:10.1016/j.jaac.2016.12.014.

[27] Meruelo A. D., Castro N., Cota C. I., Tapert S. F. Cannabis and alcohol use, and the developing brain. *Behav Brain Res.* 2017;325(Pt A):44–50. doi:10.1016/j.bbr.2017.02.025.

[28] Meier M. H., Caspi A., Ambler A., et al. Persistent cannabis users show neuropsychological decline from childhood to midlife. *Proc Natl Acad Sci USA.,* 2012. Oct 2; 109(40) E2657-64 doi 10.1073/pnas. 1206820109. Epub 2012 Aug 27.

[29] Silins, E., Horwood, L. J., & Patton, G. C. (2014). Young adult sequelae of adolescent cannabis use: An integrative analysis. *The Lancet Psychiatry,* 1(4), 286-293. doi:10.1016/s2215-0366(14)70307-4.

[30] Di Forti, M., Quattrone, D., & Freeman, T. (2019). The contribution of cannabis use to variation in the incidence of psychotic disorder across Europe (EU-GEI): A

multicenter case-control study. *The Lancet Psychiatry,* 6(5), 427-436. doi:10.1016/S2215-0366(19)30048-3.

[31] Lopez-Quintero C., Perez de los Cabos J., Hasin D. S. (2011). Probability and predictors of transition from first use to dependence on nicotine, alcohol, cannabis, and cocaine: results of the National Epidemiologic Survey on Alcohol and Related Conditions (NESARC). *Drug Alcohol Dependence.* 115(1-2):120-130.

[32] Jones, C. M., & McCance-Katz, E. F. (2019). Relationship Between Recency and Frequency of Youth Cannabis Use on Other Substance Use. *Journal of Adolescent Health,* 64(3), 411-413. doi:10.1016/j.jadohealth.2018.09.017.

[33] Meier M. H., Docherty M., Leischow S. J., Grimm K. J., Pardini D. Cannabis Concentrate Use in Adolescents. *Pediatrics.* 2019 Sep;144(3). pii: e20190338. doi: 10.1542/peds.2019-0338.

[34] Maia J., Midão L., Cunha S.C., Almada M., Fonseca B. M., Braga J., Gonçalves D., Teixeira N., Correia-da-Silva G. Effects of cannabis tetrahydrocannabinol on endocannabinoid homeostasis in human placenta. *Arch Toxicol.* 2019 Mar;93(3):649-658. doi: 10.1007/s00204-019-02389-7. Epub 2019 Jan 18.

[35] Petrangelo A., Czuzoj-Shulman N., Balayla J., Abenhaim H. A. Cannabis Abuse or Dependence During Pregnancy: A Population-Based Cohort Study on 12 Million Births. *J Obstet Gynaecol Can.* 2019 May;41(5):623-630. doi: 10.1016/j.jogc.2018.09.009. Epub 2018 Nov 15.

Chapter 2

Evaluation of Potential Hazards during Harvesting and Trimming Cannabis at an Indoor Cultivation Facility*

Michael P. Grant, ScD, CIH
Douglas M. Wiegand, PhD
Brett J. Green, PhD
and Angela R. Lemons, MS

Keywords: North American Industry Classification System (NAICS) 111419 (other food crops grown under cover), Colorado, Cannabis, cultivation, agriculture, fungus, endotoxin, psychosocial, Delta-9 Tetrahydrocannabinol, Delta-9 Tetrahydrocannabinol Acid, Cannabidiol, Cannabinol, THC, THCA, Cannabinoids, CBD, CBN, noise, particles, musculoskeletal, ergonomics

Introduction

Request

Management at an indoor cultivation facility requested a health hazard evaluation of potential hazards during harvesting and trimming of cannabis crops.

---

* This is an edited, reformatted and augmented version of Health Hazard Evaluation Program Report No. 2019-0152-3381, dated February 2022.

In: Marijuana
Editor: Charles M. Edmond
ISBN: 979-8-88697-869-8

Workplace

The facility was a single, large building with two floors. Immediately inside the entrance was a two-floor lobby with space for visitors and employees to wait or take breaks. Offices and a conference room were on the second floor of the lobby area. The cultivation space of the facility was separated into two sides that cultivated and harvested cannabis separately for each of two brand names owned by the same parent company. The facility had a basement, but we were informed that the company did not use that space.

To learn more about the workplace, go to Section A in the Supporting Technical Information

Our Approach

The evaluation was broad in scope, designed to characterize potential hazards among employees harvesting and trimming cannabis plants. Job titles for these employees included grow technicians, cultivation managers, facility managers, and trimming employees. We visited the facility in July and September 2019 and completed the following activities:

- Observed work processes, work practices, and conditions.
- Measured employee exposures to endotoxins in air.
- Sampled surfaces for cannabinoids including delta-9 tetrahydrocannabinol (Δ9-THC), delta-9 tetrahydrocannabinol acid (Δ9-THCA), cannabidiol (CBD), and cannabinol (CBN).
- Measured area exposures to fungi in air.
- Measured particulates in air during trimming and harvesting activities.
- Measured sound levels throughout the cultivation and trimming areas of the facility.
- Completed confidential medical interviews with employees who did cultivation, harvesting, and trimming activities.

To learn more about our methods, go to Section B in the Supporting Technical Information

Our Key Findings

Employees Were Exposed to Endotoxins in the Air

- Employees were exposed to endotoxins in the air that were greater than the Dutch Expert Committee on Occupational Safety occupational exposure limit.
- Endotoxins were detected in the air during harvesting and repotting activities where soil and plant matter was disturbed.

Employees Were Concerned About Their Potential Exposures at Work

- Cultivation and harvesting employees reported health and safety concerns about noise, lights that were too bright, and pesticide exposure.
- Trimming employees reported health and safety concerns about indoor environmental quality, use of alcohol to clean workstations, pesticide exposure, ozone exposure, and communication issues.
- Employees from both groups reported allergic, irritant, and musculoskeletal symptoms they believed were associated with their work.

Trimming Employees Had Exposures to Highly Repetitive Work That Increased Their Risk of Musculoskeletal Disorders

- Trimming employees had exposures to highly repetitive and forceful work, most notably during hand trimming activities.
- Trimming employees spend long periods of time sitting at tables performing manual tasks.

To learn more about our results, go to Section B in the Supporting Technical Information

Our Recommendations

The Occupational Safety and Health Act requires employers to provide a safe workplace.

	Benefits of Improving Workplace Health and Safety:		
↑	Improved employee health and well-being	↑	Enhanced image and reputation
↑	Better workplace morale	↑	Superior products, processes, and services
↑	Easier employee recruiting and retention	↑	May increase overall cost savings

The recommendations below are based on the findings of our evaluation. For each recommendation, we list a series of actions you can take to address the issue at your workplace. The actions at the beginning of each list are preferable to the ones listed later. The list order is based on a well-accepted approach called the "hierarchy of controls." The hierarchy of controls groups actions by their likely effectiveness in reducing or removing hazards. In most cases, the preferred approach is to eliminate hazardous materials or processes and install engineering controls to reduce exposure or shield employees. Until such controls are in place, or if they are not effective or practical, administrative measures and personal protective equipment (PPE) might be needed. Read more about the hierarchy of controls at https://www.cdc.gov/niosh/topics/hierarchy/.

We encourage the company to use a health and safety committee to discuss our recommendations and develop an action plan. Both employee representatives and management representatives should be included on the committee. Helpful guidance can be found in *Recommended Practices for Safety and Health Programs* at https://www.osha.gov/shpguidelines/index.html.

Recommendation 1: Reduce Exposures to Endotoxins in the Workplace

Why? Endotoxins are toxic substances located inside the cell walls of some types of bacteria and are found throughout agricultural environments. Employees can be exposed to endotoxins when soil and plant matter are disturbed. Studies have shown that individuals can have acute and chronic respiratory health effects when exposed to high concentrations of endotoxin.
We found four employees on each side of the facility were exposed to endotoxins in the air greater than the Dutch Expert Committee on Occupational Safety occupational exposure limit. The main soil and plant-disturbing activities that employees did during sampling were harvesting and repotting.

How? At your workplace, we recommend these specific actions:

Use wet methods or high efficiency particulate air (HEPA) filter vacuums instead of dry sweeping.

- Train employees in the proper methods to use while cleaning. Wet methods (e.g., mops or surface wipes) and HEPA-filtered vacuums are preferred when cleaning up soil and debris left on the floor after harvests or repotting activities.

Use tools to move and mix soil when repotting plants.

- Hand tools will reduce the amount of bending and direct contact with soil by employees when repotting. Less direct contact and less bending could reduce potential endotoxin exposure.
- Slowing the pace of work will also help reduce the amount of soil disturbance when repotting plants.

Encourage employees to report any symptoms they believe are work-related to their supervisor.

- Supervisors should refer employees to an occupational health physician or their primary care provider to discuss their individual health concerns and questions about work- related symptoms.

Recommendation 2: Reduce Dermal Exposures to Cannabinoids in the Workplace

Why? Occupational exposures to cannabinoids are thought to be mostly through skin absorption and ingestion. The long-term health effects of these occupational exposure routes are currently unknown. We expect to see cannabinoids in production areas but not in nonproduction areas. In this type of facility, cannabinoids found in nonproduction areas are likely brought out of the production areas on gloves and hands. It is important to practice good hand hygiene and cleaning practices in nonproduction areas to prevent unnecessary exposures. We detected cannabinoids on production and nonproduction surfaces. Employees could be exposed through dermal contact or hand to mouth actions (e.g., eating or drinking).

How? At your workplace, we recommend these specific actions:

Train employees about the importance of removing gloves and washing hands before using the bathroom, eating, drinking, or smoking.

- Instruct employees on proper handwashing techniques and when to wash their hands (e.g., before going on break, at the end of the workday, before using the restroom).
- Ensure access to soap, clean running water, and paper towels or hand dryers in all break areas.
- Require that employees always remove gloves before leaving production areas.
- Incorporate this training into new employee and annual refresher training.

Clean break area surfaces once per shift to reduce potential exposures to cannabinoids.

- Choose an employee or employees to use wet cleaning methods (e.g., 70% alcohol surface wipes) to wipe down high-contact surfaces (e.g., microwave face, refrigerator handles) at least once per shift.
- Incorporate this practice into standard operating procedures and into new employee and annual refresher training.

Encourage cultivation and harvesting employees to wear long sleeves when working.

- Train employees about the importance of protecting themselves from exposures to cannabinoids when touching plants.
- Supply long sleeve scrub options for employees. Other technologies may also be appropriate (e.g., athletic arm sleeves). Ensure that employees understand that all shirts, scrubs, or other sleeve technologies worn during cultivation and harvesting tasks should be laundered regularly.

Recommendation 3: Reduce Potential Exposures to Ozone, Light, and Noise in the Workplace

Why? Low concentrations of ozone may produce a sharp, irritating odor even during brief exposures. Symptoms of ozone exposure include eye irritation, nose and throat dryness, and cough. At higher ozone concentrations, more severe symptoms may develop including headache, pain or tightness in the chest, and shortness of breath or tiredness. Exposures from grow lights in cultivation facilities have not been widely studied. There is a potential for exposure to ultraviolet (UV) light from many types of lightbulbs used in these types of facilities. Overexposures to UV light can cause a number of health effects including skin cancer and eye damage. Noise-induced hearing loss is an irreversible condition that progresses with noise exposure. Unlike some other types of hearing disorders, noise- induced hearing loss cannot be treated medically. Noise-exposed workers can develop substantial noise-induced hearing loss before it is clearly recognized.

We learned that employees had health and safety concerns about exposures to ozone, bright lights, and noise. Ozone generators were attached to analog timers which would be affected by power outages. The ozone generators were intended to be run overnight when no employees were in the building. Employees told us that past power outages led to ozone generation during working hours. Cultivation and harvesting employees worked under grow lights almost continuously throughout their shifts. Loud music was played in production areas and many employees were observed wearing earbud headphones while working in these areas.

How? At your workplace, we recommend these specific actions:

Adjust the current ozone generation practices to reduce the chance of accidental ozone generation with employees present.

- Use ozone generators that have a built-in timer. Leaving the current generator set to be continuously "on" and controlling the electricity with the analog timer is not how the generator was designed to be operated.
- Unplug the ozone generators at the start of each day—if keeping the current setup using analog timers—to prevent the accidental generation of ozone during the shift. Plug the generators in at the end of the shift and ensure the analog timer settings are correct.

Supply employees with the right protective eyewear for the specific wavelengths emitted by the bulbs in the facility.

- Train employees about the importance of protecting themselves from exposures to UV light and why wavelength-specific protection is needed.

Encourage cultivation and harvesting employees to wear long sleeves when working.

- Train employees about the importance of protecting themselves from exposures to UV light.
- Provide long sleeve scrub options for employees. Other technologies may also be appropriate (e.g., UV-protective athletic arm sleeves). Ensure that employees understand that all shirts, scrubs, or other sleeve technologies worn during cultivation and harvesting tasks should be laundered regularly.

Reduce noise exposures in production areas.

- Monitor the volume of the music being played in production areas. Playing music (on a speaker or in headphones) adds to the employees' cumulative noise exposure'. No longer playing music in production areas or reducing the volume at which it is played may help address

potential overexposures from headphones being used in the workplace.
- Suggest employees keep their headphone volumes at a lower level, which will be easier to do if there is no competing noise from the shared speakers.

Offer hearing protection to employees who wish to use it.

- Train employees upon hiring and at least annually about the hazards of noise exposure.
- Give training about the proper use for the type of hearing protection provided (e.g., earplugs, earmuffs).
- Ensure adequate supplies of hearing protection are available for employees to use.

Recommendation 4: Reduce Risks for Musculoskeletal Disorders

Why? Musculoskeletal disorders are conditions that involve the nerves, tendons, muscles, and supporting structures of the body. They can be characterized by chronic pain and limited mobility. A substantial body of data shows strong evidence of an association between musculoskeletal disorders and certain work-related factors (physical, work organizational, and psychosocial). The preferred method for preventing and controlling work-related musculoskeletal disorders is to design tasks, workstations, and tools and other equipment to match the physiological, anatomical, and psychological characteristics and capabilities of the employee. Our observations indicate that employees had exposures to highly repetitive and forceful work, most notably during hand trimming and harvesting activities. These exposures increase the risk of musculoskeletal disorders. Trimming employees spent long periods sitting at tables performing their manual tasks. Improving workstations will reduce lower back, shoulder, and neck strain for these employees. Harvesting employees also experienced repetitive work with frequent bending and reaching to access plastic trellis netting and stems on the lower parts of the plants.

How? At your workplace, we recommend these specific actions:
Rotate job tasks for employees performing highly repetitive work.

- Develop a job rotation plan to move employees working in high hand and finger motion frequency tasks to other jobs that require using different muscle-tendon groups. An effective job rotation plan will reduce the risk of musculoskeletal disorders.
- Provide frequent breaks for employees working in high hand and finger motion frequency tasks such as hand trimming.

Provide employees with clean, sharp tools.

- Discuss equipment needs with harvesting and trimming employees regularly and replace or maintain tools as needed.
- Develop a cleaning schedule to remove cannabinoids from work and tool surfaces.
- Train employees to clean, lubricate, sharpen, and maintain their tools according to manufacturer recommendations.

Improve the workstations for trimming employees.

- Supply adjustable and comfortable seating for trimming employees.
- Add padded elbow rests to the edges of the trimming tables or otherwise ensure that there are no hard, sharp edges on the trimming tables.
- Include several standing workstations with anti-fatigue mats to allow employees variation and choice of posture during trimming tasks.

Raise all cultivation beds and other ground-level work areas to reduce bending and awkward postures during cultivation and harvesting activities.

- Raising all cultivation beds off the ground allows employees to access the lower parts of the plants and plastic trellis netting with less bending and reaching. This will help employees avoid unnecessary bending when setting up the plastic trellis netting,
- de-leafing and caring for the plants, and harvesting.
- Raising the children's pool of soil further off the ground when repotting plants and adding an elevated work surface (e.g., washable

folding table) to the cleaning area will help employees avoid unnecessary bending during these tasks.

Provide employees with longer-handled brushes for cleaning pots.

- Longer handles will reduce the amount of reaching and bending required during cleaning tasks. Longer handles will also reduce the chance that cleaning produce gets splashed on employees.

Recommendation 5: Obtain Regular Input from Employees about Workplace Safety and Health Issues and Use This Input to Improve Conditions

Why? Monitoring employee concerns, satisfaction, and well-being is useful for finding areas of focus for intervention and improvement. Engaging employees and asking for their input about work builds trust and morale when they feel their input is valued and useful for improving working conditions. We learned that employees had safety and health concerns related to the physical working environment (lighting, noise, potential exposures), work organization (e.g., practices and policies), and psychosocial environment (e.g., communication). Exploring these concerns in greater detail may lead to organizational change and improvement based on employee input. Employee safety and health concerns may change over time, so frequent communication is important, especially during times when new or different practices and procedures are implemented.

How? At your workplace, we recommend these specific actions:

Use employee input to guide efforts in improving worker safety, health, and well-being.

- Develop or use existing tools (survey, interview, or focus group questions/topics) to obtain employee input about workplace safety and health and use the results to inform the development or revision of interventions, policies, and practices in the workplace to improve employee safety and health.
- An example tool is the National Institute for Occupational Safety and Health (NIOSH) Well-Being Questionnaire or WellBQ. WellBQ is a

survey tool developed to assess employee well-being across multiple areas, including work evaluation and experience, workplace policies and culture, workplace physical environment and safety culture, health status, and home, family, and society. The WellBQ and instructions are available at www.cdc.gov/niosh/twh/wellbq.

- Use the interview results from this health hazard evaluation (Tables C6 through C8) as a baseline to guide and monitor improvement efforts in areas of concern to employees.

Recommendation 6: Address Other Health and Safety Issues We Identified During Our Evaluation

Why? A workplace can have multiple health hazards that cause employee illness or injury. Similar to the ones identified above, these hazards can potentially cause serious health symptoms, lower morale and quality of life for your employees, and possibly increase costs to your business. We saw the following potential issues at your workplace:

- No respiratory protection program was provided for pesticide applicators, although pesticide applicators were certified to apply pesticides by the state Department of Agriculture.
- Incorrect respirator cartridges were being used for the chemical exposures during pesticide application.
- The trimming machine safety switch was taped so that it could be operated with the cover in an open position.
- No eye wash stations were located near the pesticide/nutrient preparation areas.
- Goggles or face shields were not available for employees working with the hydrogen peroxide to wash pots from harvested plants.
- High-percentage alcohol was being sprayed directly onto surfaces in the trimming areas causing many employees to report discomfort from strong odors when performing those tasks.
- Powder-free latex gloves were available in some parts of the facility, latex is a potential allergen source.

Although they were not the focus of our evaluation, these hazards could cause harm to your employees' health and safety and should be addressed.

How? At your workplace, we recommend these specific actions:
Develop a respiratory protection program.

- Contact your local Occupational Safety and Health Administration (OSHA) consultation program for free help in developing your respiratory protection program, addressing questions about PPE, and other safety concerns. Additional information can be found at https://www.osha.gov/html/RAmap.html.
- Ensure that the respiratory protection program also complies with the Environmental Protection Agency (EPA) Agricultural Worker Protection Standard.

Use the correct respirator cartridges for the chemical exposures during pesticide application.

- We learned that pink P100 cartridges were used for pesticide and nutrient application. P100 cartridges are designed to protect against exposures to particulates or fibers, not chemical vapors. Organic vapor (OV) or combination OV and P100 cartridges would be appropriate for the pesticide and nutrient application.
- Consider using the NIOSH MultiVapor™ tool or the OSHA Respiratory Protection eTool to assist with cartridge selection.

Operate the trimming machine according to manufacturer's instructions.

- Do not tape down the safety switch. Operate the machine with the cover in a closed position to prevent getting fingers or clothing caught in moving machinery.
- Use a tool to move the cannabis around inside the machine when the cover is open.

Install plumbed eye wash stations and emergency showers in each of the pesticide/nutrient preparation areas.

- Ensure that eye wash stations and emergency showers are accessible, provide adequate flow of tepid water, and not blocked by equipment.
- Provide training to employees so that they know the locations and how to operate the eye wash and emergency shower and report incidents where the eye wash or shower needed to be used.

- Incorporate this procedure into new employee and annual refresher training.

Provide goggles (not safety glasses) or face shields to employees who wash pots after harvesting.

- Goggles and face shields should be compliant with the American National Standards Institute Standard Z87.1-2015, "American National Standard for Occupational and Educational Personal Eye and Face Protection Devices."
- Face shields should be at least ¾-length or full-length. Smaller-sized shields are not acceptable.

Adjust the cleaning procedures and training for the trimming areas.

- Purchase cleaning wipes to avoid spraying cleaning products.
- If the current practice of spraying cleaning products is kept, reduce the alcohol concentration to 70% alcohol for cleaning hard, nonporous surfaces.
    - Train employees to spray the alcohol directly onto paper towels and then use those paper towels to wipe down surfaces.
    - Provide to training about proper handling of flammable liquids to employees using high-percentage alcohol for cleaning. Training should cover potential fire hazards and instruction about safe handling and storage of flammable liquids.
- Incorporate this procedure and training into new employee and annual refresher training.

Remove powder-free latex gloves from the facility.

- Continue to provide non-latex gloves for employees. Consider using the OSHA guidance publication on PPE: Personal Protective Equipment.

Supporting Technical Information: Evaluation of Potential Hazards During Harvesting and Trimming Cannabis at an Indoor Cultivation Facility, HHE Report No. 2019-0152-3381 February 2022

Section A: Workplace Information

Background

According to the National Conference of State Legislatures, 37 states and 4 territories allow for medical or non-medical adult use of cannabis products as of February 2, 2022. These legal changes have given rise to a rapidly growing industry. As of January 2021, the cannabis industry employed about 321,000 full-time equivalent jobs in 37 states in the United States [Barcott et al. 2021]. Understanding the nature of work and potential hazards involved in the growth, harvesting, processing, and packaging of cannabis products are important steps in improving occupational safety and health for this fairly new industry.

The National Institute for Occupational Safety and Health (NIOSH) has completed two previous health hazard evaluations [NIOSH 2017, 2019] in this regard.

Building

The facility was a single building that housed office and operations areas for two brand names of cannabis that were owned by the same parent company (Side A and Side B). Each brand grew, harvested, dried, trimmed, and packaged bulk product in separate areas of the facility.

Employee Information

Each side of the facility employed cultivation and harvesting employees who worked full time. The facility also had a contract with a staffing agency to supply trimming employees for each side of the facility. All employees worked a single, 8-hour shift and were not unionized. Trimming did not occur every day, so those employees were not always at the facility. We visited the facility when trimming operations were occurring in addition to cultivating and harvesting. Additionally, trimming staffing varied due to availability and scheduling dictated by the staffing agency that managed this pool of employees.

Process Description

This facility cultivated, harvested, trimmed, and packaged bulk cannabis. The bulk product was either sold to other companies or moved to further processing facilities. The health hazard evaluation (HHE) request did not extend to other processing facilities. Employees and management told us that production levels and conditions we observed were representative of normal operations at this facility.

Employees in this type of environment may be exposed to a variety of plant-derived materials (e.g., leaves, buds, sap/exudate, flowers, and pollen) when handling the plant during cultivation and processing procedures. They can also encounter cannabinoids and other contaminant- and plant-pathogen sources such as bacteria and fungi.

Cultivation

The cultivation process began in the clone room where employees removed cuttings from mature donor plants to create clones, or seedlings. The clones grow to be new individual plants that were genetically identical to the donor plants. As the clones grow larger, they were moved out of the clone room and into the cultivation areas where they were cared for until mature and ready for harvest. There were two large, open areas of the facility where cultivation took place. In each area, multiple sets of plants were being grown. Each set had dozens of plants of the same type that were cloned and grown together at the same time.

In the cultivation areas, employees performed a variety of tasks aimed to promote growth and inhibit pests during the cultivation cycle. Employees removed leaves from plants so that the plant would dedicate energy into producing flowers instead of leaves. When the plants reached certain heights, plastic trellis netting was attached to the grow areas to promote vertical growth and prevent plants from falling over when top-heavy. Nutrients and pesticides were applied according to a proprietary schedule and according to manufacturer's recommendations.

Harvesting

Once a set of plants reached maturity, they were harvested. Harvesting involved cutting the plastic trellis nets that held up the plants and removing large stems containing the cannabis flowers from the plants. The stems were hung on garment racks in preparation for transfer to the drying room. After harvesting was complete, the harvesting crew cleaned the area in preparation for a new set of plants to be grown.

Drying

After harvest, the stems of flowers were transferred to the drying rooms. Stems were hung to dry before trimming in two drying rooms on each side of the facility. An ozone generator was used to generate ozone in the drying rooms periodically throughout the drying process. The ozone generation was used to prevent microbial growth on the plants while they were drying.

Trimming

After the flowers were dried, employees removed the stems from the drying room and trimmed the flowers from the stems by hand. The trimmed flowers were packaged in bulk and brought to the vault for storage before leaving the facility. There was an ozone generator in the vault that was used in a similar way to the ones in the drying rooms.

Section B: Methods, Results, and Discussion

The objectives of this evaluation were to observe work practices, measure employee exposures to potential hazards, and learn about employees' general safety and health concerns to provide recommendations for improving employee safety, health, and well-being in the cannabis industry.

Methods: Observations of Work Processes, Practices, and Conditions

During our two visits to the facility, we observed the work processes, PPE use, and workplace conditions of employees as they performed cultivating, harvesting, drying, and trimming tasks.

Results: Observations of Work Processes, Practices, and Conditions

Cultivation

All cultivation and harvesting employees changed into employer-provided scrubs prior to entering the cultivation areas of the facility. Scrubs were laundered by the employer. All employees were given sunglasses as eye protection from the grow lights. This facility used high pressure sodium (HPS) grow lights throughout the cultivation areas. During our first visit, we noticed that the sunglasses being provided to employees were not specifically chosen based on their ability to filter out the specific wavelengths of light produced by the grow lights. We recommended that the company purchase sunglasses that were appropriate for protection from grow lights. During our second visit, the company had purchased hydroponics grow room light glasses for employees. The packaging for the glasses stated that the glasses provided UV light protection, reduced glare, and were "perfect for using under HPS… lighting systems." We were unable to determine whether the claims of the manufacturer were accurate. There was no testing information available on the manufacturer's website to support these claims.

During leaf removal, some employees wore long sleeve shirts under their scrubs and told us it was to protect their skin from contacting the plants while removing leaves. The employer did not provide the long sleeve shirts. We were told that nutrients and pesticides were added periodically to the plants according to the manufacturer's recommendations. There was a table posted near the nutrient and pesticide storage areas that included information about each product (e.g., concentration, protective equipment during application).

We did not observe pesticide application during our visits. We learned that all pesticide application was performed by employees who were certified to apply pesticides by the state Department of Agriculture. We were told by employees and management that pesticides were only applied after normal business hours. Employees were issued one elastomeric full-face respirator by the company and were responsible for cleaning and maintenance. The company relied on the state Department of Agriculture pesticide applicator certification and did not have a respiratory protection program (i.e., did not provide medical clearance, fit testing, or training about respiratory protection to employees). We observed respirators hung on the wall near the pesticide/nutrient mixing area in between uses. We saw both P100 and OV cartridges in the facility. No combination P100/OV cartridges were evident. There was no changeout schedule for cartridges. After our first visit, we recommended that the company improve respiratory protection practices, including creating a written program. During the second visit, the company had improved storage practices for the elastomeric full-face respirators.

We noted the lack of eye wash stations near the pesticide/nutrient mixing areas during our first visit. During our second visit, the company had purchased eye wash bottles to place in the two pesticide/nutrient mixing areas.

We observed employees repotting plants during one of our visits. During this task, soil was placed in a children's pool elevated about 12–18 inches off the ground. The pool was placed on a wooden pallet that was on top of overturned pots. Empty pots and plants were staged around the pool. Employees were observed rapidly placing the plants into the pots and filling the pots with soil from the pool. To accomplish this task, employees were bent over to access the soil and used their hands and forearms to quickly scoop soil into the pot (Figure B1).

On both sides of the facility were several large ventilation units that ran continuously to mix the air inside the facility. These units were large, ductless, open-building heating and cooling equipment. We were informed that the units were intended only to mix and condition the air within the facility, not to filter contaminants. The units appeared to contain large filter banks. A handwritten note on the side of the units indicated 44 filters, sized 20 inches × 20 inches × 2 inches, and 22 filters, sized 20 inches × 12 inches × 2 inches; however, we were informed that filters were not used in these units.

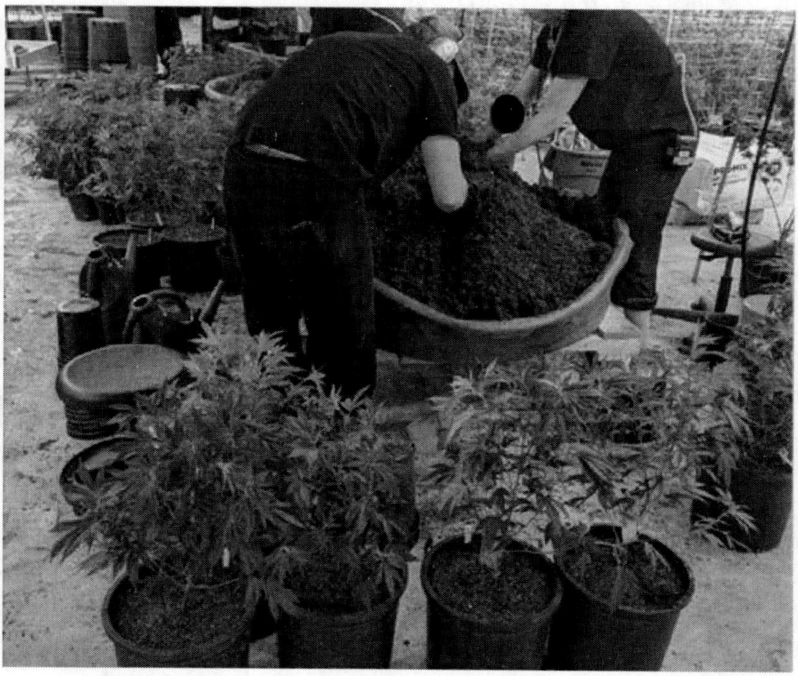

Figure B1. Employees repotting plants using soil from an elevated children's pool. Photo by NIOSH.

We learned that the employer washed the intake grates periodically but had never bought filters for the units.

Harvesting

The plastic trellis netting needed to be cut away from the plants before and periodically during the harvesting process. The cut plastic was placed on the ground wherever it was cut, presenting a tripping hazard for employees. During the harvesting process, employees cut several large stems off the plants and brought them to a folding table for weighing. Employees were observed repeatedly bending over to access the lower parts of the plastic trellis netting and the lower stems on the plants. The harvest we observed was for plants with pots placed directly on the ground. Other sets of plants were on raised cultivation beds. We were told that there was no difference between the cultivation setups, and that some sections of the facility just had raised cultivation beds. The stems were hung on a garment rack after being weighed and logged into the computer system. Once the harvest was complete, the garment racks were moved into the drying rooms.

After the harvest, multiple steps were involved in cleaning up the area previously occupied by the plants. First, the plastic trellis netting was placed in trash cans. Then the growing pots, still full of soil, were placed on a cart and brought to another area of the facility where they were emptied. The pile of soil from the pots was either reused for future planting or disposed of, depending on the condition. We observed employees dry sweeping the floor to clean up dirt and debris from the harvesting activities.

Harvesting did not occur every day, and the harvest we observed did not last the full shift.

After the growing pots were emptied of soil, they were brought to another area of the facility to be washed and rinsed in preparation to be reused. Employees who were washing the pots were wearing work scrubs, latex or nitrile gloves, and sunglasses. The cleaning product contained 34% hydrogen peroxide. Employees were observed pouring the cleaning product into the pots and scrubbing them with short-handled brushes. Employees needed to reach their hands into the pots when scrubbing. Pots were rinsed out with clean water from a hose and all runoff was captured by a drain in the floor. The scrubbing and rinsing tasks produced visible splashes periodically during the process.

Drying

Each drying room had an ozone generator inside. The generator was operated by plugging it in and then turning a knob to start the generation. The knob could be turned to run for a specific period, or it could be set to be continuously operational. The process we observed involved all generators set to continuously operate. The generators were plugged into an analog electrical timer that turned the generator on for a set amount of time overnight and turned it off before employees arrived for their shift the following day. We learned from employees that power outages could inadvertently cause the timer to be inaccurate (i.e., the analog timer did not account for power outages). When this occurred, employees told us that the ozone generators would run while employees were in the building instead of overnight. It was unclear how often this occurred, but many employees were concerned about potential ozone exposures.

Trimming

The trimming rooms were set up with multiple eight-foot folding tables situated around the room (Figure B2). Each table had chairs arranged around it. The contractors who were assigned to trimming tasks either stood or sat around the table and used hand cutters to trim the flowers from the stems. Stems were discarded in one pile while the trimmed flowers were placed in a tote. The trimming process was a highly repetitivetask where most trimming employees were continuously snipping flowers from stems and placing them into the tote. Employees had a 45-minute lunch break and two scheduled 15-minute personal breaks per shift. None of the chairs or tables had adjustable heights and the trimming employees varied considerably in height. When trimming employees were standing at the tables, many needed to bend over to pick up stems and again to place flowers into the totes. When trimming employees were seated, many would rest their forearms on the edges of the tables. The table edges were square (i.e., not rounded) and did not have padding along the edges where trimming employees would rest their forearms and elbows.

At the end of each shift, trimming employees used 90% isopropyl alcohol solutions to clean work surfaces. The alcohol was applied using a spray bottle and then paper towels were used to wipe the sprayed surfaces. Employees told us that they were concerned about their exposures to alcohol vapors during the cleaning process.

When the flower tote was full or when the trimming employees were done with their allotted stems, employees brought the tote to a supervisor at a table in the corner for the product to be weighed and logged into the system. There was also one trimming machine that could be used to process the trimmed flowers (Figure B3). When in use, we noted that the safety switch was taped down so the machine would run when the cover was not closed. We were informed that the employees needed to be able to see the flowers and to move the flowers around while the machine was in operation. This process required employees to stick their hands into the machine while it was rotating.

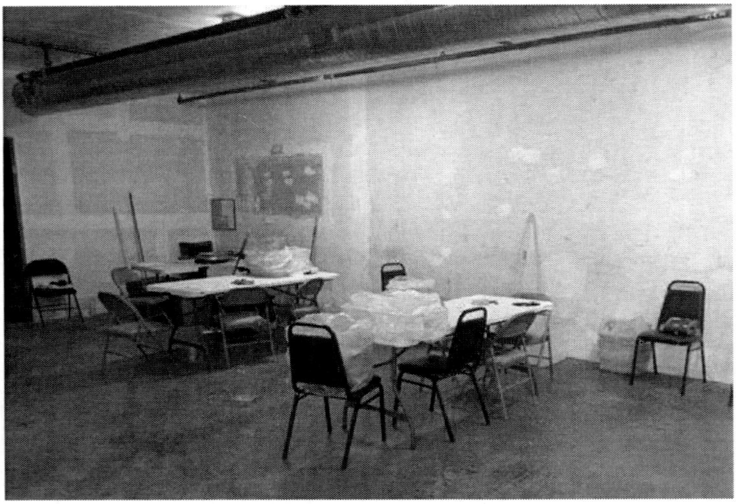

Figure B2. One of the trimming areas. Each table can accommodate four to six trimming employees. Photo by NIOSH.

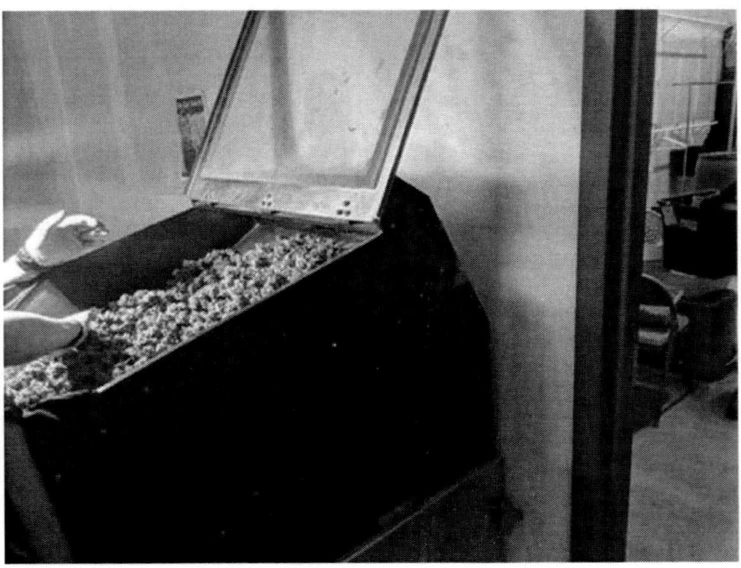

Figure B3. An employee operating the trimming machine with the lid opened while the machine is operating. Photo by NIOSH.

We were not permitted to step into the vault during our visits, but we were able to observe that there was an ozone generator in the vault. We learned that this ozone generator was used in a similar manner to the ones in the drying rooms. The generator was attached to an analog electrical timer that turned the generator on for a set amount of time overnight and turned it off before employees arrived for their shift the following day.

Methods: Exposure Assessment

Endotoxin

We collected personal air samples on cultivation and harvesting employees using three-piece, 37-millimeter-diameter close-faced cassettes with 0.45-micrometer (μm) pore size preloaded polycarbonate filters. The sampling pumps were calibrated at a flow rate of 2 liters of air per minute. Each sample was analyzed for endotoxin using a recombinant Factor C assay method (HyGlos EndoZyme® rFC Assay). The assay was a quantitative endpoint florescence test used to measure gram- negative bacterial endotoxin.

We collected personal air samples for endotoxin on 20 employees during their entire work shift (10 employees from each side of the facility). All cultivation and harvesting employees were invited to participate in the sampling. Samples were paused and pumps removed from employees during breaks. For these analyses, the reporting limit was 0.40 endotoxin units (EU) per sample.

Cannabinoids

Surface wipe samples were collected in production and nonproduction areas of the facility and analyzed for Δ9-THC, Δ9-THCA, CBD, and CBN. Where possible, two samples were taken in each location.

The second sample was taken directly adjacent to the first sample whenever possible. Each sample was taken with a cotton twill wipe moistened with 3 milliliters of isopropanol. All samples were taken using a disposable 100-square-centimeter (100 cm2) template. If the template was not feasible (e.g., the surface was an irregular shape that did not lend itself to using the template), approximately 100 cm2 of surface was wiped for the sample.

Each pair of samples were analyzed using two methods, one for each sample. One sample was analyzed for Δ9-THC using a contract laboratory's internal method. The method used high performance liquid chromatography and tandem mass spectrometry with a limit of detection of 5 nanograms (ng) per sample. The second sample was analyzed for Δ9-THC, Δ9-THCA, CBD, and CBN using a modified method [Ambach et al. 2014]. The modified method used high performance liquid chromatography with diode-array detection with a limit of detection of 2 micrograms (μg) per sample for each analyte.

Fungi

Genomic DNA Extraction from Air Samples

General area air samples (n = 14) were collected using the NIOSH BC251 two-stage air sampler: 7 samples from each side (Side A and Side B) of the facility. All samples were processed for fungal DNA extraction using the Roche High Pure Polymerase Chain Reaction (PCR) Template kit as previously described in earlier studies [Green et al. 2017; Green et al. 2018]. Each stage obtained from the NIOSH two-stage sampler was combined. The after filter was sectioned into six pieces and placed into a 2-milliliter (mL) reinforced tube containing 300 milligrams of glass beads. We placed the tubes in liquid nitrogen for 30 seconds and processed two times in a bead mill homogenizer for 30 seconds. The Roche kit lysis buffer (650 microliters [μL]) was then sequentially added to the first and second stage tubes and vortexed to collect the deposited bioaerosols. The lysis buffer was then added to the 2 mL reinforced tube containing the macerated filter material. We processed the tubes again in a bead mill homogenizer for 30 seconds and then centrifuged for 1 minute at 20,000 × g, a measure of relative centrifugal force. We collected the supernatant and incubated with 40 μL Cell Lytic B lysis reagent (Sigma Aldrich) for 15 minutes at 37°C. We mixed the sample with the Roche kit binding buffer (200 μL) and proteinase K solution (40 μL) and incubated at 70°C for 10 minutes. We washed and eluted the genomic DNA from the samples as recommended by the manufacturer.

Fungal ITS Region Amplification, Cloning, and Sanger Sequencing

We amplified the fungal Internal Transcribed Spacer (ITS) regions using a procedure modified from methods that were described in previous studies [Green et al. 2017; Green et al. 2018]. Briefly, the fungal ITS1 region sequences were amplified with the primer pair ITS1F (CTTGGTCATTTAGAGGAAGTAA) and ITS2aR (GCTGCGTTCT TCATCGATGC) using Platinum Taq DNA polymerase (Invitrogen) and 5 μL of genomic DNA template. Three replicate PCR reactions (50 μL) were run for each sample and were then combined and purified with a Qiagen PCR purification kit according to the manufacturer's instructions.

We cloned the fungal amplicons into the pDRIVE vector using a Qiagen PCR cloning kit and then generated clone libraries by transforming cloned plasmids into chemically competent Escherichia coli cells as previously described [Green et al. 2017]. Based on the fungal gDNA yield, we selected 12–48 positive colonies per air sample (as determined colorimetrically by the inactivation of the lacZ gene) and cultured the colonies for 16 hours at 37°C in liquid Luria-Bertani media containing 100 μg/mL of ampicillin. The cells were centrifuged at 1800 × g (relative centrifugal force) for 10 minutes and the pellets were resuspended in 200 μL of 15% glycerol and sent to Genewiz, Inc., for Sanger sequencing of the fungal ITS1 insert.

Inserts were sequenced in both directions, allowing for sequence analysis of the full ITS1 region. We downloaded the sequencing results as ".ab1" trace files and the forward and reverse sequences were trimmed and assembled using Biomatters Geneious R7 Software. Sequence data were then clustered into operational taxonomic units with MOTHUR software version 1.32.1 using a 97% similarity cutoff as described previously [Green et al. 2017]. Sequences representative of each operational taxonomic unit were then used in a Basic Local Alignment Search Tool search against the National Center for Biotechnology Information sequence database.

Particulates

We measured particulates in three areas of the facility for a full shift using DustTrak™ DRX 8533 Aerosol Monitors (TSI, Inc.). Two monitors were in the trimming rooms, one on a table near the trimming machine on Side A, and one near the middle of the trimming room on Side B. The third monitor was on a folding table that was temporarily set up during a harvest. All monitors were set to log particle concentrations every 60 seconds in different size groups: particulate matter (PM) smaller than 1 μm (PM_1), PM smaller than 2.5 μm ($PM_{2.5}$), respirable (less than 4 μm), PM smaller than 10 μm (PM_{10}), and total PM (less than 100 μm).

Noise

We measured area noise levels in different parts of the production areas using a Quest 3M Model 2400 calibrated, battery-operated, type-2 sound level meter. We focused on areas where employees were working, including close to the ventilation units, in the trimming rooms, and in areas where music was being played by a portable speaker.

Results: Exposure Assessment

Endotoxin

Endotoxin was detected in all samples (Table C1). On Side A, exposures ranged 6–980 endotoxin units per cubic meter of air (EU/m^3). On Side B, exposures ranged 11–660 EU/m^3. Four employees (40%) from each side were exposed to endotoxin above the Dutch Expert Committee on Occupational Standards (DECOS) limit of 90 EU/m^3 [DECOS 2010]. The United States does not have an occupational exposure limit (OEL) for endotoxin. The DECOS limit is the most relevant available OEL for our results.

Cannabinoids

Surface wipe samples for cannabinoids were collected using two methods in eight locations throughout the facility (Table C2). One method analyzed samples for Δ9-THC only. The second method analyzed samples for multiple cannabinoids simultaneously (Δ9-THC, Δ9-THCA, CBD, and CBN).

For the Δ9-THC only method, all surface wipe samples had detectable levels of Δ9-THC. The surface wipe results ranged 1–91 micrograms per 100-square-centimeters ($\mu g/100\ cm^2$) in production areas and from 0.035–0.93 $\mu g/100\ cm^2$ in nonproduction areas.

For the method analyzing samples for multiple cannabinoids simultaneously, three of five surface wipe samples in production areas had detectable levels of Δ9-THC (range: not detected–110 $\mu g/100\ cm^2$). Δ9-THCA was detected in all samples taken in production areas (range: 25–1,000 $\mu g/100\ cm^2$) and in two of three samples taken in nonproduction areas (range: not detected–15 $\mu g/100\ cm^2$). CBD and CBN were detected in low amounts in production areas. We did not detect Δ9-THC, CBD, or CBN in nonproduction areas using this method.

Fungi

A total of 226 fungal DNA sequences that clustered into 87 operational taxonomic units were identified in the 14 area air samples. There was low to no fungal DNA yield in the field and media blanks. As shown in Figure B4, the identified fungi were placed into three major fungal phlya: Ascomycota (56%), Basidiomycota (43%), and Zygomycota (1%). The most prevalent fungal orders in the phylum Ascomycota were Erysiphales (19%), plant pathogens often referred to as powdery mildews, and Eurotiales (12%), containing ubiquitous fungi, like *Aspergillus* and *Penicillium* species (Figure

4B). Within the phylum Basidiomycota, 13% of the fungi were placed in the order Sporidiobolales (Figure 4B), with most belonging to the genus *Rhodotorula* (Table C3). The most abundant species making up almost 20% of all fungal sequences detected in the area samples was *Golovinomyces spadiceus*, a powdery mildew in the order Eryisiphales, followed by species in the genera *Rhodotorula*, and *Penicillium* (Table C3). *Cladosporium* species, often encountered in outdoor environments, were also prevalent in some samples.

More fungal DNA was obtained from area samples collected from Side A of the facility (169 of the 216 sequences) than those collected from Side B. The samples with the highest number of fungal sequences identified were obtained near the trim room tables and the grow area closest to harvesting procedures (Table C4).

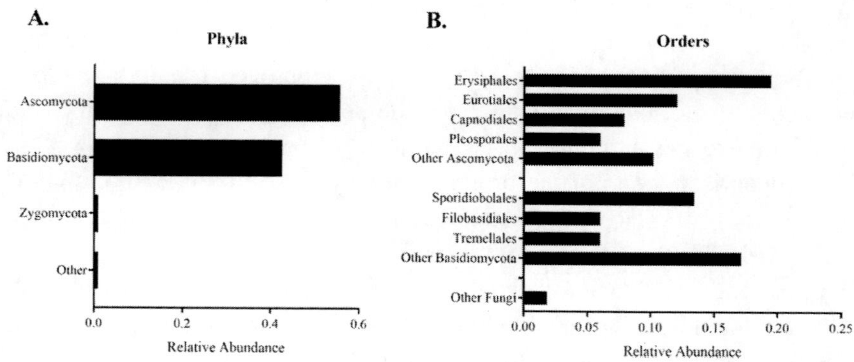

Figure B4. Relative abundance of fungal phyla (A) and orders (B) identified in area air samples.

Particulates

Particle mass concentrations were low in all three areas, across all size ranges (Table C5). Respirable dust ranged 0.014–0.15 milligrams per cubic meter of air (mg/m3) on the Side A harvest table, 0.015–0.13 mg/m3 in the Side A trimming area, and 0.012–0.11 mg/m3 in the Side B trimming area.

Noise

We made area sound measurements while work was being performed in the cultivation and trimming areas of the facility. The ventilation units were operating, and music was being played in both trimming rooms and where harvesting was taking place. Many employees were observed wearing earbud headphones while working in these areas. The Side A cultivation area ranged 75–83 decibels,

A-weighted (dBA). The Side A trimming room averaged 83 dBA. The Side B cultivation area ranged 73–83 dBA. The Side B trimming room averaged 74 dBA. The measured exposures cannot be compared to OELs since they are not personal exposure measurements collected as full-shift time-weighted averages. However, the upper end of the sound levels we measured were slightly below the NIOSH recommended exposure limit (REL) of 85 dBA and the OSHA action level (AL) of 85 dBA.

Methods: Confidential Medical Interviews

We completed semi-structured, confidential medical interviews with employees performing cultivation and harvesting duties and employees performing trimming. The results of these employee groups are reported separately (i.e., no comparisons are made between groups) in this report due to the differences in job roles, tasks, and work locations).

Supervisors coordinated bringing employees one by one to a low traffic area in the workplace which had been identified as suitable for maintaining privacy during the interviews. When an employee arrived, we explained the purpose of the HHE and asked if they would like to participate in a confidential interview about workplace safety and health. Those who refused were thanked for their time and returned to work. Interviews averaged about 15 minutes each.

The interviews included questions to assess the following:

- Job tasks (cultivation and harvesting employees only): Employees were read a list of tasks common to the cultivation and harvesting of cannabis and were asked to indicate (yes/no response) whether they performed each task as part of their job duties. Employees were also given the opportunity to identify additional tasks not on the list (open-ended response format).
- PPE use: Cultivation and harvesting employees were asked, “If you mix and/or apply pesticides as part of your duties, what type of PPE do you wear?” (open-ended response format). Trimming employees were asked, “What kind of PPE do you regularly wear on the job?” (open-ended response format).

- Health and safety concerns: Employees were asked, "Do you have any work-related health or safety concerns?" (yes/no response), followed by, "If yes, describe" (open-ended response format).
- Health symptoms: Employees were read a list asking them to indicate whether they had experienced any work-related health symptoms over the past 4 weeks (yes/no response). Employees were also given the opportunity to identify additional symptoms not on the list (open-ended response format).
- Perceptions of physical working conditions and psychosocial factors: We used a combination of items from an occupational health survey [Weel and Fortuin 1998] and items developed specifically for this HHE to ask if employees had concerns about physical working conditions and psychosocial factors at work (yes/no response).
- Job stress: Employees were read the following definition of job stress: "NIOSH defines job stress as the harmful physical and emotional responses that occur when the requirements of the job do not match the capabilities, resources, or needs of the worker." They were then asked to rate their overall level of job stress on a scale from 0 (no stress at all) to 10 (severe stress). Responses of 0–3 indicated low job stress, 4–6 indicated moderate job stress, and scores of 7 or greater indicated high job stress [Clark et al. 2011]. Employees were then asked to identify major sources of job stress (open-ended response format).

Employee responses were transcribed onto paper, which were later recorded in a spreadsheet maintained on a secure server at NIOSH. Employee names were not recorded to protect confidentiality. All employee responses to interview questions are protected to the greatest extent possible by the Privacy Act of 1974 and the Freedom of Information Act.

Results: Confidential Medical Interviews

Employee Information

We interviewed 25 of 25 (100%) cultivation and harvesting employees present during our visit. Of these, 24 (96%) were male. The average age was 30 years (range: 22–47 years), the average amount of time working at the facility was 1 year, 4 months (range: 2 days–5 years), and the average number of hours worked a week was 37 hours (range: 30–45 hours).

We interviewed 25 of 30 (83%) trimming employees present during our visit. Of these, 19 (76%) were male. The average age of these employees was 31 years (range: 21–60 years), the average amount of time working at the facility was 10 months (range: 2 days–2.5 years), and the average number of hours worked a week was 31 hours (range: 5–40 hours).

Job Tasks

Cultivation and harvesting employees had job titles of grow technician, cultivation manager, and facility manager. We asked these employees to indicate whether a list of common job tasks was part of their responsibilities. These tasks included cultivation (n = 24; 96%); harvesting (n = 23; 92%); topping (n = 23; 92%); transplanting (n = 23; 92%); examining plants (n = 23; 92%); staking plants; (n = 23; 92%); waste disposal (n = 22; 88%); pest control (n = 22; 88%); feeding (n = 22; 88%); cloning (n = 21; 84%); pesticide application (n = 20; 80%); flushing plants (n = 16; 64%); inventory (n = 10; 40%); and maintenance (n = 16; 64%). When asked an open-ended question about "other" job tasks, some employees reported trimming and super-cropping of plants.

A supervisor informed us that all trimming employees had the same job title of "trimmer" and were expected to complete the same job tasks, which included trimming flowers from stems, fanning and bucking plants, quality control, and cleaning tools and workspaces.

Personal Protective Equipment

Of the 20 cultivation and harvesting employees who reported mixing or applying pesticides, all (100%) reported wearing a Tyvek® suit, nitrile and rubber gloves, booties, a head sock, respirator, and face shield during these tasks. Some employees reported that they wore personal sunglasses to reduce light exposure on the floor. Also, some employees reported wearing earbud headphones to drown out the noise of the ventilation unit(s).

All 25 (100%) of the trimming employees reported wearing nitrile gloves, 16 (64%) reported wearing a bandanna or dust mask, and 6 (24%) reported wearing scrubs while working.

Work-Related Safety Concerns

Of the 25 cultivation and harvesting employees interviewed, 10 (40%) indicated that they had work- related safety concerns. They included noise (n = 6; 24%); bright lights (n = 4; 16%); and exposure to pesticides (n = 3; 12%).

Other concerns were reported by two or fewer employees and are not described to maintain employee confidentiality.

Seventeen of 25 (68%) trimming employees indicated they had work-related safety concerns. They included indoor air quality (n = 6; 24%); exposure to pesticides (n = 4; 16%); using alcohol to clean workstations (n = 4; 16%); exposure to ozone (n = 3; 12%); and communication concerns (n = 3; 12%). Other concerns were reported by two or fewer employees and are not described to maintain employee confidentiality.

Work-Related Health Symptoms

Table C6 includes the frequency and percentage of employees who reported "yes" to experiencing work-related health symptoms in the past 4 weeks. The five most frequently reported symptoms among cultivation and harvesting employees were stuffy nose or sinus problems (n = 10; 40%); runny nose (n = 9; 36%); back pain (n = 9; 36%); rash on skin (n = 7; 28%); and red or irritated eyes (n = 6; 24%).

The five most frequently reported symptoms among trimming employees were stuffy nose or sinus problems (n = 18; 72%); back pain (n = 15; 60%); headaches (n = 13; 52%); runny nose (n = 12; 48%); and hand/wrist pain (n = 11; 44%).

Physical Working Conditions and Psychosocial Factors

Table C7 includes the physical working conditions that employees indicated made them uncomfortable at work. The most frequently reported conditions that made cultivation and harvesting employees uncomfortable at work were bright light (n = 18; 72%); dust/dirt (n = 17; 68%); and heat (n = 12; 48%). The most frequently reported conditions that made trimming employees uncomfortable at work were dust/dirt (n = 16; 64%); lack of fresh air (n = 15; 60%); lengthy periods of being in the same physical position (n = 14; 56%); bad smells/odors (n = 13; 52%); and loud noise (n = 13; 52%).

Table C8 shows the number of employees who responded "yes" to the psychosocial items. Overall, most cultivation and harvesting employees reported positive perceptions of psychosocial factors at work. Some areas that may need improvement among these employees are related to the responses to "is your work made more difficult due to other people not doing their job properly?" (n = 19; 79%); "do you regularly work under short deadlines?" (n = 12; 48%); "is your work made more difficult by other people being absent?" (n = 9; 36%); and "do you have a lot of say or get to make many decisions as part of your job?" (n = 9; 36%).

Overall, most trimming employees reported positive perceptions of psychosocial factors at work. Some areas that may need improvement among these employees are related to the responses to "is your work made more difficult due to other people not doing their job properly?" (n = 19; 76%); "is your work well organized?" (n = 14; 56%); "do you have a lot of say or get to make many decisions as part of your job?" (n = 8; 32%); "do you believe you were trained well for your job?" (n = 16; 64%); and "do you have enough variation in your work?" (n = 16; 64%).

Job Stress

The average job stress score for cultivation and harvesting employees was 2.6 (range: 0–7, n = 25), indicating low job stress overall. On the basis of individual stress scores, 16 (64%) employees indicated low job stress, 8 (32%) indicated moderate job stress, and one (4%) indicated high job stress. Eighteen (72%) provided an open-ended response about major sources of job stress. The most frequently reported sources of job stress were the growth of the company (n = 4; 16%); increased responsibilities (n = 4; 16%); and being concerned about the plants (n = 3; 12%). Other stressors were reported by two or fewer employees and are not described to maintain employee confidentiality.

The average job stress score for trimming employees was 3.1 (range: 0–7; n = 25), indicating low job stress overall. On the basis of individual stress scores, 13 (54%) employees indicated low job stress, 9 (38%) indicated moderate job stress, and 2 (8%) indicated high job stress. Twenty-two (88%) provided an open-ended response about major sources of job stress. The most frequently reported sources of job stress were changes in procedures (n =10; 40%); communication issues (n = 7; 28%); perceived poor product quality (n = 4; 16%); lack of proper equipment (n = 4; 16%); working with inexperienced coworkers (n = 3; 12%); and perceived lack of trust from the company (n = 3; 12%).

Other stressors were reported by two or fewer employees and are not described to maintain employee confidentiality.

Discussion

Exposures to airborne endotoxin come from soil- and plant-disturbing activities. During our evaluation we observed employees dry sweeping after a harvest, rapidly moving soil into pots when repotting, and bending over the pool of soil as they used their hands and forearms to move soil while repotting.

All of these activities, in addition to trimming, removing leaves, and harvesting, will increase the chance of exposure to airborne endotoxin. When disturbed soil or plants can release endotoxin-containing bacteria into the air. Some potential opportunities to reduce endotoxin exposures would be to eliminate or minimize dry sweeping and reduce soil disturbance when repotting plants.

The airborne endotoxin concentrations at the facility were similar to those found at an indoor flower greenhouse (range: 0.84–1,100 EU/m3) but much lower than those found in other agricultural settings. These settings include two indoor herb processing plants (median endotoxin concentration: 3 × 105 EU/m3); four peppermint and nine chamomile herb farm indoor processing operations (median for endotoxin peppermint farms: 1 × 106 EU/m3; median endotoxin for chamomile farms: 1.8 × 104 EU/m3); and an indoor hemp processing plant (mean endotoxin concentration: 1.9 × 104 EU/m3) [Dutkiewicz et al. 2001; Fishwick et al. 2001; Skórska et al. 2005; Thilsing et al. 2015].

The main way cannabinoids are differentiated is by the degree of their psychoactivity. Δ9-THCA, CBD, and CBN are not psychoactive substances, meaning they do not change a person's mental state by affecting the way the brain and nervous system work. Δ9-THC is the psychoactive component of cannabis. The long-term health effects of occupational exposures are currently unknown. The differences between occupational exposures to psychoactive cannabinoids and non-psychoactive cannabinoids are also unknown.

We detected cannabinoids on both production and nonproduction surfaces, though nonproduction surfaces had lesser concentrations detected. Cannabinoids are expected to be found in production areas. Detecting cannabinoids in nonproduction areas indicates that cleaning and hand hygiene could be improved to prevent contaminating nonproduction areas when leaving production areas. While collecting surface wipe samples, efforts were made to ensure that the majority of samples were adjacent. However, because of presumed unequal distribution of cannabinoids across surfaces, even when directly adjacent, we cannot directly compare results between the two methods. Δ9-THCA concentrations were higher than Δ9-THC concentrations in all surface wipe samples except for one sample collected on the surface of a table in the lobby of the building. A previous NIOSH HHE report suggested that in cannabis cultivation workplaces, Δ9-THCA concentrations would be present in higher concentrations than Δ9-THC concentrations because the Δ9-THCA would not have been decarboxylated through heat or aging [NIOSH 2017]. This facility was focused on the cultivation, harvest, and trimming of cannabis and not on further processing, so these surface wipe results are consistent with other evaluations in similar workplaces.

The most abundant fungal species detected at the trim room table was Golovinomyces spadiceus on Sides A and B of the facility. G. spadiceus is a plant pathogen that causes powdery mildew on several plants, such as okra [Moparthi et al. 2018], goldenstar [Trigiano et al. 2017], Coreopisis 'Full Moon' [Dugan 2013], and wild sunflowers [Félix-Gastélum et al. 2019]. G. spadiceus, along with other Golovinomyces species such as G. cichoracearum, have also been known to cause powdery mildew on Cannabis sativa plants [Pépin et al. 2018; Punja et al. 2019; Szarka et al. 2019]. In addition, Pencillium olsonii, which was among the penicillium species detected in area samples, has also been shown to cause bud rot on C. sativa [Punja et al. 2019]. Golovinomyces species were detected in previous Cannabis grow facilities, although not as abundantly as was detected in the current facility, along with other plant pathogens like Botrytis cinerea that belong to the same Leotiomycetes class [Green et al. 2018]. The health effects following exposure to Golovinomyces species have not been studied.

Our results from particulate monitoring indicate that there are dust exposures during trimming and harvesting activities, but there are no specific OELs that can be used to evaluate these exposures. OELs exist for general dust, but those limits are intended for nuisance dust that is known to not contain harmful components. Additionally, area samples cannot be compared to OELs since OELs are based on personal exposure levels. In this evaluation, we sampled areas where we expected work processes may produce particulates, and we were able to confirm that this was the case. The particulates produced during these tasks are likely a major mechanism by which endotoxin and cannabinoids are released when soil and plant matter is disturbed.

Area noise measurements indicated that at times the sound levels we measured reached levels approaching the NIOSH REL and OSHA AL levels of 85 dBA. If noise levels increased in these work areas the possibility of noise overexposure would likewise increase. We found that noise levels were greater near the ventilation units and in areas where loud music was playing. If an employee works in one of these areas and is also wearing headphones to listen to music during work, the noise exposures from those headphones could exceed exposure limits because the volume of the headphones would likely need to be raised to compete with the external noise. Further, our measurements were short-term, area measurements and cannot accurately capture individual exposures. Our goal was to characterize noise levels across these work areas and identify whether there was potential for overexposure to noise.

Many of the tasks we observed included repetitive motion and awkward postures. When repotting plants employees were observed to be bending over the pool of soil to add soil to the pots. Employees then added a plant and more soil to completely fill the pot before moving it to the floor and beginning the process again. Additionally, when removing leaves, employees needed to bend over to reach those on the lower parts of the plants, increasing the risk for lower back injury. Our observations and findings indicate that the trimming employees have exposures to highly repetitive work, most notably during hand trimming activities. These exposures increase their risk of musculoskeletal disorders. The trimming area also does not have adjustable tables or chairs, further increasing the risk for musculoskeletal disorders.

The confidential medical interview results provide a "snapshot" of employee safety and health concerns during our evaluation. It is important to communicate and receive input about work and well-being from employees on a regular basis, especially during times of change or company growth when policies and procedures may be in fluctuation. Assessing, understanding, and monitoring employee well-being and work concerns can help employees and employers work together to design work and employment conditions in a way that will prioritize safety and improve physical and psychological outcomes.

Additional information on policies, programs, and practices that integrate protection from work-related safety and health hazards with promotion of injury and illness-prevention efforts to advance worker well-being can be found through the NIOSH Total Worker Health™ program at www.cdc.gov/niosh/twh.

Limitations

This evaluation was subject to several limitations. Industrial hygiene sampling could only document exposures and conditions in the locations evaluated and on the days which the evaluation occurred. These results may not have been representative of conditions during other days. Medical interviews were also subject to similar limitations. We were only able to document concerns and symptoms that were reported to us during our evaluations by current employees who chose to participate. We were not able to include information from employees who had left the workforce or were not present at the facility at the time of the evaluation. Interviews may have been impacted by selection, recall, and social desirability biases.

Conclusion

Employees were concerned about potential exposures to ozone, bright lights, and pesticides, among others. Our air sampling found that employees were exposed to endotoxins. We also found that trimming employees have exposure to highly repetitive work that increases their risk for musculoskeletal disorders. We recommended that the workplace reduce exposures to endotoxins, cannabinoids, ozone, light, and noise. We also recommended that they reduce the risk of musculoskeletal disorders and obtain regular input from employees about workplace safety, health, and well-being issues.

Section C: Tables

Table C1. Personal air sample results for endotoxin exposures

Job title	**Sample duration (minutes)**	**Endotoxin concentration (EU/m^3)**	**Exceeds occupational exposure limit?**
Side A			
Cultivator 1	333	220	Yes
Cultivator 2	347	56	No
Cultivator 3	355	85	No
Cultivator 4	329	6	No
Cultivator 5	333	980	Yes
Cultivator 6	365	110	Yes
Cultivator 7	331	430	Yes
Cultivator 8	329	12	No
Cultivator 9	339	16	No
Cultivator 10	39*	17	No
Side B			
Cultivator 11	341	140	Yes
Cultivator 12	333	61	No
Cultivator 13	335	63	No
Cultivator 14	336	11	No
Cultivator 15	339	120	Yes
Cultivator 16	328	150	Yes
Cultivator 17	335	660	Yes
Cultivator 18	340	16	No
Cultivator 19	61*	46	No
Cultivator 20	343	78	No
DECOS limit		90	

*These employees left work early.

Table C2. Surface wipe sampling for cannabis compounds (μg/100 cm^2)

Location	Δ9-THC only method		Cannabinoid method*		
	Δ9-THC	Δ9-THC	Δ9-THCA	CBD	CBN
Side A Production area					
Trimming room supervisor desk	56	71	530	ND	[4.2]
Table near harvest activities	3.7	ND	140	[3.4]	8.5
Side B Production area					
Trimming room table	91	110	1,000	[2.9]	17
Table outside of trimming room	18	25	280	[3.2]	[4.2]
Table near repotting activities	1	ND	25	ND	ND
Nonproduction areas					
Table in lobby sitting area	0.035	ND	ND	ND	ND
Breakroom countertop	0.45	ND	15	ND	ND
Breakroom refrigerator handle†	0.93	ND	12	ND	ND

ND = not detected

[ ] = values in brackets are between the limit of detection and limit of quantification. This means there is more uncertainty associated with these values.

*The limit of detection was 2 μg and the limit of quantification was 6.7 μg per sample.

†The disposable 100 cm^2 template could not be used so an estimated 100 cm^2 was sampled.

Table C3. The common fungal species identified in area air samples collected on Side A and Side B of the facility

Species	All area samples		Side A		Side B	
	# Clones	% Total fungi	# Clones	% Total fungi	# Clones	% Total fungi
Golovinomyces spadiceus	41	18.98	38	22.49	3	6.38
Rhodotorula spp.	27	12.50	24	14.20	3	6.38
Penicillium spp.	22	10.19	18	10.65	4	8.51
Cladosporium spp.	14	6.48	8	4.73	6	12.77

Table C4. Detection of fungal clones and *Golovinomyces spadiceus* in various areas of the facility

Area sample	Sample size	Total fungal clones (range)*	*Golovinomyces spadiceus*	
			# Clones (range)*	% Total fungi (range)*
Side A				
Trim room table	2	38.5 (38–39)	19 (17–21)	49.4 (43.6–55.3)
Grow area, close to harvest	1	43	0	0
Grow area, away from harvest	3	11.3 (9–14)	0	0
Harvest check table	1	15	0	0

Area sample	Sample size	Total fungal clones (range)*	*Golovinomyces spadiceus*	
			# Clones (range)*	% Total fungi (range)*
Side B				
Trim room table, weighing product	1	17	3	17.6
Grow area, near repotting	1	8	0	0
Grow area, away from repotting	4	5 (0–8)	0	0
Dry/cure room	1	2	0	0

*Averages (range) are presented for those areas where multiple air samples were collected.

Table C5. Particle monitoring results for three locations (mg/m^3)

Location			Particle size		
	PM1	PM2.5	Respirable	PM10	Total
Side A - Harvest					
Average	0.026	0.027	0.028	0.039	0.061
Minimum	0.012	0.13	0.014	0.016	0.018
Maximum	0.12	0.12	0.15	0.31	0.61
Side A - Trim room					
Average	0.025	0.025	0.027	0.038	0.064
Minimum	0.14	0.014	0.015	0.016	0.016
Maximum	0.12	0.12	0.13	0.22	0.54
Side B - Trim room					
Average	0.03	0.03	0.032	0.043	0.077
Minimum	0.011	0.012	0.012	0.014	0.018
Maximum	0.1	0.11	0.11	0.21	0.53

Table C6. Symptoms believed to be work-related reported by employees over the last 4 weeks

Symptom	Cultivation/harvesting employees (n = 25) Frequency (%)	Trimming employees (n = 25) Frequency (%)
Stuffy nose or sinus problems	10 (40)	18 (72)
Runny nose	9 (36)	12 (48)
Back pain	9 (36)	15 (60)
Rash on skin	7 (28)	8 (32)
Red or irritated eyes	6 (24)	9 (36)
Difficulty hearing	6 (24)	6 (25)*
Fatigue	5 (20)	7 (28)
Hand or wrist pain	5 (20)	11 (44)
Hives	5 (20)	2 (8)

Table 6. (Continued)

Symptom	Cultivation/harvesting employees (n = 25) Frequency (%)	Trimming employees (n = 25) Frequency (%)
Shoulder pain	5 (20)	8 (32)
Leg pain	4 (16)	4 (16)
Foot pain	4 (16)	4 (16)
Lightheadedness	4 (16)	9 (36)
Respiratory problems	4 (16)	8 (32)
Anxiety	3 (12)	8 (32)
Chest tightness	3 (12)	3 (13)*
Shortness of breath	3 (12)	3 (12)
Headaches	3 (12)	13 (52)
Changes in appetite	1 (4)	1 (4)
Sore throat	1 (4)	7 (28)
Frequent changes in mood	1 (4)	2 (8)*
Difficulty concentrating	0 (0)	2 (8)
Depression	0 (0)	4 (16)
Difficulty sleeping	0 (0)	3 (12)
Unexplained fevers	0 (0)	0 (0)

*N = 24 (due to lack of response).

Table C7. Frequency of affirmative responses to physical working conditions items during confidential medical interviews

Working conditions items	Cultivation/harvesting employees (n = 25) Frequency (%)	Trimming employees (n = 25) Frequency (%)
During your work, are you made uncomfortable by:		
Bright light	18 (72)	10 (40)
Dust/dirt?	17 (68)	16 (64)
Heat?	12 (48)	7 (28)
Changes in temperature?	9 (36)	8 (32)
Loud noise?	9 (36)	13 (52)
Bending down regularly?	9 (36)	5 (20)
Stagnant water?	9 (36)	4 (16)
Dry air?	9 (36)	10 (40)
Damp air?	8 (32)	2 (8)
Lack of fresh air?	8 (32)	15 (60)
Lengthy periods of being in the same physical position?	7 (28)	14 (56)
Lengthy periods of performing repetitive motions?	6 (24)	10 (40)
Pests?	6 (24)	9 (36)
Lengthy standing?	5 (20)	9 (36)

Working conditions items	Cultivation/harvesting employees (n = 25) Frequency (%)	Trimming employees (n = 25) Frequency (%)
Lifting/carrying items?	4 (16)	2 (8)
Bad smells/odors?	3 (12)	13 (52)
Lengthy sitting?	1 (4)	9 (36)
Reaching up regularly	1 (4)*	2 (8)
Cold	1 (4)	10 (40)

*N = 24 (due to lack of response).

Table C8. Employee responses to psychosocial items during confidential medical interviews

Psychosocial item	Cultivation/harvesting employees (n = 25) frequency of "yes" responses (%)	Trimming employees (n = 25) frequency of "yes" responses (%)
Do your supervisors listen to what you have to say?	25 (100)	19 (76)
Do you need to spend a lot of time being alert at work?	24 (96)	14 (56)
Do you feel free to report health or safety concerns at work?	24 (96)	19 (76)
Can you take a break if you need to?	24 (96)	18 (72)
Is it clear to you what your responsibilities are at work?	24 (96)	24 (96)
Do you normally enjoy your work?	24 (96)	24 (96)
Do you have enough variation in your work?	24 (96)	16 (64)
Do you believe you were trained well for your job?	24 (96)	16 (64)
Are you well-informed about the goals and results of your work?	23 (92)	20 (80)
Does your employer encourage you to stay home if you are ill?	22 (88)	23 (92)
Can you usually manage to take a day off easily?	21 (88)*	21 (84)
Is your work usually well organized?	21 (84)	14 (56)
Is your work highly physical?	20 (80)	3 (12)
Is your work made more difficult due to other people not doing their job properly?†	19 (79)*	19 (76)
Does this work offer you sufficient job security?	19 (79)*	17 (71)*
Do you always have the tools necessary to complete your work?	19 (76)	20 (80)
Do you trust your employer to look out for your well-being?	19 (76)	19 (76)
Does your work require a lot of thinking?	15 (60)	2 (8)
Do you regularly work under short deadlines?†	12 (48)	8 (32)
Is your work made more difficult due to other people being absent?†	9 (36)	8 (32)
Do you have a lot of say or get to make many decisions as part of your job?	9 (36)	8 (32)

Table C8. (Continued)

Psychosocial item	Cultivation/harvesting employees (n = 25) frequency of "yes" responses (%)	Trimming employees (n = 25) frequency of "yes" responses (%)
Do you often have to do something which isn't part of your job description?†	5 (20)	10 (40)
Does your work interfere with your private or family life?†	4 (16)	1 (4)
Do you have poor relations with any of your coworkers?†	1 (4)	2 (8)
Do you have poor relations with any of your supervisors?†	0 (0)	4 (16)

*N = 24 (due to lack of response).
†Item has negative connotation.

Section D: Occupational Exposure Limits

NIOSH investigators refer to mandatory (legally enforceable) and recommended OELs for chemical, physical, and biological agents when evaluating workplace hazards. OELs have been developed by federal agencies and safety and health organizations to prevent adverse health effects from workplace exposures. Generally, OELs suggest levels of exposure that most employees may be exposed to for up to 10 hours per day, 40 hours per week, for a working lifetime, without experiencing adverse health effects.

However, not all employees will be protected if their exposures are maintained below these levels. Some may have adverse health effects because of individual susceptibility, a preexisting medical condition, or a hypersensitivity (allergy). In addition, some hazardous substances act in combination with other exposures, with the general environment, or with medications or personal habits of the employee to produce adverse health effects. Most OELs address airborne exposures, but some substances can be absorbed directly through the skin and mucous membranes.

Most OELs are expressed as a time-weighted average (TWA) exposure. A TWA refers to the average exposure during a normal 8- to 10-hour workday. Some chemical substances and physical agents have recommended short-term exposure limits (STEL) or ceiling values. Unless otherwise noted, the STEL is a 15-minute TWA exposure. It should not be exceeded at any time during a workday. The ceiling limit should not be exceeded at any time.

In the United States, OELs have been established by federal agencies, professional organizations, state and local governments, and other entities. Some OELs are legally enforceable limits; others are recommendations.

- OSHA, an agency of the U.S. Department of Labor, publishes PELs [29 CFR 1910 for general industry; 29 CFR 1926 for construction industry; and 29 CFR 1917 for maritime industry]. These legal limits are enforceable in workplaces covered under the Occupational Safety and Health Act of 1970.
- NIOSH RELs are recommendations based on a critical review of the scientific and technical information and the adequacy of methods to identify and control the hazard. NIOSH RELs are published in the *NIOSH Pocket Guide to Chemical Hazards* [NIOSH 2007]. NIOSH also recommends risk management practices (e.g., engineering controls, safe work practices, employee education/training, PPE, and exposure and medical monitoring) to minimize the risk of exposure and adverse health effects.
- Another set of OELs commonly used and cited in the United States include the threshold limit values or TLVs, which are recommended by the American Conference of Governmental Industrial Hygienists (ACGIH®). The ACGIH TLVs are developed by committee members of this professional organization from a review of the published, peer-reviewed literature. TLVs are not consensus standards. They are considered voluntary exposure guidelines for use by industrial hygienists and others trained in this discipline "to assist in the control of health hazards" [ACGIH 2021].

Outside the United States, OELs have been established by various agencies and organizations and include legal and recommended limits. The Institut für Arbeitsschutz der Deutschen Gesetzlichen Unfallversicherung (Institute for Occupational Safety and Health of the German Social Accident Insurance) maintains a database of international OELs from European Union member states, Canada (Québec), Japan, Switzerland, and the United States. The database, available at https://www.dguv.de/ifa/gestis/gestis-stoffdatenbank/index-2.jsp, contains international limits for more than 2,000 hazardous substances and is updated periodically.

OSHA (Public Law 91-596) requires an employer to furnish employees a place of employment free from recognized hazards that cause or are likely to cause death or serious physical harm. This is true in the absence of a specific OEL. It also is important to keep in mind that OELs may not reflect current health-based information.

When multiple OELs exist for a substance or agent, NIOSH investigators generally encourage employers to use the lowest OEL when making risk assessment and risk management decisions.

Endotoxin

Endotoxins are found throughout the agricultural environment. Endotoxins are located in the cell wall of Gram-negative bacteria and are released when the bacterial cell is lysed (broken down) or when it is multiplying. In experimental studies, human volunteers exposed via inhalation to high levels of endotoxin experienced airway and alveolar inflammation as well as chest tightness, fever, and malaise, and have an acute reduction in lung function, as measured by the forced expiratory volume in one second [Castellan 1995]. Airborne endotoxin exposures between 45 and 400 EU/m3 have been associated with acute airflow obstruction, mucous membrane irritation, chest tightness, cough, shortness of breath, fever, and wheezing [Thorne and Duchaine 2007]. Chronic health effects that have been associated with airborne endotoxin exposures include asthma, chronic bronchitis, bronchial hyperreactivity, chronic airway obstruction, hypersensitivity pneumonitis, and organic dust toxic syndrome [Duquenne et al. 2013; Rylander 2006]. Some studies suggest that high environmental and occupational endotoxin exposures may protect exposed individuals from developing atopic sensitization [Rylander 2006]. Rylander and Jacobs [1997] have suggested an occupational threshold concentration for endotoxin equivalent to 100 EU/m3 of air to prevent airway inflammation.

No accepted OELs for endotoxins have been developed in the United States because of the variability of sampling and analytical methods, and because of a lack of data showing a consistent dose-response relationship [AIHA 2005; Duquenne et al. 2013]. In 2010, DECOS recommended a health-based OEL for airborne endotoxin of 90 EU/m3 as an 8-hour TWA [DECOS 2010].

Δ9-THC

Δ9-THC is the psychoactive component of cannabis. There is no OEL for Δ9-THC. Occupational exposures to cannabinoids are thought to be mostly through skin absorption and ingestion. The long- term health effects of these occupational exposure routes are currently unknown. Past Δ9-THC and health effects research has focused primarily on inhalation in nonoccupational settings. Short term effects may include cannabis intoxication, which is characterized by symptoms such as impaired motor coordination, euphoria, anxiety, sensation of slowed time, impaired judgement, social withdrawal [American Psychiatric Association 2013]. These symptoms occur during or within 2 hours of cannabis use [American Psychiatric Association 2013]. The National Institute on Drug Abuse [2016] also characterizes mood changes, diminished memory, and disorientation as short-term health effects of an effective dose of cannabis. Some studies have associated chronic exposure to firsthand cannabis smoke with social anxiety disorder, depressive disorders, psychosis, and respiratory symptoms [National Academies of Sciences, Engineering, and Medicine 2017].

The adverse health effects associated with nonmedicinal and chronic consumption of Δ9-THC derived from C. sativa and Cannabis indica have been extensively studied and reviewed [Hall and Degenhardt 2014; Volkow et al. 2014]. In contrast, the short-term and long-term health effects of occupational exposure to Cannabis species material are not well described in the literature.

Δ9-THCA, CBD, and CBN

Δ9-THCA, CBD, and CBN are several other of more than 60 cannabinoids found in small quantities in cannabis. These are not psychoactive substances, meaning they do not change a person's mental state by affecting the way the brain and nervous system work. Unlike Δ9-THC, these cannabinoids do not cause intoxication or a "high." There are currently no OELs for Δ9-THCA, CBD, or CBN.

Hemp

Hemp, also derived from Cannabis sativa, is used for a variety of purposes including fiber, rope, paper composites, food, and oil and oil-based products [United States Department of Agriculture 2000].

Occupational hemp exposure can result in a variety of clinical symptoms including sinusitis, byssinosis, and reductions in lung function [Zuskin et al. 1990; Zuskin et al. 1992; Zuskin et al. 1994]. Employees who directly handle the plant are particularly at risk [Barbero and Flores 1967; Valić et al. 1968; Zuskin et al. 1990; Zuskin et al. 1994]. There is no OEL for hemp. Transdermal applications of medicinal cannabis demonstrate that occupational dermal absorption is a potential exposure route [Goldsmith et al. 2015]. Other studies have demonstrated dermal reactions such as an urticarial rash (hives) in subjects who directly contact cannabis [Basharat et al. 2011; Ozyurt et al. 2014]. Urticaria has also occurred in forensic specialists and law enforcement officers following the handling of cannabis [Herzinger et al.

2011; Majmudar et al. 2006; Mayoral et al. 2008; Williams et al. 2008]. Several of these plant components have recently been shown to produce high molecular weight proteins that can result in the allergic sensitization following personal exposure [Nayak et al. 2013].

Ozone

Ozone is a colorless to blue gas with a pungent odor. Exposure to ozone may cause headaches, coughing, dry throat, shortness of breath, a heavy feeling in chest, and fluid in the lungs. Higher levels of exposure can lead to more severe symptoms. Chronic exposure may lead to asthma. Workers may be harmed from exposure to ozone. The level of exposure depends upon the dose, duration, and work being done [NIOSH 2019]. The NIOSH REL for ozone is 0.1 ppm and is to be evaluated as a ceiling limit, and the current OSHA PEL for ozone is 0.1 ppm [NIOSH 2007]. The current ACGIH TLV is based on the amount of physical exertion or work load required for the job and is to be averaged over an 8–hour period. The TLV is 0.1 ppm for jobs requiring light physical exertion, 0.08 ppm for moderate physical exertion, 0.05 ppm for heavy physical exertion. A separate TLV for ozone is 0.2 ppm for heavy, moderate, or light work loads less than or equal to 2 hours in duration [ACGIH 2021].

Noise

Noise-induced heating loss (NIHL) is an irreversible condition that progresses with noise exposure. It is caused by damage to the nerve cells of the inner ear and, unlike some other types of hearing disorders, cannot be treated medically [Berger et al. 2003]. More than 22 million U.S. workers are estimated to be exposed to workplace noise levels above 85 dBA [Tak et al. 2009]. NIOSH estimates that workers exposed to an average daily noise level of 85 dBA over a 40-year working lifetime have an 8% excess risk of material hearing impairment. This excess risk increases to 25% for an average daily noise exposure of 90 dBA [NIOSH 1998]. NIOSH defines material hearing impairment as an average of the hearing threshold levels for both ears that exceeds 25 dB at frequencies of 1,000 Hz; 2,000 Hz; 3,000 Hz; and 4,000 Hz.

Although hearing ability commonly declines with age, exposure to excessive noise can increase the rate of hearing loss. In most cases, NIHL develops slowly from repeated exposure to noise over time, but the progression of hearing loss is typically the greatest during the first several years of noise exposure. NIHL can also result from short-duration exposures to high noise levels or even from a single exposure to an impulse noise or a continuous noise, depending on the intensity of the noise and the individual's susceptibility to NIHL [Berger et al. 2003]. Noise-exposed workers can develop substantial NIHL before it is clearly recognized. Even mild hearing losses can impair a person's ability to understand speech and hear many important sounds. In addition, some people with NIHL also develop tinnitus.

Tinnitus is a condition in which a person perceives sound in one or both ears, but no external sound is present. Persons with tinnitus often describe hearing ringing, hissing, buzzing, whistling, clicking, or chirping like crickets. Tinnitus can be intermittent or continuous and the perceived volume can range from soft to loud. Currently, there is no cure for tinnitus.

The preferred unit for reporting noise measurements is dBA. A-weighting is used because it approximates the "equal loudness perception characteristics of human hearing for pure tones relative to a reference of 40 dB at a frequency of 1,000 Hz" and is considered to provide a better estimation of hearing loss risk than using unweighted or other weighting measurements [Berger et al. 2003].

Employees exposed to noise should have baseline and yearly hearing tests to evaluate their hearing thresholds and determine whether their hearing has changed over time. Hearing testing should be done in a quiet location, such as an audiometric test booth, where background noise does not interfere with accurate measurement of hearing thresholds. In workplace hearing conservation programs, hearing thresholds must be measured at 500 Hz; 1,000 Hz; 2,000 Hz; 3,000 Hz; 4,000 Hz; and 6,000 Hz. Additionally, NIOSH recommends testing at 8,000 Hz [NIOSH 1998].

The OSHA hearing conservation standard requires analysis of changes from baseline hearing thresholds to determine if the changes are substantial enough to meet OSHA criteria for a standard threshold shift (STS). OSHA defines an STS as a change in hearing threshold (relative to the baseline hearing test) of an average of 10 dB or more at 2,000 Hz; 3,000 Hz; and 4,000 Hz in either ear [29 CFR 1910.95]. If an STS occurs, the company must determine if the hearing loss also meets the requirements to be recorded on the OSHA Form 300 Log of Work-Related Injuries and Illnesses [29 CFR 1904.1]. In contrast to OSHA, NIOSH defines an STS as a change in the hearing threshold level of 15 dB or more (relative to the baseline hearing test) at any test frequency in either ear measured twice in succession [NIOSH 1998].

The NIOSH REL for noise is 85 dBA as an 8-hour TWA. For calculating exposure limits, NIOSH uses a 3-dB time/intensity trading relationship, or exchange rate. Using the NIOSH criterion, an employee can be exposed to 88 dBA for no more than 4 hours, 91 dBA for 2 hours, 94 dBA for 1 hour, 97 dBA for 0.5 hours, etc. Exposure to impulsive noise should never exceed 140 dBA. For extended work shifts, NIOSH adjusts the REL to 84.5 dBA for a 9-hour shift, 84.0 dBA for a 10-hour shift, 83.6 dBA for an 11-hour shift, and 83.2 dBA for a 12-hour work shift. NIOSH recommends the use of hearing protection and the implementation of a hearing loss prevention program when noise exposures exceed the REL [NIOSH 1998].

The OSHA noise standard specifies a PEL of 90 dBA and an AL of 85 dBA, both as 8-hour TWAs. OSHA uses a less conservative 5-dB exchange rate for calculating the PEL and AL. Using the OSHA criterion, an employee may be exposed to noise levels of 95 dBA for no more than 4 hours, 100 dBA for 2 hours, 105 dBA for 1 hour, 110 dBA for 0.5 hours, etc. Exposure to impulsive or impact noise must not exceed 140 dB peak noise level. OSHA does not adjust the PEL for extended work shifts. However, the AL is adjusted to 84.1 dBA for a 9-hour shift, 83.4 dBA for a 10-hour shift, 82.7 dBA for an 11-hour shift, and 82.1 dBA for a 12-hour work shift. OSHA requires implementation of a hearing conservation program when noise exposures exceed the AL [29 CFR 1910.95].

Section E: References

Background

Barcott B, Whitney B, Bailey J [2021]. Leafly Jobs Report 2021. Seattle, WA: Leafly Holdings, Inc., https://leafly-cms-production.imgix.net/wp-content/uploads/2021/02/13180206/Leafly-JobsReport- 2021-v14.pdf.

NIOSH [2017]. Evaluation of potential hazards during harvesting and processing cannabis at an outdoor organic farm. By Couch J, Victory K, Lowe B, Burton N, Green B, Nayak A, Lemons A, Beezhold D. Cincinnati, OH: U.S. Department of Health and Human Services, Centers for Disease Control and Prevention, National Institute for Occupational Safety and Health, Health Hazard Evaluation Report 2015-0111-3271, http://www.cdc.gov/niosh/hhe/reports/pdfs/2015-0111- 3271.pdf.

NIOSH [2019]. Evaluation of a medicinal cannabis manufacturing facility with an indoor and outdoor grow operation. By Couch J, Wiegand D, Grimes GR, Green BJ, Lemons AR, Glassford E, Zwack L, Jackson SR, Beezhold D. Cincinnati, OH: U.S. Department of Health and Human Services, Centers for Disease Control and Prevention, National Institute for Occupational Safety and Health, Health Hazard Evaluation Report 2016-0090-3317, https://www.cdc.gov/niosh/hhe/reports/pdfs/2016-0090-3317revised082019.pdf.

Confidential Medical Interviews

Clark MM, Warren BA, Hagen PT, Johnson BD, Jenkins SM, Werneburg BL, Olsen KD [2011]. Stress level, health behaviors, and quality of life in employees joining a wellness center. *Am. J. Health Promot.* *26*(1):21–25, http://doi.org/10.4278/ajhp.090821-QUAN-272.

Weel ANH, Fortuin RJ [1998]. Design and trial of a new questionnaire for occupational health surveys in companies. *Occup. Med.* *48*(8):511–518, https://doi.org/ 10.1093/occmed/48.8.511.

Discussion

Dugan FM [2013]. Golovinomyces spadiceus causing powdery mildew on Coreopsis hybrid 'Full Moon' (Heliantheae, Asteraceae) in Washington State. *N. Am. Fungi* 8:1–3, https://doi.org/10.2509/naf2013.008.001.

Dutkiewicz J, Krysińska-Traczyk E, Skórska C, Sitkowska J, Prazmo Z, Golec M [2001]. Exposure to airborne microorganisms and endotoxin in herb processing plants. *Ann. Agric. Environ. Med.* 8(2):201– 211.

Félix-Gastélum R, Olivas-Peraza DD, Quiroz-Figueroa FR, Leyva-Madrigal KY, Peñuelas-Rubio O, Espinosa-Matías S, Maldonado-Mendoza IE [2019]. Powdery mildew caused by Golovinomyces spadiceus on wild sunflower in Sinaloa, Mexico. Can J Plant Pathol 41(2):301–309, https://doi.org/10.1080/07060661.2019.1577916.

Fishwick D, Allan LJ, Wright A, Curran AD [2001]. Assessment of exposure to organic dust in a hemp processing plant. *Ann. Occup. Hyg.* 45(7):577–583, http://doi.org/10.1093/annhyg/45.7.577.

Green BJ, Couch J, Lemons AR, Burton N, Victory KR, Nayak AP, Beezhold DH [2018]. Microbial hazards during harvesting and processing at an outdoor United States cannabis farm. *J. Occup. Environ. Hyg.* 15(5):430–440, https://doi.org/10.1080/15459624.2018.1432863.

Moparthi S, Bradshaw M, Frost K, Hamm PB, Buck JW [2018]. First report of powdery mildew caused by Golovinomyces spadiceus on okra in the United States. Plant Dis 102(8):1664, https://doi.org/10.1094/PDIS-01-18-0179-PDN.

NIOSH [2017]. Evaluation of potential hazards during harvesting and processing cannabis at an outdoor organic farm. By Couch J, Victory K, Lowe B, Burton N, Green B, Nayak A, Lemons A, Beezhold D. Cincinnati, OH: U.S. Department of Health and Human Services, Centers for Disease Control and Prevention, National Institute for Occupational Safety and Health, Health Hazard Evaluation Report 2015-0111-3271, http://www.cdc.gov/niosh/hhe/reports/pdfs/2015-0111- 3271.pdf.

Pépin N, Punja ZK, Joly DL [2018]. Occurrence of powdery mildew caused by Golovinomyces cichoracearum sensu lato on Cannabis sativa in Canada. *Plant Disease* 102(12):2664, https://doi.org/10.1094/PDIS-04-18-0586-PDN.

Punja ZK, Collyer D, Scott C, Lung S, Holmes J, Sutton D [2019]. Pathogens and molds affecting production and quality of Cannabis sativa L. *Front Plant. Sci.* 10(1120):1–23, https://doi.org/10.3389/fpls.2019.01120.

Skórska C, Sitkowska J, Krysińska-Traczyk E, Cholewa G, Dutkiewicz J [2005]. Exposure to airborne microorganisms, dust and endotoxin during processing of peppermint and chamomile herbs on farms. *Ann. Agric. Environ. Med.* 12(2):281–288.

Szarka D, Tymon L, Amsden B, Dixon E, Judy J, Gauthier N [2019]. First report of powdery mildew caused by Golovinomyces spadiceus on industrial hemp (Cannabis sativa) in Kentucky. *Plant Dis.* 103(7):1773, https://doi.org/10.1094/PDIS-01-19-0049-PDN.

Thilsing T, Madsen AM, Basinas I, Schlünssen V, Tendal K, Bælum J [2015]. Dust, endotoxin, fungi, and bacteria exposure as determined by work task, season, and type of plant in a flower greenhouse. *Ann. Occup. Hyg.* 59(2):142–157, http://doi.org/10.1093/annhyg/meu090.

Trigiano RN, Boggess SL, Bernard EC [2017]. First report of powdery mildew caused by Golovinomyces spadiceus on green and gold (Chrysogonum virginianum) in the United States. *Plant Dis.* 102(1):252, https://doi.org/10.1094/PDIS-08-17-1292-PDN.

Exposure Assessment

Ambach L, Penitschka F, Broillet A, Konig S, Weinmann W, Bernhard W [2014]. Simultaneous quantification of delta-9-THC, THC-acid A, CBN, and CBD in seized drugs using HPLC-DAD. *Forensic Sci. Int. 243*(Suppl C):107–111, https://doi.org/10.1016/j.forsciint.2014.06.008.

DECOS [2010]. Endotoxins: health-based recommended occupational exposure limit. The Hague, Netherlands: Health Council of The Netherlands, Dutch Expert Committee on Occupational Standards, Publication no. 2010/04OSH, https://www.healthcouncil.nl/documents/advisory-reports/2010/07/15/endotoxins-health-based-recommended-occupational-exposure-limit.

Green BJ, Lemons AR, Park Y, Cox-Ganser JM, Park JH [2017]. Assessment of fungal diversity in a water-damaged office building. *J. Occup. Environ. Hyg. 14*(4):285–293, https://doi.org/10.1080/15459624.2016.1252044.

Green BJ, Couch J, Lemons AR, Burton N, Victory KR, Nayak AP, Beezhold DH [2018]. Microbial hazards during harvesting and processing at an organic U.S. cannabis farm. J Occup Environ Hyg *15*(5):430–440, https://doi.org/10.1080/15459624. 2018. 1432863.

Noise

Berger EH, Royster LH, Royster JD, Driscoll DP, Layne M, eds. [2003]. The noise manual. 5th rev. ed. Fairfax, VA: American Industrial Hygiene Association.

NIOSH [1998]. Criteria for a recommended standard: occupational noise exposure (revised criteria 1998). Cincinnati, OH: U.S. Department of Health and Human Services, Centers for Disease Control and Prevention, National Institute for Occupational Safety and Health, DHHS (NIOSH) Publication No. 98-126, http://www.cdc.gov/niosh/docs/98-126/pdfs/98-126.pdf.

Tak S, Davis RR, Calvert GM [2009]. Exposure to hazardous workplace noise and use of hearing protection devices among U.S. workers—NHANES, 1999–2004. *Am. J. Ind. Med. 52*(5):358–371, http://doi.org/10.1002/ajim.20690.

Occupational Exposure Limits

ACGIH [2021]. 2021 TLVs® and BEIs®: threshold limit values for chemical substances and physical agents and biological exposure indices. Cincinnati, OH: American Conference of Governmental Industrial Hygienists.

AIHA [2005]. Field guide for the determination of biological contaminants in environmental samples. 2nd ed. Falls Church, Virginia: American Industrial Hygiene Association.

American Psychiatric Association [2013]. Diagnostic and statistical manual of mental disorders. 5th ed. Arlington, VA: American Psychiatric Association.

Barbero A, Flores R [1967]. Dust disease in hemp workers. *Arch. Environ. Health 14*(4):529–532, https://doi.org/10.1080/00039896.1967.10664789.

Basharat P, Sussman G, Beezhold D, Leader N [2011]. Hypersensitivity reactions to marijuana. J Allergy Clin Immunol 127(2):AB178, .http://doi.org/10.1016/j.jaci.2010.12.707.

Castellan RM [1995]. Respiratory health effects of inhaled endotoxins: byssinosis and beyond. In: McDuffie H, Dosman J, Semchuk K, Olenchock S, eds. Agricultural health and safety—workplace, environment, sustainability. Boca Raton, FL: CRC Press, pp. 97–100.

CFR [2021]. Code of Federal Regulations. Washington, DC: U.S. Government Printing Office, Office of the Federal Register.

DECOS [2010]. Endotoxins: health-based recommended occupational exposure limit. The Hague, Netherlands: Health Council of The Netherlands, Dutch Expert Committee on Occupational Standards, Publication no. 2010/04OSH, .https://www.healthcouncil.nl/documents/advisory-reports/2010/07/15/endotoxins-health-based-recommended-occupational-exposure-limit.

Duquenne P, Marchand G, Duchaine C [2013]. Measurement of endotoxins in bioaerosols at workplace: a critical review of literature and a standardization issue. *Ann. Occup. Hyg. 57*(2):137–172, http://doi.org/10.1093/annhyg/mes051.

Goldsmith RS, Targino MC, Fanciullo GJ, Martin DW, Hartenbaum NP, White JM, Franklin P [2015]. Medical marijuana in the workplace: challenges and management options for occupational physicians. *J Occup. Environ. Med. 57*(5):518–525, http://doi.org/10.1097/JOM.0000000000000454.

Hall W, Degenhardt L [2014]. The adverse health effects of chronic cannabis use. Drug Test Anal *6*(1– 2):39–45, http://doi.org/10.1002/dta.1506.

Herzinger T, Schöpf P, Przybilla B, Ruëff F [2011]. IgE-mediated hypersensitivity reactions to cannabis in laboratory personnel. *Int. Arch. Allergy Immunol. 156*(4):423–426, http://doi.org/10.1159/000324444.

Majmudar V, Azam NA, Finch T [2006]. Contact urticaria to *Cannabis sativa*. Contact Dermatitis *54*(2):127, http://doi.org/10.1111/j.0105-1873.2006.0560h.x.

Mayoral M, Calderón H, Cano R, Lombardero M [2008]. Allergic rhinoconjunctivitis caused by Cannabis sativa pollen. J Investig Allergol Clin Immunol *18*(1):73–74.

National Academies of Sciences, Engineering, and Medicine [2017]. The health effects of cannabis and cannabinoids: the current state of evidence and recommendations for research. Washington, DC: The National Academies Press; .https://dx.doi.org/10.17226/24625.

National Institute on Drug Abuse [2016]. DrugFacts: marijuana. Rockville, MD: U.S. Department of Health and Human Services, National Institutes of Health, National Institute on Drug Abuse, https://www.drugabuse.gov/publications/drugfacts/marijuana.

Nayak AP, Green BJ, Sussman G, Berlin N, Lata H, Chandra S, ElSohly MA, Hettick JM, Beezhold DH [2013]. Characterization of *Cannabis sativa* allergens. Ann Allergy Asthma Immunol *111*(1):32–37e4, http://doi.org/10.1016/j.anai.2013.04.018.

NIOSH [2007]. NIOSH pocket guide to chemical hazards. Cincinnati, OH: U.S. Department of Health and Human Services, Centers for Disease Control and Prevention, National Institute for Occupational Safety and Health, DHHS (NIOSH) Publication No. 2005-149, http://www.cdc.gov/niosh/npg/.

NIOSH [2019]. Ozone. Cincinnati, OH: U.S. Department of Health and Human Services, Centers for Disease Control and Prevention, National Institute for Occupational Safety and Health, https://www.cdc.gov/niosh/topics/ozone.

Ozyurt S, Muderrisoglu F, Ermete M, Afsar F [2014]. Cannabis-induced erythema multiforme-like recurrent drug eruption. *Int. J. Dermatol.* *53*(1):e22–e23, http://doi.org/10.1111/j.1365- 4632.2011.05318.x.

Rylander R [2006]. Endotoxin and occupational airway disease. *Curr. Opin. Allergy Clin. Immunol.* *6*(1):62–66, http://doi.org/10.1097/01.all.0000202356.83509.f7.

Rylander R, Jacobs RR [1997]. Endotoxin in the environment: a criteria document. *Int. J. Occup. Environ. Health* *3*(1):S1–S48.

Thorne PS, Duchaine C [2007]. Airborne bacteria and endotoxin. In: Hurst CJ, Crawford RL, Garland JL, Lipson DA, Mills AL, Stetzenbach LD, eds. Manual of environmental microbiology. 3rd ed. Washington, DC: American Society for Microbiology Press, pp. 989–1004.

United States Department of Agriculture [2000]. Industrial hemp in the United States: status and market potential. United States Drug Administration, Economic Research Service, https://www.ers.usda.gov/publications/pub-details/?pubid=41757.

Valić F, Žuškin E, Walford J, Keršić W, Pauković R [1968]. Bysinnosis, chronic bronchitis, and ventilatory capacities in workers exposed to soft hemp dust. *Br. J. Ind. Med.* *25*(3):176–186, https://doi.org/10.1136/oem.25.3.176.

Volkow ND, Baler RD, Compton WM, Weiss SR [2014]. Adverse health effects of marijuana use. *N. Engl. J. Med.* *370*(23):2219–2227, http://doi.org/10.1056/ NEJMra 1402309.

Williams C, Thompstone J, Wilkinson M [2008]. Work-related contact urticaria to *Cannabis sativa*. Contact Dermatitis *58*(1):62–63, http://doi.org/10.1111/j.1600-0536.2007.01169.x.

Zuskin E, Kanceljak B, Pokrajac D, Schachter EN, Witek TJ Jr. [1990]. Respiratory symptoms and lung function in hemp workers. *Br. J. Ind. Med.* *47*(9):627–632, https://doi.org/10.1136/oem.47.9.627.

Zuskin E, Kanceljak B, Schachter EN, Witek TJ, Maayani S, Goswami S, Marom Z, Rienzi N [1992]. Immunological findings in hemp workers. *Environ. Res.* *59*(2):350–361, https://doi.org/10.1016/s0013- 9351(05)80041-6.

Zuskin E, Mustajbegovic J, Schachter EN [1994]. Follow-up study of respiratory function in hemp workers. *Am. J. Ind. Med.* *26*(1):103–115, https://doi.org/10.1002/ajim.4700260109.

Chapter 3

Talking with Your Teen about Marijuana: Keeping Your Kids Safe*

Substance Abuse and Mental Health Service Administration

Another telling sign is the presence of drug paraphernalia—any equipment, product, or material of any kind that is modified for making, using, or concealing a controlled substance.

Examples of drug paraphernalia include the following:

- Rolling paper (a specialty paper used for making a marijuana cigarette);
- Cigar (hollowed out and filled with marijuana to make what is referred to as a "blunt");
- Pipe (a device to smoke marijuana);
- Bong (a filtration device to smoke marijuana);
- Roach clip (a metal clip used to hold a marijuana cigarette);
- Electronic cigarette (a device to smoke marijuana extracts); and
- Grinder (a tool that breaks marijuana up into smaller bits).

---

* This is an edited, reformatted and augmented version of Substance Abuse and Mental Health Service Administration Publication.

In: Marijuana
Editor: Charles M. Edmond
ISBN: 979-8-88697-869-8

Take Action

Use these tips to talk with your teen:

- Check in frequently to see how they are doing;
- Choose informal times to talk, such as in the car, during dinner, or while watching TV;
- Be clear and consistent about your expectations regarding marijuana and other drug use;
- Establish family agreements together for social and extracurricular activities;
- Let them know you care and are always there for them; and
- Continue talking with your teens as they get older.

Help your teen create an "exit plan" in case he or she is offered or faced with a difficult decision about marijuana. Peer pressure can be powerful, so coming up with realistic action steps and practicing them together in a safe environment will prepare and empower your teen to make good choices when it matters.

Research suggests that one of the most influential factors when a teen is growing up is a strong, open relationship with a parent or caregiver.

For more information about how to talk with your teen about marijuana, visit www.underagedrinking.samhsa.gov and www.samhsa.gov.

It's never too late to start talking with your teen about the risks of marijuana use. As teens age, they make more decisions on their own and face greater temptation and peer pressure. Though it may not seem like it, teens really do hear your concerns. It's important you help them understand what marijuana is, and why they shouldn't use it.

What Is Marijuana?

Marijuana refers to the dried leaves, flowers, stems, and seeds from the Cannabis sativa or Cannabis indica plant. It is a psychoactive drug that contains close to 500 chemicals, including THC, a mind-altering compound that causes harmful health effects. Marijuana use is prevalent among teens and young adults, and according to SAMHSA's 2019 National Survey on Drug Use and Health, an estimated 3.3 million youths ages 12-17 reported using marijuana in the past year.

Marijuana use tends to increase with age. While 2.5 percent of youths ages 12–13 reported consuming marijuana in the past year, that number increased to 11.7 percent of those ages 14–15 and 25.3 percent by ages 16–17.

Why Are Young People Using Marijuana?

Teens and young adults use marijuana for many reasons, including curiosity, peer pressure, and wanting to fit in with friends. Some use it to cope with anxiety, stress, and even depression. Ultimately, many things factor into why some people decide to use marijuana, including their environment at home, at school, and in the community.

The perception of the dangers of marijuana use is declining and, increasingly, young people today do not consider marijuana use a risky behavior.

This is partially due to the changes to some states' policies on the legalization of marijuana and recreational use. Marijuana remains illegal at the federal level, even though many states have legalized its use.

Make sure your teen understands that marijuana is addictive. In fact, research shows that 1 in 6 youths who start using the drug before the age of 18 can become addicted.

How Are Young People Using Marijuana?

Marijuana can be consumed in a variety of ways—including smoking, vaping, oils, teas, and edibles. Edibles have become popular because people can mix marijuana into their favorite foods, such as brownies, cookies, and candy. However, edibles are dangerous because they can lead to accidental ingestion or overconsumption. Since it takes longer to digest edibles and feel their effects, people may consume more at one time to expedite that process.

Know the Risks and Harms of Marijuana Use

Marijuana use among teens and young adults can harm brain development and cause other negative impacts. Additionally, the amount of THC in marijuana has steadily climbed; today's marijuana has three times the concentration of THC compared to 25 years ago, increasing the impact on the brain. Make sure you know the risks of marijuana use and are prepared to talk with your teen about them.

Common risks include, but are not limited to:

- Issues with attention, concentration, problem solving, learning, and memory;
- Poor academic and job performance;
- Lack of balance and coordination;
- Poor judgment and decision-making;
- Less life satisfaction;
- Relationship problems;
- Increased risk of mental issues; and
- Potential for addiction.

Identify the Signs

Recognizing signs of marijuana use can be difficult if you don't know what to look for. Be aware of any noticeable changes in your teen's behavior, as it might indicate he or she is using marijuana.

Common signs include, but are not limited to:

- Unusual laughing, coordination issues, or forgetfulness;
- Bloodshot eyes or repeated use of eye drops;
- Strange smelling clothes or bedroom;
- Frequent use of incense and other deodorizers;
- Drug-themed clothing, jewelry, or décor; and
- Unexplained lack of money or frequent requests for money.

Chapter 4

Preventing Marijuana Use among Youth*

Substance Abuse and Mental Health Services Administration (SAMHSA)

Abstract

Marijuana use among youth and young adults is a major public health concern. Early youth marijuana use is associated with:

- Neuropsychological and neurodevelopmental decline
- Poor school performance
- Increased school drop-out rates
- Increased risk for psychotic disorders in adulthood
- Increased risk for later depression
- Suicidal ideation or behavior

As policy and legalization efforts evolve and the availability of legal marijuana increases, communities and families need guidance to support the prevention of marijuana use among youth.

This chapter covers programs and policies to prevent marijuana use among youth aged 12 to 17, including:

- Environmental strategies, such as regulating the price of marijuana products, where these products are sold, the products themselves, and their promotion and advertising.
- School- and community-based substance use prevention programs to implement along with environmental interventions as part of a comprehensive prevention strategy.

---

* This is an edited, reformatted and augmented version of Substance Abuse and Mental Health Services Administration (SAMHSA), Publication No. PEP21-06-01-001, dated 2021.

In: Marijuana
Editor: Charles M. Edmond
ISBN: 979-8-88697-869-8

The guide provides considerations and strategies for key stakeholders (including policy makers, community coalitions, businesses, school administrators, educators, and other community members), states, and the prevention workforce to prevent and reduce marijuana use among youth.

Foreword: Evidence-Based Resource Guide Series Overview

The Substance Abuse and Mental Health Services Administration (SAMHSA), and specifically, its National Mental Health and Substance Use Policy Laboratory (Policy Lab), is pleased to fulfill the charge of the 21st Century Cures Act to disseminate information on evidence-based practices and service delivery models to prevent substance misuse and help people with substance use disorders (SUD), serious mental illnesses (SMI), and serious emotional disturbances (SED) get the treatment and support they need.

Prevention of, treatment for, and recovery from SUD, SMI, and SED can vary based on several factors, including geography, socioeconomics, culture, gender, race, ethnicity, and age. This can complicate evaluating the effectiveness of services, treatments, and supports. Despite these variations, however, there is substantial evidence to inform the types of resources that can help prevent and reduce substance use, lessen symptoms of mental illness, and improve quality of life.

The Evidence-Based Resource Guide Series is a comprehensive set of modules with resources to improve health outcomes for people at risk for, experiencing, or recovering from mental and/or substance use disorders. It is designed for practitioners, administrators, community leaders, and others considering an intervention for their organizations or communities.

A priority topic for SAMHSA is preventing marijuana use among youth. This chapter reviews the related literature and science, examines emerging and best practices, identifies gaps in knowledge, and discusses challenges and strategies for implementation.

Expert panels of federal, state, and non-governmental participants provided input for each guide in this series. The panels included accomplished scientists, researchers, service providers, community administrators, federal and state policy makers, and people with lived experience.

Members provided input based on their knowledge of healthcare systems, implementation strategies, evidence-based practices, provision of services, and policies that foster change.

Research shows that implementing new programs or policies requires a comprehensive, multi-pronged approach. This chapter is one piece of an overall approach to implement and sustain change. Readers are encouraged to review the SAMHSA website for additional tools and technical assistance opportunities.

Content of the Chapter

This chapter contains a foreword and five sections. The sections stand alone and do not need to be read in order. Each section is designed to be brief and accessible to anyone working to prevent and reduce youth marijuana use.

The goal of this chapter is to review the literature on prevention of marijuana use among youth, distill the research evidence into recommendations for practice, and provide examples of the ways stakeholders can implement the recommendations.

FW	*Evidence-Based Resource Guide Series Overview* Introduction to the series.
1	*Issue Brief* Overview of current approaches and challenges to reducing marijuana use among youth.
2	*What Research Tells Us* Current evidence on effectiveness of prevention strategies to address youth marijuana use.
3	*Guidance for Selecting and Implementing Evidence-Based Policies and Programs* Practical information to consider when selecting and implementing programs and policies to address marijuana use among youth.
4	*Examples of Interventions for Prevention of Marijuana Use Among Youth* Descriptions of programs and policies that address marijuana use among youth.
5	*Resources for Evaluation and Quality Improvement* Guidance and resources for evaluating implementation of prevention strategies and programs, monitoring outcomes, and improving quality.

Focus of the Guide

Marijuana use among youth and adolescents is a major public health concern. In 2019, about 1 in 8 adolescents aged 12 to 17 (13 percent) used marijuana in the past year, about 3.3 million people.

Marijuana use during adolescence, a period when the brain is still developing, is associated with: negative impacts on brain development; poor school performance; increases in drop-out rates; increased risk for psychotic disorders and depression in adulthood; and suicidal ideation or behavior.[1,2,3]

As policy and legalization efforts evolve and availability of legal marijuana increases, communities and families need guidance to support the prevention of marijuana use among youth. For this chapter, the terms "youth" and "adolescents" are individuals aged 12 to 17.

The purpose of this Evidence-Based Resource Guide is to provide strategies for preventing youth marijuana use to states, communities, the prevention workforce, and other stakeholders. Youth are the focus, as significant evidence suggests early initiation is associated with some of the most serious harms. This chapter discusses programs and policies key stakeholders (including policy makers, community coalitions, businesses, school administrators, educators, and other community members) can implement to prevent and reduce marijuana use among youth and young adults.

The framework below provides an overview of this chapter and prevention efforts that have been implemented and evaluated among youth. The review of these policies and programs in Section 2 includes specific outcomes, stakeholders, and delivery settings for the interventions.

---

[1] Substance Abuse and Mental Health Services Administration. (2020). *Key substance use and mental health indicators in the United States: Results from the 2019 National Survey on Drug Use and Health.* Retrieved from https://www.samhsa.gov/data/release/2019-national- survey-drug-use-and-health-nsduh-releases.

[2] D'Souza, D. C., Radhakrishnan, R., Sherif, M., Cortes-Briones, J., Cahill, J., Gupta, S., ... Ranganathan, M. (2016). Cannabinoids and Psychosis. *Current Pharmaceutical Design, 22*, 6380-6391.

[3] Jacobus J, Tapert SF. (2014). Effects of cannabis on the adolescent brain. *Current Pharmaceutical Design, 20*(13):2186-2193. doi:10.2174/13816128113199990426.

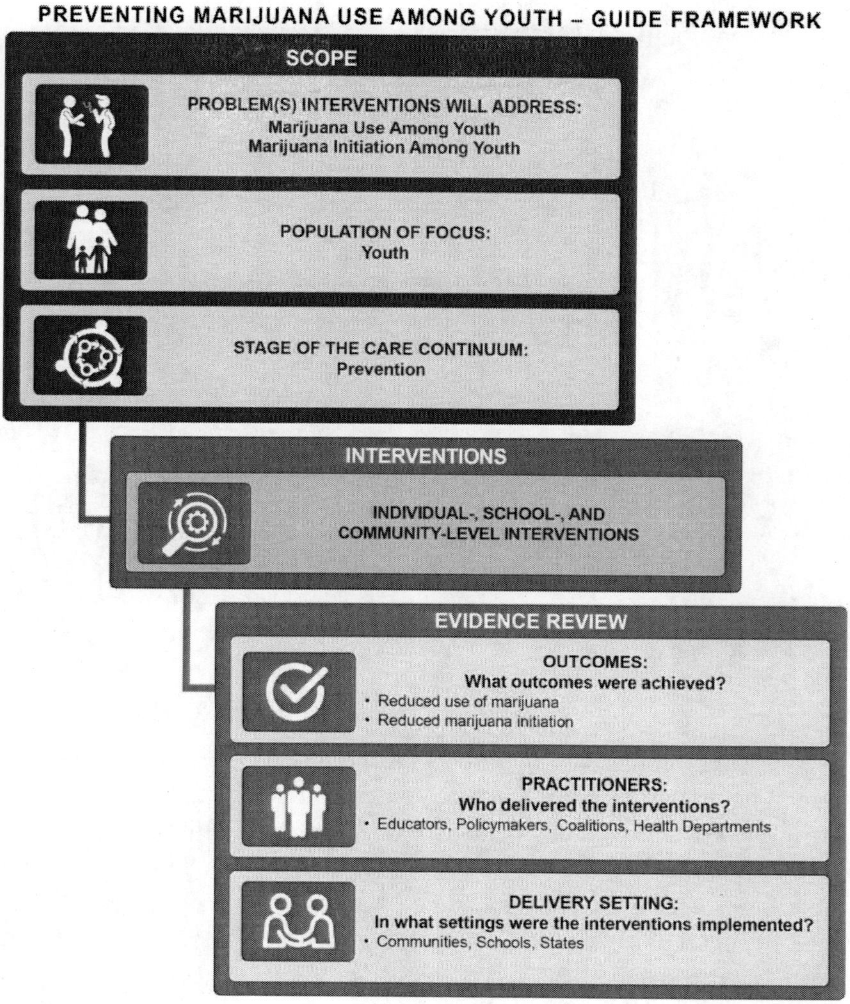

Section 1. Issue Brief

Addressing marijuana use among youth is a major public health concern. Some studies suggest early use can cause disruptions to adolescent brain development that may result in negative consequences, such as cognitive impairment and delayed maturation of the brain areas responsible for decision-making [2].

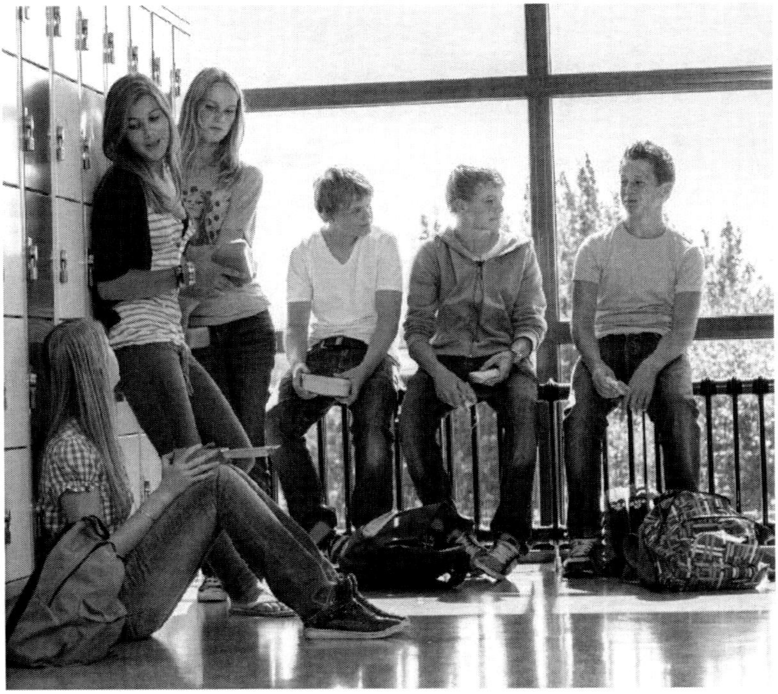

Research on long-lasting effects has produced mixed results. However, there is increasing evidence that heavy and/or regular (e.g., daily or near daily) marijuana use among young people may be associated with cognitive deficits, such as impaired learning [2]. Other concerning risks include physical changes in the brain areas responsible for attention and memory, and increased risk for and early onset of psychiatric conditions and SUDs, such as schizophrenia and marijuana use disorder [9].

Youth marijuana use is also correlated with suicidal ideation and behavior [10], poor school performance, increased high school dropout rates [12], and negative effects on male fertility [14-15].

Terminology

The terms "marijuana" and "cannabis" are often used interchangeably, although there are historical and scientific distinctions [4-5]. This document primarily uses the term "marijuana," including when speaking about use disorders.

The full scope of long-term health and social effects of youth marijuana use is still unknown, particularly among those who may be using marijuana regularly or daily [12].

The high prevalence of youth marijuana use is concerning, with rates of daily use among 8th and 10th graders increasing between 2018 and 2019 (although rates of daily use remained relatively constant between 2010 and 2020) [7, 16]. Daily use rates rise rapidly by the ages of 18 to 22, and marijuana use among this age group is currently at a 35-year high [17].

National estimates indicate more than 3 million youth aged 12 to 17 used marijuana in the past year and 1.9 million in the past month; more youth reported using marijuana than any other illicit drug [6-7].

Several factors impact the growing use of marijuana. For example:

- Widespread availability of marijuana via illegal market sources and state-regulated retail sales
- Increasing legalization of medical and non-medical adult use of marijuana across the country, despite remaining illegal at the federal level
- Mass commercialization of higher potency marijuana, and the availability of an array of consumer-friendly products that often appeal to youth (e.g., candy and baked goods infused with marijuana)
- High and frequent rates of youth use, with increases in the number of people initiating marijuana use each year

These factors, combined with marijuana's clear evidence of harm, makes preventing initiation of its use among youth a public health priority.

The purpose of this Evidence-Based Resource Guide is to provide states, communities, the prevention workforce, and other stakeholders with strategies for preventing youth marijuana use. The population of focus is youth aged 12 to 17, as significant evidence suggests initiation of marijuana use at a young age is associated with some of the most serious harms [18-19].

The guide reflects regulatory structures that currently exist in the country, including states where non-medical (i.e., recreational) or medical use of marijuana is considered legal. It is important to note that no state has legalized non-medical marijuana use for people under the age of 21.

To fully recognize the nature and consequences of youth marijuana use, it is important to first understand the different types of marijuana, its potency (THC content), and how methods of use have evolved in the 21st century.

What Is Marijuana?

Under the Controlled Substances Act (CSA), cannabis (family Cannabaceae) falls into two categories— marijuana and hemp—but, in fact, both come from the same group of plants. Marijuana refers to the cannabis plant, or derivative products that contain more than 0.3 percent of the chemical compound delta-9-tetrahydrocannabinol (THC), the main psychoactive component responsible for the plant's intoxicating effects. The term "hemp" denotes a cannabis plant that contains THC levels no more than 0.3 percent or less.

Marijuana Types [1]

Plant form or "flower": The most known form of marijuana; the dried flowers of the cannabis plant.

Sinsemilla: Seedless flowers from unfertilized female plants; contain more THC than other marijuana plant parts or fertilized flowers.

Hashish: Historically produced by a manual process of compressing dried cannabis flowers through screens to amass trichomes—the part with the most THC—resulting in a dried resin-type substance more potent than dried flowers.

Concentrates/Extracts: The modern process of extracting cannabinoids, especially THC, from the entire marijuana/cannabis plant with solvents or carbon dioxide extraction processes. The plant body is mostly discarded, leaving a more potent product (akin to grain alcohol). Concentrates may not smell like marijuana, depending on how refined the extraction is. Commonly used terms for concentrates include dabs, budder/badder, wax, shatter, crystalline, distillate, crumble, and sift.

Learn more about the different types of marijuana here and here.

Composition and characteristics vary across marijuana plants and products. Marijuana plants contain more than 100 cannabinoids (chemical substances unique to the cannabis plant), in addition to many other chemicals (e.g., terpenes and flavonoids) found in other plant species. THC is the principal psychoactive constituent of marijuana, producing psychotropic or mind-altering effects, with high misuse potential [1]. The other chemical constituents present in marijuana have minor effects relative to THC, and, therefore, the potency of marijuana is related to its THC content. Cannabidiol [1] (CBD), the second most common ingredient in marijuana, does not produce a high.

Specific pharmaceutical CBD and THC formulations have approval from the U.S. Food and Drug Administration (FDA) for the treatment of defined health conditions. For example, these include seizures, nausea from cancer treatments, and acquired immunodeficiency syndrome (AIDS) wasting syndrome.

The following FDA-approved medications are available through a pharmacy via prescription written by a licensed healthcare provider:

- Epidiolex® contains cannabis-derived CBD and is approved for the treatment of seizures associated with Lennox-Gastaut syndrome, Dravet syndrome, or tuberous sclerosis complex in patients one year of age and older.
- Marinol® and Syndros® (dronabinol) are synthetic THC and are indicated for treating anorexia associated with weight loss in patients with AIDS and for nausea and vomiting associated with cancer chemotherapy.
- Cesamet® (nabilone) is a synthetic THC analogue approved for nausea and vomiting associated with cancer chemotherapy [20].

These FDA-approved products are distinct from non-FDA-approved medical marijuana products, which consumers acquire from a state-run marijuana dispensary rather than a pharmacy.

> Medical marijuana is the use of the whole, unprocessed marijuana plant or its basic extracts to treat symptoms of illness as recommended by an authorized practitioner in a state with a medical marijuana law. The FDA does not recognize or approve the marijuana plant as medicine; only the two synthetic and one derivative product described above are approved for medical use.

Sold under a variety of names, such as Spice and K-2, other synthetic cannabinoids are also available on illicit commercial markets. These products activate the same cannabinoid receptors in the human brain as THC [21].

However, they are 10 to 200 times more potent than THC, and, therefore, have the potential to cause serious adverse events, including psychosis and fatal overdose [22].

Evolution of the Marijuana Market: Increasing Potency and Product Diversification

Variation in the content of THC and CBD, as well as how it is consumed (e.g., inhaled, orally ingested, or topically applied) heavily influences its effects. In recent decades, the marijuana products in both state-run legal markets and illicit marijuana markets have been increasingly diverse with respect to route of administration, formulation, and dose. Marijuana from both markets is increasingly available, has higher THC content, has flavors and flavor-sounding names, and greater marketing and promotion. All of these factors may have significant impact on youth initiation and use [13].

> Slang terms for marijuana include ganja, pot, weed, boom, bud, gangster, grass, green, hash, herb, kush, loud, reefer, skunk, dope, Mary Jane, hooch, brew, and greens.

Furthermore, the emergence of the legal marijuana industry has led to a wide range of new products, many composed of extracts or concentrates, including vaping products, other oils and resins, edibles, and topical products.

The amount of THC in marijuana flowers has increased from an average of 3 to 4 percent in the early 1990s to 14 percent currently [23-25], though some marijuana flowers can have THC concentrations of up to about 30 percent [23, 26]. Marijuana concentrates typically have THC concentrations of 40 to 90 percent or greater [24] Overall, the market has been rapidly shifting to products with increased THC concentrations and higher THC:CBD ratios, with no pre-market evaluation of safety [25, 27].

Four primary concerns regarding increased THC concentration are:

1) It is difficult to know how much THC is inhaled or otherwise being ingested.
2) Use of marijuana products with higher THC concentrations is associated with greater risk of marijuana use disorder [28].

3) Use of high potency products is associated with greater risk of psychosis [29].
4) State adult-use laws limiting sales of these products generally use weight-based measures rather than potency-based measures (the amount of money spent per milligram of THC is lower for concentrates). This allows people to purchase a small amount of high potency products, with potentially high levels of intoxicating effects. The National Institutes of Health (NIH) currently has an initiative working to establish a standard unit for THC, currently asking researchers to use 5 milligrams as the standard unit for consistency [30].

How Is Marijuana Used?

How people use marijuana has changed substantially over the years. In addition to smoking traditional marijuana cigarettes, a vast array and combinations of manufactured products have evolved. These include edibles, marijuana-infused beverages, topical applications, and various devices for inhalation. There has also been an increase in people using products originally designed for nicotine/tobacco for marijuana, such as blunts, vaporizing devices, and e-cigarettes [31]. Youth are using marijuana via all of these routes, especially edibles and concentrates [32].

The graphic below shoes the variety of ways people can consume marijuana.

In 2018, among U.S. 12th grade students who used marijuana in the past year, 89 percent reported smoking it, 34 percent reported vaping it, and 40 percent ingested it in food [16]. Youth who ingest edibles are at increased risk of adverse events in part because the THC concentration can vary across products and batches of a single product. Consumption also has a delayed rate of absorption compared to other routes of administration [16]. As a result, youth may not know how the amount of THC will affect the body. This is relevant because of the variability in how much and how quickly THC is absorbed in the body.

Foods and beverages can be infused with THC, including products such as brownies and cookies, candies such as gummies and lollipops, sodas, and alcoholic beverages such as wine and beer. Edible marijuana products are especially attractive to youth, as their packaging often look very similar to that of non-marijuana products. Although some states prohibit such packaging, there is little evidence of enforcement [33]. Marijuana-infused beverages, often with sweet flavors such as orange soda, are similar to alcopops that are often marketed in the form of juices, sodas, lemonade, and iced tea, which are known to attract teens, especially girls [34].

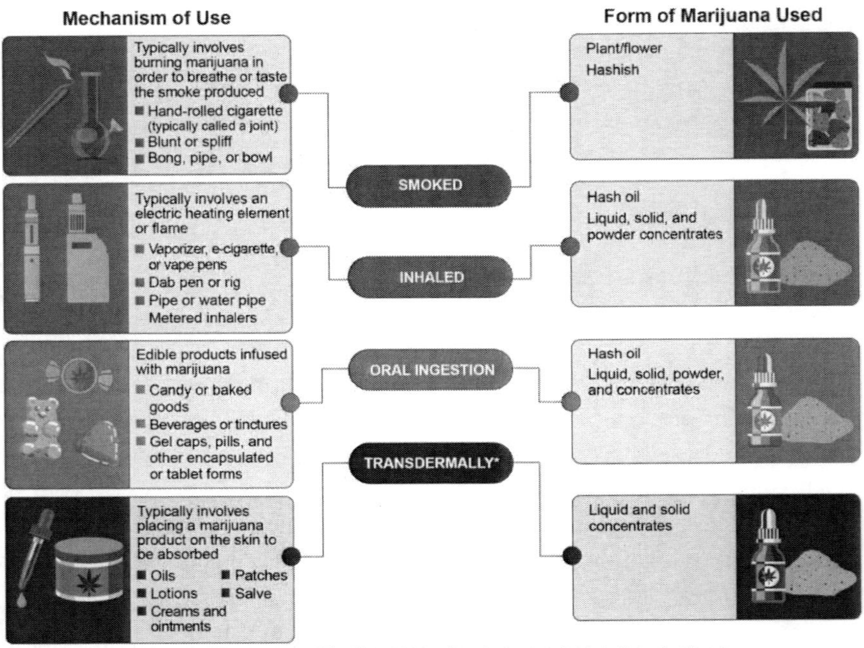

*Transdermal use of marijuana has low misuse potential and has not been shown to cause acute intoxication or impairment.

Of note, the timing of a THC high from edibles is different from that of inhaled/smoked sources; it can take 1 to 2 hours to feel an effect from edibles, and peak effects occur later and may last for several hours. When the high is felt and how long it lasts depends on a user's metabolism, the product formulation, what the person ate, and the dose consumed. Overconsumption can lead to severe intoxication and overdose [35].

Vaping liquid marijuana products can lack the characteristic smell of marijuana, making detection of use difficult. Vaping devices are also packaged in ways that resemble memory sticks or other non-drug paraphernalia devices [36-37]. Detection-free use may be one reason why vaping marijuana has become increasingly popular among youth [38].

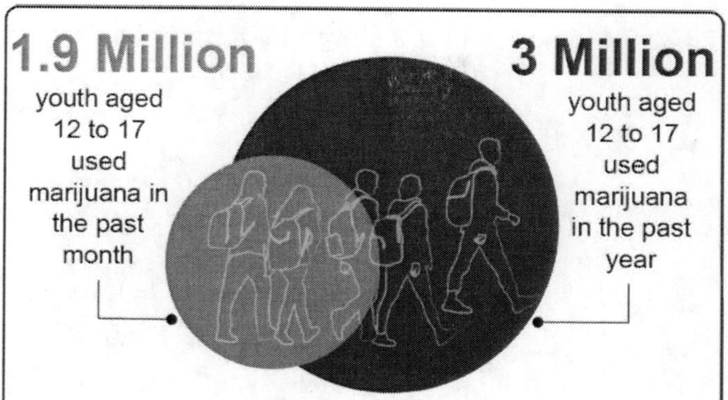

Source: Center for Behavioral Health Statistics and Quality. (2020). *Results from the 2019 National Survey on Drug Use and Health: Detailed tables*. Rockville, MD: Substance Abuse and Mental Health Services Administration. Retrieved from https://www.samhsa.gov/data/

Marijuana products, such as vaping concentrates or hemp wrappers used for blunts, may be flavored. This is a strategy well documented to attract youth to tobacco products and is associated with over 80 percent of youth tobacco initiation [39-41]. Marijuana products also frequently use names implying fruit or other flavors (e.g., grape, peanut butter cup, or pineapple haze), even if that fruit/flavor is not present.

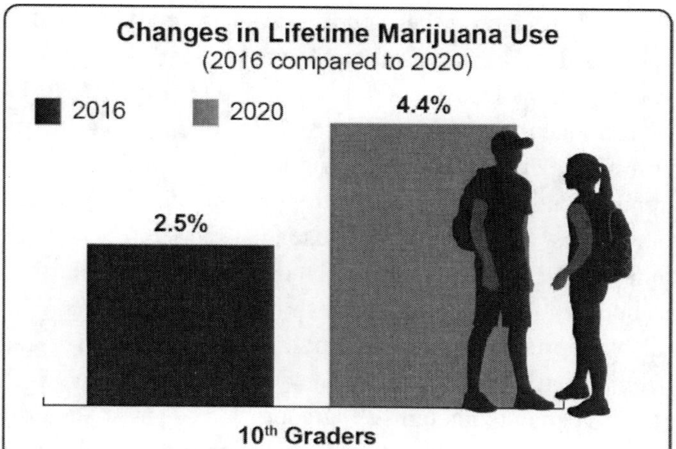

Source: National Institute on Drug Abuse. (2019). *Monitoring the Future 2019 Survey Results: Overall Findings*. National Institutes of Health, U.S. Department of Health and Human Services.

Changes in Past Month Marijuana Use
(2016 compared to 2020)

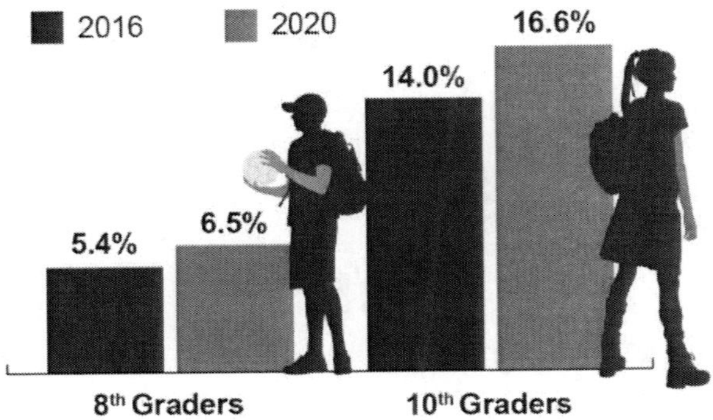

Source: National Institute on Drug Abuse. (2019). *Monitoring the Future 2019 Survey Results: Overall Findings*. National Institutes of Health, U.S. Department of Health and Human Services.

Prevalence of Marijuana Use among Youth

Overall Prevalence

According to the 2019 National Survey on Drug Use and Health (NSDUH), marijuana was the most commonly used substance after alcohol among 12- to 17-year-olds [7]. Among the youth surveyed, 16, 13, and 7 percent, respectively, reported having used marijuana within their lifetime, within the past year, and within the past month [7]. In this age group, 16- to 17-year-olds had the highest rates of marijuana use; 31 percent reported using marijuana in their lifetime, 25 percent reported using marijuana in the past year, and 14 percent reported using marijuana in the past month. Those aged 12 to 13 reported the lowest rates of marijuana use [7, 17].

Data from the 2019 Monitoring the Future Survey further highlight concerns about youth marijuana use as shown in the following graphics:

It is also important to look at how past month use increases across the age groups, from 7 percent among 8th graders to 17 percent among 10th graders and up to 21 percent among 12th graders [16]. These data suggest that prevention at younger ages is critical to reducing marijuana use among older adolescents.

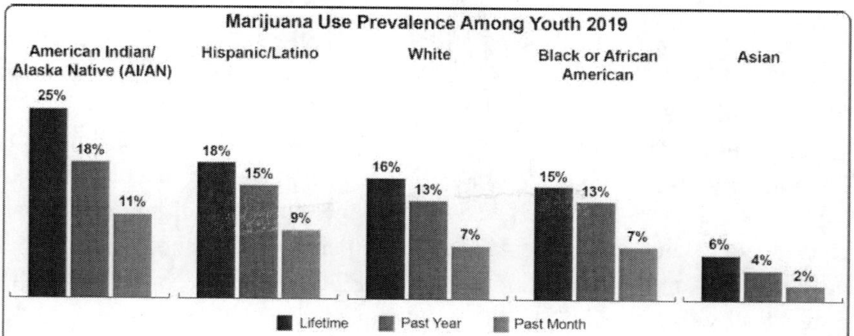

Source: Center for Behavioral Health Statistics and Quality. (2020). *Results from the 2019 National Survey on Drug Use and Health: Detailed tables.* Rockville, MD: Substance Abuse and Mental Health Services Administration. Retrieved from https://www.samhsa.gov/data/

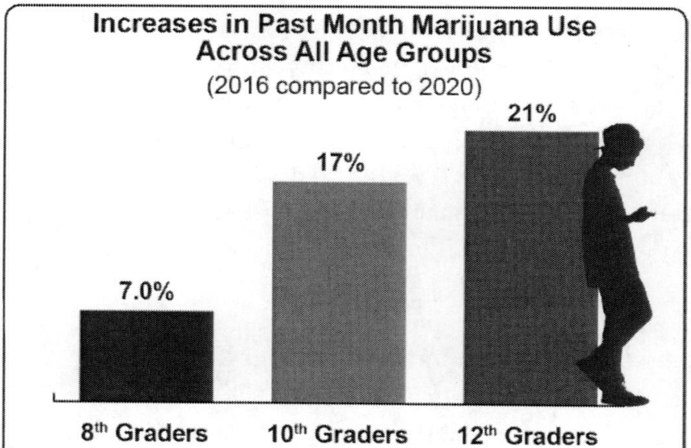

Source: Miech, R. A., Johnston, L. D., O'Malley, P. M., Bachman, J. G., Schulenberg, J. E., & Patrick, M. E. (2021). Monitoring the Future national survey results on drug use, 1975–2020: Volume I, Secondary school students. Ann Arbor: Institute for Social Research, The University of Michigan. Available at http://monitoringthefuture.org/pubs.html#monograph

Prevalence of Marijuana Use by Specific Population Groups

Nationally, the prevalence of youth marijuana use varies across demographic groups. In the general population, males report higher rates of marijuana use compared to females. However, among 12- to 17-year-olds, female and male youth report lifetime, past year, and past month marijuana use at comparable rates nationwide [7].

Rates of marijuana use also vary by race and ethnicity. American Indian/Alaska Native youth reported the highest rates of lifetime, past year, and past month marijuana use, while Asian youth reported the lowest. A breakdown of marijuana use prevalence by race and ethnicity is shown in the graphic that follows below [6].

For past month use, youth who identify as sexual and gender minorities are 1.6 times more likely to report recent marijuana use than heterosexual youth [42] and marijuana use is 2.5 times higher among transgender compared to cisgender youth [43]. These differences persist in adulthood, and lesbian, gay, bisexual, transgender, and queer (LGBTQ) youth are more likely to be diagnosed with a marijuana use disorder as adults.44 Research suggests this difference may be due to greater exposure to stressful life events, discrimination, and stigma among LGBTQ youth as compared to their heterosexual peers [42, 44-45].

Among sexual minority youth (i.e., whose sexual orientation, gender identity, or sexual characteristics are different from the presumed majority of the population), those assigned male at birth demonstrate greater rates of recent and lifetime marijuana use, despite comparable rates between male and female youth at the national level [46]. These data underscore the importance of culturally specific marijuana prevention strategies for populations who experience disparities in marijuana use prevalence.

Harms Associated with Youth Marijuana Use

Youth may experience substantial harm resulting from marijuana use, especially heavy and chronic use. Frequent or intensive (e.g., daily or near-daily) marijuana use is strongly associated with higher risks of experiencing many adverse health and social outcomes [11].

Effects of Marijuana Use on the Brain

Human brain development continues well into an individual's twenties and several genetic and environmental factors can influence this process [47]. Findings from animal studies show chemicals (e.g., cannabinoids) in marijuana bind to the brain's own endocannabinoid system, disrupting the body's normal levels of naturally occurring cannabinoids [24]. The important role of the endocannabinoid system in neurodevelopment may explain why youth are particularly susceptible to the effects of marijuana. Exposure to marijuana during this time can alter the brain's normal communication mechanisms and epigenetic (how behaviors and environment can cause changes that affect the way genes work) development [47]. THC attaches to cannabinoid receptors in the brain, like a key to a lock, which in part activates the brain's reward pathway, resulting in the intoxicating effects when people use marijuana.

In addition to intoxication, flooding the brain with large amounts of THC may impact normal functions for short or long periods of time, including:

- Learning, memory, and other cognitive processes critical to learning
- Pleasure/reward
- Appetite
- Motion/motor control
- Sleep
- Reproduction/fertility

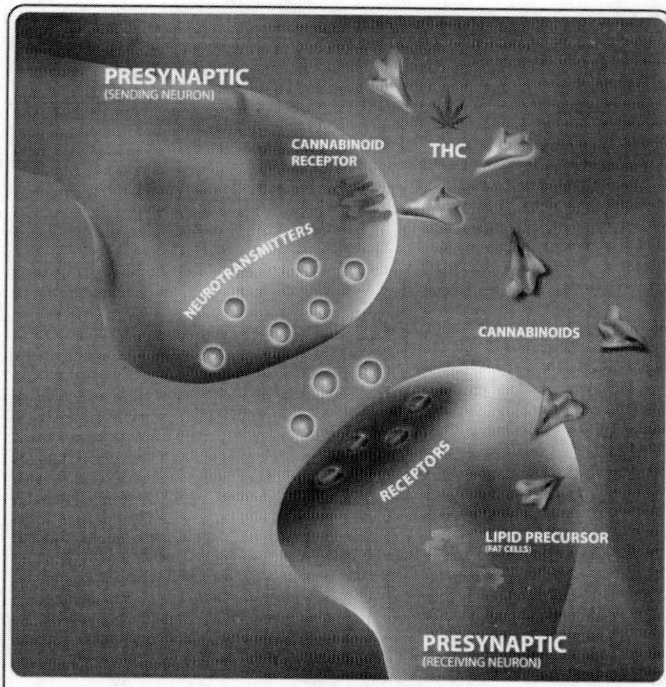

Source: Jacobus, J., & F Tapert, S. (2014) Effects of cannabis on the adolescent brain. *Current Pharmaceutical Design, 20(*13), 2186-2193.

Other possible effects can include altered senses, changes in mood, and hallucinations [48-49].

THC can also result in disruption of cognitive processes that are important for academic performance and activities like driving and sports [50, 51]. In some studies, chronic, long-term marijuana use has been associated with altered brain structure and impaired cognitive functioning [50]. There is debate about the clinical significance of these changes and whether they reverse with abstinence. Collectively, these studies suggest a potential risk associated with adolescent marijuana use related to brain development [52]. It is important to note that much of this information comes from preclinical studies, meaning more research with larger populations is needed.

Short- and Long-Term Adverse Effects of Marijuana Use

Common Short-Term Adverse Effects

- Brief periods of: increased heart rate; altered sense of time; increased anxiety/paranoia; slow reaction time; problems with balance and coordination; impaired driving; increased appetite; difficulty with thinking and problem solving; memory impairment [1]. The likelihood of adverse effects increases with increasing doses of marijuana [53].

Less Common Short-Term Adverse Effects

- Increased heart rate, which may increase the risk of a heart attack; nausea and vomiting [54]; panic attacks; psychosis (losing touch with reality); hallucinations (seeing or hearing things that are not really there); delusions (believing something that is not true) [55].

Long-Term Effects

- Lung and breathing problems (particularly when smoked and often among those who also smoke cigarettes), though these problems often manifest later in life; stroke, poor academic performance [56]; truancy [57]; increased risk for social anxiety [58]; suicidal ideation [2], attempts, and completion [59].
- Babies exposed to marijuana during pregnancy are exposed to similar harms. Specifically, prenatal marijuana use is associated with poor birth outcomes such as low birth weight and brain development

delays, which may have longer term effects on the adolescent brain [60-61].

- Chronic marijuana use is also associated with a condition called "cannabinoid hyperemesis syndrome," characterized by repeated and severe instances of nausea and vomiting [54].

Marijuana Use Disorder

- People who begin using marijuana at or before the age of 18 are 4 to 7 times more likely to develop a marijuana use disorder than adults who did not use under age 18 [62]. Three in 10 people who used marijuana developed a marijuana use disorder between 2012 and 2013 [63].
- Those who have a marijuana use disorder may experience withdrawal symptoms (anxiety, insomnia, depression) [64], which may create acute discomfort and an incentive to continue marijuana use [65].
- Most individuals who seek treatment for marijuana use disorder fail to achieve sustained abstinence (one study reported 8 percent of their sample had sustained abstinence); rates of successful quitting are comparable to those for individuals who use tobacco [66-67]. Other substance use disorders show success rates between 20 and more than 50 percent, though research suggest an average of approximately 18 percent sustained abstinence [68].

Psychotic Symptoms and Disorders

- Marijuana use is associated with higher risk and worsening outcomes of later psychotic disorder, such as schizophrenia, for those with the disorder, but causality remains unclear [2, 29].
- Youth who have psychoses or psychotic symptoms and who use marijuana typically have an earlier age of first-episode psychosis [69].
- Evidence supports that stopping marijuana use can reduce the onset and occurrence of psychotic symptoms [70].

Personal Harms

- Frequent marijuana use between the ages of 14 to 21 is associated with lower high school completion and college graduation [71], subsequent lower income at age 25, and lower levels of relationship and life satisfaction [72].

- Daily or near-daily marijuana use is associated with financial difficulties, antisocial behavior in the workplace, and more interpersonal relationship conflict. This is particularly true among those who reported a longer history of marijuana use and development of a marijuana use disorder [73-74].
- Recent studies suggest marijuana use is associated with higher rates of depression and suicide, especially among youth [75-77].
- Initiation of marijuana use before the age of 18 is also a predictor of opioid use disorder in adulthood [78].
- Marijuana has been found to be contaminated with bacteria, viruses, and metals that can negatively impact health, particularly among immunocompromised youth [79].

> The fat-soluble nature of THC is why a person can test THC-positive for days, and sometimes weeks, after use. This is also why blood levels of THC are not a reliable way of indicating impairment from marijuana the way blood alcohol content is used to measure impairment from alcohol.
>
> Practically, this means there is not currently a mechanism to test marijuana impairment, which presents challenges for workplace policies and driving under the influence. Research is being done to develop devices to address this challenge.

Overdoses

- THC does not typically shut down core bodily functions like breathing as other substances such as opioids may. With uncommon exceptions of some severe pediatric ingestions, there are no reports of fatal overdoses directly tied to marijuana use [80].
- Uncomfortable side effects can result from excess consumption of edibles, use of high potency products, or accidental ingestion. These result in a variety of effects from psychosis to anxiety, and large increases in marijuana-associated emergency room visits [81-82].

Risk and Protective Factors for Youth Marijuana Use

Several factors place some youth at higher risk of initiating and continuing marijuana use, while other factors protect them from adopting this behavior. Both types of factors are present at multiple levels across the socio-ecological model (SEM), including those with a direct effect on an individual as well as indirect neighborhood and community factors. Additionally, these risk and protective factors can, and should, be considered within the context of social determinants of health, which recognize the broader social and community context of marijuana use across each of the SEM levels [83].

What is the Socio-Ecological Model?

The socio-ecological model (SEM) defines the complex relationship between individual/peer, family, school, and community factors that protect or put individuals at risk.[68] This guide uses a version of this model to frame the discussion of risk and protective factors for marijuana use, as well as the marijuana use prevention strategies discussed in **Chapter 2**.

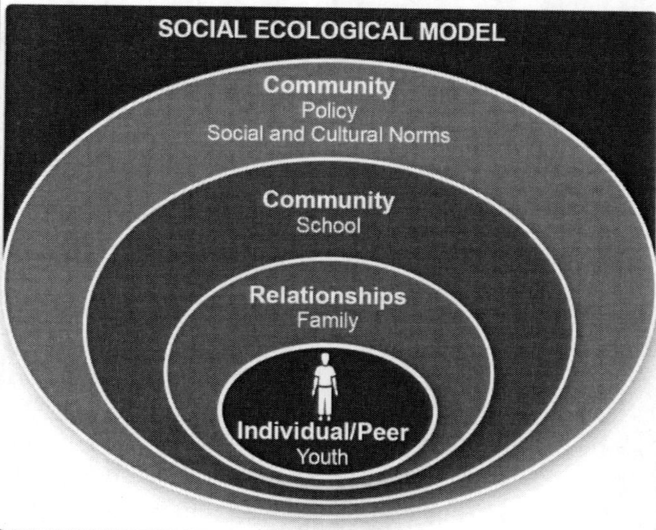

Individual and Peer Risk and Protective Factors

At the individual level, risk factors include current behavior, such as sensation seeking and aggression, whereas protective factors include having college aspirations and self-confidence to say no to substances. As with other SUDs, neurobiology and genetics contribute to marijuana use and use disorders [84-85]. Recent studies show distinction between genetic hereditability to marijuana use and developing a marijuana use disorder [86]. Youth thinking that their peers are using marijuana is associated with their own decisions to use. However, perceived level of peer use among students aged 12 to 17 is greater than the actual rate of use among peers [6]. Alternatively, peer disapproval can be a protective factor [87]. A large percentage of students also reported that they believe close friends would strongly disapprove or somewhat disapprove of trying marijuana (78 percent) or using marijuana once a month or more (79 percent) [6, 7].

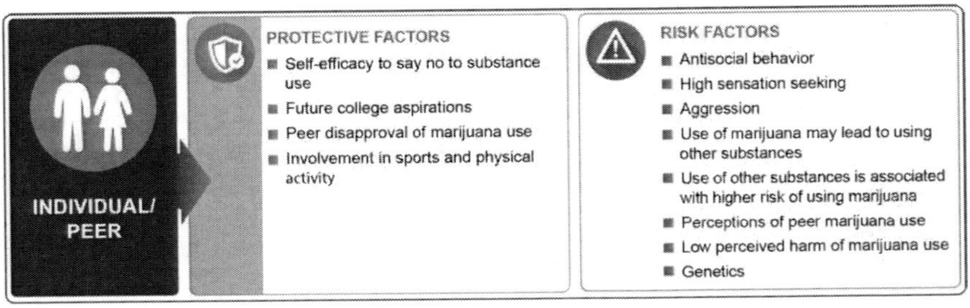

Family Risk and Protective Factors

Family factors associated with increased risk of youth marijuana use include home environments characterized by family conflict and poor relationships with parents/caregivers [88-89]. Parental use and beliefs about marijuana use also strongly influence youth behavior; youth whose parents have ever used marijuana are about three times more likely to use marijuana than youth whose parents have never used marijuana. Youth whose parents do not believe marijuana use is risky are 1.5 times more likely to use when compared with youth whose parents hold more negative beliefs [90-91].

Conversely, families can play a protective role in preventing youth marijuana use by fostering a supportive family environment and monitoring and prohibiting youth marijuana use. Positive family factors such as identifying with one's parents/caregiver, maternal affection displayed toward child, and perceived parental trust have been found to play a protective role in preventing youth marijuana use [91-92]. No tolerance rules around youth marijuana use and greater parental monitoring are also associated with decreased marijuana use [93].

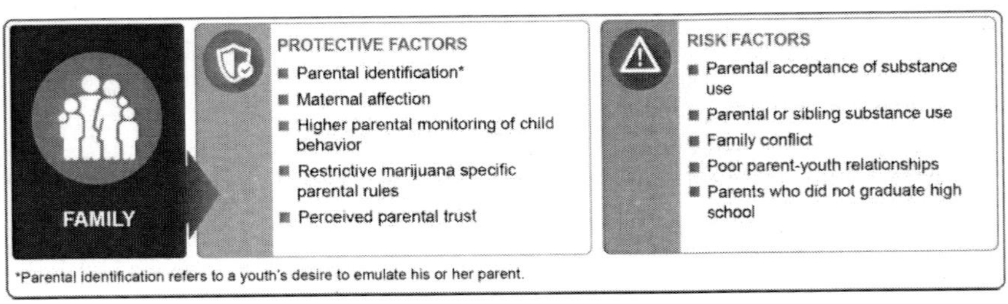

School Risk and Protective Factors

Rates of marijuana use vary at the school level, and research has identified a variety of related factors associated with marijuana use among students [94-97]. Authoritative school environments characterized by fair disciplinary practices and mutual respect between teachers and students have shown lower levels of marijuana use among students [97-98]. Less predictable school environments where rules are not clearly articulated nor consistently enforced tend to have higher rates of use [98-99]. A school's substance use disciplinary policies also influence marijuana use; more remedial approaches to violations, such as counseling, have been found to result in less marijuana use when compared with more punitive measures, such as expulsion [99].

It is also important to consider students' relationships to the school environment in understanding marijuana use risk. The level of connection students feel to their school, fellow students, and academics is associated with student marijuana use [96]. Researchers hypothesize that greater school connectedness creates a sense of shared identity and belonging that reduces the role of marijuana use in achieving social status, thereby decreasing students' likelihood of using marijuana [96, 100]. A student's involvement in school activities, such as clubs and sports, also serves as a protective factor [95, 101-102].

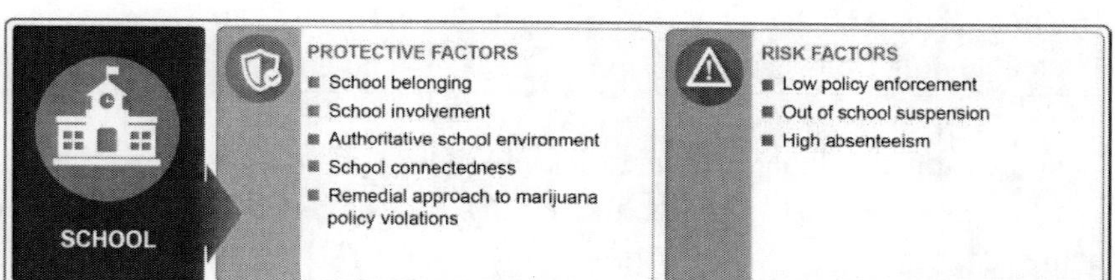

Community Risk and Protective Factors

The laws and ordinances that govern a neighborhood, city, county, state, or tribal community have a direct effect on a youth's ability to access and use substances. In the case of marijuana, community-level risk factors include the availability of the product (either medically or illegally), product marketing (primarily relevant in states where marijuana is legal at the state or local level for non-medical or medical use), community disorganization, economic deprivation, and other social determinants of health.[83,103-105] For each of these risk factors, the opposite can be considered important as a protective factor that can reduce or prevent youth marijuana use.

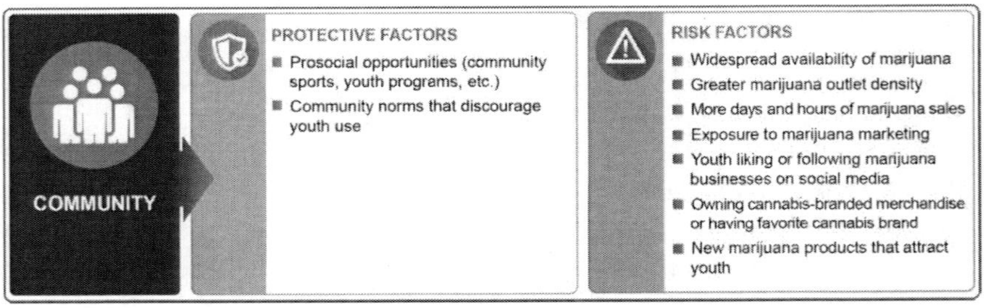

Challenges to Prevention Efforts

This chapter focuses on prevention interventions for youth marijuana use, considering the different regulatory structures that currently exist in the country, including states where the sale of marijuana remains illegal and states where recreational or medical use is considered legal. The rapidly evolving policy landscape at the state level poses significant challenges for preventing marijuana use by youth. Greater public acceptance, declining perception of risk, increasing availability, product diversification, pervasive marketing, and other trends may contribute to an increase in youth marijuana use.

> The Controlled Substances Act (CSA) [104] places all substances regulated under federal law into five schedules. Under the CSA, marijuana is a Schedule I substance, meaning it has a high potential for misuse [105].

According to federal regulations, marijuana is considered a controlled substance, as defined by the Controlled Substances Act (CSA) [106]; however, many state regulations vary from the CSA [107]. As of February 2021, legislation to allow the medical use of marijuana has been passed in 36 states plus the District of Columbia, Guam, Puerto Rico, and the U.S. Virgin Islands. Legislation permitting the legalized, non-medical use of marijuana for adults age 21 and older has been passed in 17 states and territories [108].

As a result, legally produced marijuana is not considered a controlled substance by states that allow use for medical and/or non-medical purposes, but it remains subject to violations that may result in federal prosecution [107, 109-110]. Many states still have penalties for possession of marijuana by youth under the legal age.

States vary widely in how they regulate legalized marijuana. Every state with some form of legalized marijuana use for non-medical purposes thus far has banned sales to persons under 21 years old. Other restrictions on legalized marijuana may include:

- Limits on the amount of marijuana an individual can purchase each day or possess
- Restrictions on advertisements, potency, or product design
- Requirements for quality standards and health warnings
- Limits on the number or types of businesses allowed to sell the product
- Restrictions on whether delivery from the retailer is allowed [13]

The term "legalization" is often used rather broadly. However, at the state level, marijuana can be divided into four distinct legal categories:

1) Non-medical legalization
2) Medical legalization
3) Decriminalization
4) Illegal [111]

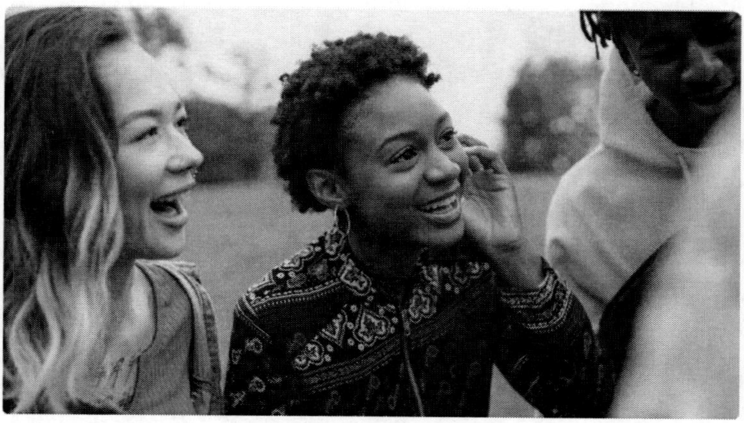

The table that follows below briefly describes each of these terms [112].

Even within states which have legalized, considerable local variation may exist between cities or counties that allow legal sale and those that do not [36].

Despite the variation in public policy and regulation, stakeholders can implement prevention programs and strategies to reduce risk and increase protective factors associated with youth marijuana use. These activities may target the individual or community environment. The next section provides information on what constitutes an evidence-based intervention and provides examples of prevention programs and policies that have demonstrated decreases in substance use, and, specifically, marijuana initiation and use among youth.

Non-Medical Legalization	**Medical Legalization**	**Decriminalized**	**Illegal**
The possession of marijuana is permitted for both medical and/or non-medical purposes by the state. Non-medical use is limited to adults aged 21 and older. Also referred to as "recreational and adult use."	The possession of marijuana is permitted by the state when recommended for medical purposes only.	Decriminalization can be full or partial and means that lesser marijuana violations, such as possession of small amounts, will typically be civil infractions or misdemeanors and will not result in imprisonment.	The possession of marijuana is not permitted for any purpose and is subject to both state and federal prosecution.
It is important to note that these categories may not be mutually exclusive in every state. For example, a state may have decriminalized marijuana while it is still illegal.			

Professional Organization Statements on Marijuana and Youth

American Academy of Pediatrics (APP): "In states that have legalized marijuana for recreational purposes, the AAP strongly recommends strict enforcement of rules and regulations that limit access and marketing and advertising to youth… Although the AAP does not condone state laws that allow the sale of marijuana products, in states where recreational marijuana is currently legal, pediatricians should advocate that states regulate the product as closely as possible to tobacco and alcohol, with a minimum age of 21 years for purchase. Revenue from this regulation should be used to support research on the health risks and benefits of marijuana" [3].

American Academy of Child and Adolescent Psychiatry (AACAP): "Marijuana-related policy changes, including legalization, may have significant unintended consequences for children and adolescents. AACAP supports (a) initiatives to increase awareness of marijuana's harmful effects on adolescents, (b) improved access to evidence-based treatment for adolescents with marijuana-related problems, and (c) careful monitoring of the effects of marijuana-related policy changes on child and adolescent mental health. Finally, AACAP strongly advocates for the involvement of the medical and research community in these critical and highly impactful policy-related discussions" [8].

American Society of Addiction Medicine: "Public health efforts through evidence-based prevention programs should be strengthened to discourage people from using cannabis products due to their known potential harms. Given the particular risks to children and adolescents, cannabis products should not be distributed to anyone under the age of 21… States or jurisdictions that decide to legalize cannabis production, distribution, or sale should only do so within a strong public health-based regulatory framework that minimizes the harms related to legalization. These should include best public health practices established for tobacco control, and components which have been identified as important for minimizing harmful use of tobacco or alcohol" [11].

American Public Health Association: "With more states legalizing retail sales of marijuana and a dearth of national research on cannabis policy, [APHA] recommends state and local governments that regulate cannabis to develop and enforce policies that control access and use by youth and other vulnerable populations. Calls on all lawmakers to develop funding and monitoring mechanisms to expunge cannabis-related records, decrease arrests, support community re-entry and community development. Encourages state and local governments to work with health departments to prevent and treat cannabis abuse and dependence. Urges agencies to develop and expand the evidence base on the health effects of cannabis, as well as on the public health and safety outcomes related to its commercial regulation" [13].

APHA
AMERICAN PUBLIC HEALTH ASSOCIATION

References

[1] National Institute on Drug Abuse. (2019). *Marijuana DrugFacts.* https://www.drugabuse.gov/publications/drugfacts/marijuana.

[2] National Academies of Sciences, Engineering, and Medicine. (2017). *The health effects of cannabis and cannabinoids: The current state of evidence and recommendations for research.* National Academies Press. https://doi.org/10.17226/24625.

[3] Mikos, R. A., & Kam, C. D. (2019). Has the "M" word been framed? Marijuana, cannabis, and public opinion. *PLoS One, 14*(10). https://doi.org/10.1371/journal.pone.0224289.

[4] National Hispanic Caucus of State Legislators. (2017). *Providing a legal framework when jurisdictions decide to decriminalize, commercialize and tax cannabis*. https://nhcsl.org/resources/resolutions/2017/2017-12/.

[5] Ammerman, S., Ryan, S., & Adelman, W. P. (2015). The impact of marijuana policies on youth: Clinical, research, and legal update. *Pediatrics, 135*(3), e769-e785. https://doi.org/10.1542/peds.2014-4147.

[6] Substance Abuse and Mental Health Services Administration. (2020). *Key substance use and mental health indicators in the United States: Results from the 2019 National Survey on Drug Use and Health*. https://www.samhsa.gov/data/sites/default/files/reports/rpt29393/2019NSDUHFFRPDFWHTML/2019NSDUHFFR090120.htm.

[7] Center for Behavioral Health Statistics and Quality. (2020). *Results from the 2019 National Survey on Drug Use and Health: Detailed tables*. https://www.samhsa.gov/data/sites/default/files/reports/rpt29394/NSDUHDetailedTabs2019/NSDUHDe-tailedTabs2019.pdf.

[8] American Academy of Child and Adolescent Psychiatry. (2017). *Marijuana legalization*. https://www. aacap.org/AACAP/Policy_Statements/2014/aacap_marijuana_legalization_policy.aspx.

[9] Casadio, P., Fernandes, C., Murray, R. M., & Di Forti, M. (2011). Cannabis use in young people: The risk for schizophrenia. *Neuroscience & Biobehavioral Reviews, 35*(8), 1779-1787. https://doi. org/10.1016/j.neubiorev.2011.04.007.

[10] Price, C., Hemmingsson, T., Lewis, G., Zammit, S., & Allebeck, P. (2009). Cannabis and suicide: Longitudinal study. *Br J Psychiatry, 195*(6), 492-497. https://doi.org/10.1192/bjp.bp.109.065227.

[11] American Society of Addiction Medicine. (2020). *Public policy statement on cannabis*. https://www.asam.org/advocacy/find-a-policy-statement/view-policy-statement/public-policy-statements/2020/10/13/cannabis.

[12] Lisdahl, K. M., Wright, N. E., Medina-Kirchner, C., Maple, K. E., & Shollenbarger, S. (2014). Considering cannabis: The effects of regular cannabis use on neurocognition in adolescents and young adults. *Current Addiction Reports, 1*(2), 144-156. https://dx.doi. org/10.1007%2Fs40429-014-0019-6.

[13] American Public Health Association. (2020, October 25). *New public health policy statements adopted at APHA 2020*. https://www.apha.org/news-and-media/news-releases/apha-news-releases/2020/2020-apha-policy-statements.

[14] Hsiao, P., & Clavijo, R. I. (2018). Adverse effects of cannabis on male reproduction. *Eur Urol Focus, 4*(3), 324-328. https://doi.org/10.1016/j. euf.2018.08.006.

[15] Payne, K. S., Mazur, D. J., Hotaling, J. M., & Pastuszak, A. W. (2019) Cannabis and Male Fertility: A Systematic Review. *J Urol, 202*(4), 674-681. https://doi.org/10.1097/ju.0000000000000248.

[16] Miech, R. A., Johnston, L. D., O'Malley, P. M., Bachman, J. G., Schulenberg, J. E., & Patrick, M. E. (2021). *Monitoring the Future national survey results on drug use, 1975–2020: Volume I, secondary school students*. http://www.monitoringthefuture.org/pubs/monographs/mtf-vol1_2020.pdf.

[17] National Institute on Drug Abuse. (2019, December 18). *Monitoring the Future 2019 survey results: Overall findings*. https://www.drugabuse.gov/drug-topics/trends-statistics/infographics/monitoring-future-2019-survey-results-overall-findings.

[18] Levar, N., Francis, A. N., Smith, M. J., Ho, W. C., & Gilman, J. M. (2018). Verbal memory performance and reduced cortical thickness of brain regions along the uncinate fasciculus in young adult cannabis users. *Cannabis Cannabinoid Res, 3*(1), 56-65. https://dx.doi.org/10.1089%2Fcan.2017.0030.

[19] Sagar, K. A., & Gruber, S. A. (2018). Marijuana matters: reviewing the impact of marijuana on cognition, brain structure and function, & exploring policy implications and barriers to research. *Int Rev Psychiatry, 30*(3), 251-267. https://dx.doi.org/10.108 0%2F09540261.2018.1460334.

[20] U.S. Food and Drug Adminstration. (2020). *FDA and cannabis: Research and drug approval process*. https://www.fda.gov/news-events/public-health-focus/fda-and-cannabis-research-and-drug-approval-process.

[21] Spaderna, M., Addy, P. H., & D'Souza, D. C. (2013). Spicing things up: Synthetic cannabinoids. *Psychopharmacology, 228*(4), 525-540. https://doi. org/10.1007/s00213-013-3188-4.

[22] National Institute on Drug Abuse. (2020). *DrugFacts: Synthetic cannabinoids (K2/Spice) DrugFacts.* https://www.drugabuse.gov/publications/drugfacts/ synthetic-cannabinoids-k2spice.

[23] Cash, M. C., Cunnane, K., Fan, C., & Romero-Sandoval, E. A. (2020). Mapping cannabis potency in medical and recreational programs in the United States. *PLoS One, 15*(3), e0230167. https://doi. org/10.1371/journal.pone.0230167.

[24] National Institute on Drug Abuse. (2020). *Marijuana research report: How does marijuana produce its effects?* https://www.drugabuse.gov/publications/research-reports/marijuana/how-does-marijuana-produce-its-effects.

[25] Smart, R., Caulkins, J. P., Kilmer, B., Davenport, S., & Midgette, G. (2017). Variation in cannabis potency and prices in a newly legal market: Evidence from 30 million cannabis sales in Washington state. *Addiction, 112*(12), 2167-2177. https://doi.org/10.1111/add.13886.

[26] Burgdorf, J. R., Kilmer, B., & Pacula, R. L. (2011). Heterogeneity in the composition of marijuana seized in California. *Drug Alcohol Depend, 7*(1), 59-61. https://dx.doi.org/10.1016%2Fj. drugalcdep.2010.11.031.

[27] ElSohly, M., Chandra, S., Radwan, M., Majumdar, C., & Church, J. (2021). A comprehensive review of cannabis potency in the United States in the last decade. *Biol Psychiatry Cogn Neurosci Neuroimaging, 6*(6), 603-606. https://doi. org/10.1016/j.bpsc.2020.12.016.

[28] Van der Pol, P., Liebregts, N., Brunt, T., Van Amsterdam, J., De Graaf, R., Korf, D. J., Van den Brink, W., & Can Laar, M. (2014). Cross-sectional and prospective relation of cannabis potency, dosing and smoking behaviour with cannabis dependence: An ecological study. *Addiction, 109*(7), 1101-1109. https://doi.org/10.1111/add.12508.

[29] Di Forti, M., Quattrone, D., Freeman, T. P., Tripoli, G., Gayer-Anderson, C., Quigley, H., Rodriguez, V., Jongsma, H. E., Ferraro, L., La Cascia, C., La Barbera, D., Tarricone, I., Berardi, D., Szöke, A., Arango, C., Tortelli, A., Velthorst, E., Bernardo, M., Del-Ben, C. M.,… Murray, R. M. (2019). The contribution of cannabis use to variation in the incidence of psychotic disorder across Europe (EU-GEI): A multicentre case-control study. *The Lancet Psychiatry 6*(5), 427-436. https://doi.org/10.1016/s2215-0366(19)30048-3.

[30] Volkow, N., & Sharpless, N. (2021, May 10). *Establishing 5mg of THC as the standard unit for research.* National Institute on Drug Abuse. https://www.drugabuse.gov/about-nida/noras-blog/2021/05/establishing-5mg-thc-standard-unit-research.

[31] Seaman, E. L., Stanton, C. A., Edwards, K. C., & Halenar, M. J. (2020). Use of tobacco products/devices for marijuana consumption and association with substance use problems among U.S. young adults (2015–2016). *Addictive Behaviors, 102,* 106133. https://doi.org/10.1016/j. addbeh.2019.106133.

[32] Patrick, M. E., Miech, R. A., Kloska, D. D., Wagner, A. C., & Johnston, L. D. (2020). Trends in marijuana vaping and edible consumption from 2015 to 2018

among adolescents in the US. *JAMA Pediatrics, 174*(9), 900-902. https://doi.org/10.1001/jamapediatrics.2020.0175.

[33] O'Connor, S., Méndez, S., Bess, J., Cooper, B., Cordova-Sanchez, A., Harris, D., & Jeong, C. (2016). *Concerning cannabis-infused edibles: Factors that attract children to foods*. Cannabis Law & Policy Project, University of Washington School of Law. https://lcb.wa.gov/publications/Marijuana/Concerning-MJ-Infused-Edibles-Factors-That-Attract-Children.pdf.

[34] Metzner, C., & Kraus, L. (2008). The impact of alcopops on adolescent drinking: A literature review. *Alcohol & Alcoholism, 43*(2), 230-239. https://doi. org/10.1093/alcalc/agm148.

[35] Grotenhermen, F. (2003). Pharmacokinetics and pharmacodynamics of cannabinoids. *Clin Pharmacokinet, 42*(4), 327-360. https://doi. org/10.2165/ 00003088-200342040-00003.

[36] Silver, L. D., Naprawa, A. Z., & Padon, A. A. (2020). Assessment of incorporation of lessons from tobacco control in city and county laws regulating legal marijuana in California. *JAMA Network Open, 3*(6), e208393-e208393. https://doi.org/10.1001/jamanetworkopen.2020.8393.

[37] Ramamurthi, D., Chau, C., & Jackler, R. K. (2018). JUUL and other stealth vaporisers: Hiding the habit from parents and teachers. *Tob Control*. https://doi. org/10.1136/tobaccocontrol-2018-054455.

[38] Liu J., Ramamurthi, D., & Halpern-Felsher, B. (2021). Inside the adolescent voice: A qualitative analysis of the appeal of different tobacco products. *Tobacco Induced Diseases, 19*(February), 15. https://doi.org/10.18332/tid/132856.

[39] Ambrose, B. K., Day, H. R., Rostron, B., Conway, K. P., Borek, N., Hyland, A., & Villanti, A. C. (2015). Flavored tobacco product use among US youth aged 12-17 years, 2013-2014. *Journal of the American Medical Association, 314*(17), 1871-1873. https://doi.org/10.1001/jama.2015.13802.

[40] Villanti, A. C., Johnson, A. L., Ambrose, B. K., Cummings, K. M., Stanton, C. A., Rose, S. W., Feirman, S. P., Tworek, C., Glasser, A. M., Pearson, J. L., Cohn, A. M., Conway, K. P., Niaura, R. S., Bansal-Travers, M., & Hyland, A. (2017). Flavored tobacco product use in youth and adults: Findings from the first wave of the PATH study (2013-2014). *American Journal of Preventive Medicine, 52*(2), 139-151. https://doi.org/10.1016/j. amepre.2017.01.026.

[41] Berg, C. J. (2016). Preferred flavors and reasons for e-cigarette use and discontinued use among never, current, and former smokers. *International Journal of Public Health, 61*(2), 225-236. https://dx.doi. org/10.1007%2Fs00038-015-0764-x.

[42] Marshal, M. P., Friedman, M. S., Stall, R., King, K. M., Miles, J., Gold, M. A., Bukstein, O. G., & Morse, J. Q. (2008). Sexual orientation and adolescent substance use: A meta-analysis and methodological review. *Addiction, 103*(4), 546-556. https://doi.org/10.1111/j.1360-0443.2008.02149.x.

[43] Day, J. K., Fish, J. N., Perez-Brumer, A., Hatzenbuehler, M. L., & Russell, S. T. (2017). Transgender youth substance use disparities: Results from a population-based sample. *Journal of Adolescent Health, 61*(6), 729-735. https://doi. org/10.1016/j.jadohealth.2017.06.024.

[44] Krueger, E. A., Fish, J. N., & Upchurch, D. M. (2020). Sexual orientation disparities in substance use: Investigating social stress mechanisms in a national sample. *Am J Prev Med, 58*(1), 59-68. https://doi.org/10.1016/j.amepre.2019.08.034.

[45] Katz-Wise S. L., Sarda, V., Austin, S. B., & Harris, S. K. (2021). Longitudinal effects of gender minority stressors on substance use and related risk and protective factors among gender minority adolescents. *PLoS One, 16*(6). https://doi.org/10.1371/journal.pone.0250500.

[46] Watson, R. J., Fish, J. N., McKay, T., Allen, S. H., Eaton, L., & Puhl, R. M. (2020). Substance use among a national sample of sexual and gender minority adolescents: Intersections of sex assigned at birth and gender identity. *LGBT Health, 7*(1), 37-46. https://dx.doi.org/10.1089%2Flgbt.2019.0066.

[47] Jacobus, J., & Tapert, S. F. (2014). Effects of cannabis on the adolescent brain. *Current Pharmaceutical Design, 20*(13), 2186-2193.

[48] D'Souza, D. C., Sewell, R. A., & Ranganathan, M. (2009). Cannabis and psychosis/schizophrenia: Human studies. *European Archives of Psychiatry and Clinical Neuroscience, 259*(7), 413-431. https://doi.org/10.1007/s00406-009-0024-2.

[49] U.S. Department of Health and Human Services. (2019). *U.S. Surgeon General's advisory: Marijuana use and the developing brain.* https://www.hhs.gov/surgeongeneral/reports-and-publications/addiction-and-substance-misuse/advisory-on-marijuana-use-and-developing-brain/index.html.

[50] Albaugh, M. D., Ottino-Gonzalez, J., Sidwell, A., Lepage, C., Juliano, A., Owens, M. M., Chaarani, B., Spechler, P., Fontaine, N., Rioux, P., Lewis, L., Jeon, S., Evans, A., D'Souza, D., Radhakrishnan, R., Banaschewski, T., Bokde, A. L. W., Quinlan, E. B., Conrod, P.,... Garavan, H. (2021). Association of cannabis use during adolescenece with neurodevelopment. *JAMA Psychiatry,* e211258. https://doi.org/10.1001/jamapsychiatry.2021.1258.

[51] D'Souza, D. C., Radhakrishnan, R., Naganawa, M., Ganesh, S., Nabulsi, N., Najafzadeh, S., Ropchan, J., Ranganathan, M., Cortes-Briones, J., Huang, Y., Carson, R. E., & Skosnik, P. (2020). Preliminary in vivo evidence of lower hippocampal synaptic density in cannabis use disorder. *Mol Psychiatry.* https://doi.org/10.1038/s41380-020-00891-4.

[52] Panlilio, L. V., & Justinova, Z. (2018). Preclinical studies of cannabinoid reward, treatments for cannabis use disorder, and addiction-related effects of cannabinoid exposure. *Neuropsychopharmacology, 43*(1), 116-141. https://doi.org/10.1038/npp.2017.193.

[53] Freeman, T., & Winstock, A. (2015). Examining the profile of high-potency cannabis and its association with severity of cannabis dependence. *Psychological medicine, 45*(15), 3181-3189. https://doi.org/10.1017/s0033291715001178.

[54] Galli, J. A., Sawaya, R. A., & Friedenberg, F. K. (2011). Cannabinoid Hyperemesis Syndrome. *Curr Drug Abuse Rev, 4*(4), 241-249. https://doi.org/10.2174/1874473711104040241.

[55] Ferner, R. (2018). Disposition of toxic drugs and chemicals in man 11th edition. *Clinical Toxicology, 56*(3), 234. https://doi.org/10.1080/15563650.2017.1388920.

[56] Tu, A. W., Ratner, P. A., & Johnson, J. L. (2008). Gender differences in the correlates of adolescents' cannabis use. *Substance Use and Misuse, 43*(10), 1438-1463. https://dx.doi. org/10.1080%2F10826080802238140.

[57] Henry, K. L., Thornberry, T. P., & Huizinga, D. H. (2009). A discrete-time survival analysis of the relationship between truancy and the onset of marijuana use. *Journal of Studies on Alcohol and Drugs, 70*(1), 5-15. https://doi.org/10.15288/jsad.2009.70.5.

[58] Marmorstein, N. R., White, H. R., Loeber, R., & Stouthamer-Loeber, M. (2010). Anxiety as a predictor of age at first use of substances and progression to substance use problems among boys. *Journal of Abnormal Child Psychology, 38*(2), 211-224. https://dx.doi.org/10.1007%2Fs10802-009-9360-y.

[59] Carvalho, A. F., Stubbs, B., Vancampfort, D., Kloiber, S., Maes, M., Firth, J., Kurdyak, P. A., Stein, D. J., Rehm, J., & Koyanagi, A. (2019). Cannabis use and suicide attempts among 86,254 adolescents aged 12–15 years from 21 low-and middle-income countries. *European Psychiatry, 56*(1), 8-13. https://doi.org/10.1016/j. eurpsy.2018.10.006.

[60] Hall, W. (2014). What has research over the past two decades revealed about the adverse health effects of recreational cannabis use? *Addiction, 110*(1), 19-35. https://doi.org/10.1111/add.12703.

[61] Paul, S. E., Hatoum, A. S., & Fine, J. D. (2020). Associations between prenatal cannabis exposure and childhood outcomes. *JAMA Psychiatry, 78*(1), 64-76. https://doi.org/10.1001/jamapsychiatry.2020.2902.

[62] Winters, K. C., & Lee, C.-Y. S. (2008). Likelihood of developing an alcohol and cannabis use disorder during youth: Association with recent use and age. *Drug and Alcohol Dependence, 92*(1-3), 239-247. https://dx.doi.org/10.1016%2Fj.drugalcdep.2007.08.005.

[63] Hasin, D. S., Saha, T. D., Kerridge, B. T., Goldstein, R. B., Chou, S. P., Zhang, H., Jung, J., Pickering, R. P., Ruan, W. J., Smith, S. M., Huang, B., & Grant, B. F. (2015). Prevalence of marijuana use disorders in the United States between 2001-2002 and 2012-2013. *JAMA Psychiatry, 72*(12), 1235-1242. https://doi.org/10.1001/jamapsychiatry.2015.1858.

[64] Budney, A. J., & Hughes, J. R. (2006). The cannabis withdrawal syndrome. *Curr Opin Psychiatry, 19*(3), 233-238. https://doi.org/10.1097/01. yco.0000218592.00689.e5.

[65] Allsop, D. J., Copeland, J., Norberg, M. M., Fu, S., Molnar, A., Lewis, J., & Budney, A. J. (2012). Quantifying the clinical significance of cannabis withdrawal. *PLoS One, 7*(9), e44864. https://doi. org/10.1371/journal.pone.0044864.

[66] Hughes, J. R., Naud, S., Budney, A. J., Fingar, J. R., & Callas, P. W. (2016). Attempts to stop or reduce daily cannabis use: An intensive natural history study. *Psychol Addict Behav, 30*(3), 389-397. https://doi.org/10.1037/adb0000155.

[67] Budney, A. J., Roffman, R., Stephens, R. S., & Walker, D. (2007). Marijuana dependence and its treatment. *Addict Sci Clin Pract, 4*(1), 4-16. https://dx.doi.org/10.1151%2Fascp07414.

[68] White, W. (2012). *Recovery/remission from substance use disorders: An analysis of reported outcomes in 415 scientific reports, 1868-2011.* Philadelphia Department of Behavorial Health and Intellectial disAbility Services, Great Lakes Addiction Technology Transfer Center. https://www.naadac.org/assets/2416/whitewl2012_ recoveryremission_from_substance_abuse_ disorders.pdf.

[69] Large, M., & Sharma, S. (2011). Cannabis use and earlier onset of psychosis: A systematic meta-analysis. *Arch Gen Psychiarty, 68*(6), 555-561. https://doi.org/10.1001/archgenpsychiatry.2011.5.

[70] Kuepper, R., Van Os, J., Lieb, R., Wittchen, H., Höfler, M., & Henquet, C. (2011). Continued cannabis use and risk of incidence and persistence of psychotic symptoms: 10 year follow-up cohort study. *BMJ, 342,* d738. https://doi.org/10.1136/bmj. d738.

[71] Silins, E., Horwood, L. J., Patton, G. C., Fergusson, D. M., Olsson, C. A., Hutchinson, D. M., Spry, E., Toumbourou, J. W., Degenhardt, L., Swift, W., Cofey, C., Tait, R. J., Letcher, P. Copeland, J., & Mattick, R. P. (2014). Young adult sequelae of adolescent cannabis use: An integrative analysis. *The Lancet Psychiatry, 1*(4), 286-293. https://doi. org/10.1016/s2215-0366(14)70307-4.

[72] Fergusson, D. M., & Boden, J. M. (2008). Cannabis use and later life outcomes. *Addiction, 103*(6), 969-976. https://doi.org/10.1111/j.1360-0443.2008.02221.x.

[73] Cerdá, M., Moffitt, T. E., Meier, M. H., Harrington, H., Houts, R., Ramrakha, S., Hogan, S., Poulton, R., & Caspi, A. (2016). Persistent cannabis dependence and alcohol dependence represent risks for midlife economic and social problems: A longitudinal cohort study. *Clinical Psychological Science, 4*(6), 1028-1046. https://doi.org/10.1177/2167702616630958.

[74] Esposito, M. H., Lee, H., Hicken, M. T., Porter, L. C., & Herting, J. R. (2017). The consequences of contact with the criminal justice system for health in the transition to adulthood. *Longit Life Course Stud, 8*(1), 57-74. https://doi.org/10.14301/llcs.v8i1.405.

[75] Gobbi, G., Atkin, T., Zytynski, T., Wang, S., Askari, S., Boruff, J., Ware, M., Marmorstein, N., Cipriani, A., Dendukuri, N., & Mayo, N. (2019). Association of cannabis use in adolescence and risk of depression, anxiety, and suicidality in young adulthood: A systematic review and meta-analysis. *JAMA Psychiatry, 76*(4), 426-434. https://doi. org/10.1001/jamapsychiatry.2018.4500.

[76] Fontanella, C. A., Steelesmith, D. L., Brock, G., Bridge, J. A., Campo, J. V., & Fristad, M. A. (2021). Association of cannabis use with self-harm and mortality risk among youths with mood disorders. *JAMA Pediatrics, 175*(4), 377-384. https://doi. org/10.1001/jamapediatrics.2020.5494.

[77] Han, B., Compton, W. M., Einstein, E. B., & Volkow, N. D. (2021). Associations of suicidality trends with cannabis use as a function of sex and depression status. *JAMA Network Open, 4*(6), e2113025. https://dx.doi. org/10.1001%2Fjama networkopen.2021.13025.

[78] Wadekar, A. S. (2020). Understanding opioid use disorder (OUD) using tree-based classifiers. *Drug and Alcohol Dependence, 208*, 107839. https://doi. org/10.1016/j.drugalcdep.2020.107839.

[79] Montoya, Z., Conroy, M., Vanden Heuvel, B., Pauli, C. S., & Park, S.-H. (2020). Cannabis contaminants limit pharmacological use of cannabidiol. *Frontiers in Psychiatry, 11,* 571832. https://dx.doi. org/10.3389%2Ffphar.2020.571832.

[80] Calabria, B., Degenhardt, L., Hall, W., & Lynskey, M. (2010). Does cannabis use increase the risk of death? Systematic review of epidemiological evidence on adverse effects of cannabis use. *Drug Alcohol Depend, 29*(3), 318-330. https://doi. org/10.1111/j.1465-3362.2009.00149.x.

[81] Crane, N. A., Schuster, R. M., Fusar-Poli, P., & Gonzalez, R. (2013). Effects of cannabis on neurocognitive functioning: Recent advances, neurodevelopmental influences, and sex differences. *Neuropsychol Rev, 23*(2), 117-137. https://doi. org/10.1007/s11065-012-9222-1.

[82] Monte, A. A., Shelton, S. K., Mills, E., Saben, J., Hopkinson, A., Sonn, B., Devivo, M., Chang, T., Fox, J., Brevik, C., Williamson, K., & Abbott, D. (2019). Acute illness associated with cannabis use, by route of exposure: An observational study. *Annals of Internal Medicine, 170*(8), 531-537. https://doi. org/10.7326/m18-2809.

[83] Hyshka, E. (2013). Applying a social determinants of health perspective to early adolescent cannabis use–An overview. *Drugs: Education, Prevention and Policy, 20*(2), 110-119. https://doi.org/10.3109/09687637.2012.752434.

[84] Hindocha, C., Freeman, T. P., Schafer, G., Gardner, C., Bloomfield, M. A. P., Bramon, E., Morgan, C. J. A., & Curran, H. V. (2020). Acute effects of cannabinoids on addiction endophenotypes are moderated by genes encoding the CB1 receptor and FAAH enzyme. *Addiction Biology, 25*(3), e12762. https://doi.org/10.1111/adb.12762.

[85] Burgdorf, C. E., Jing, D., Yang, R., Huang, C., Hill, M. N., Mackie, K., Milner, T. A., Pickel, V. M., Lee, F. S., & Rajadhyaksha, A. M. (2020). Endocannabinoid genetic variation enhances vulnerability to THC reward in adolescent female mice. *Science Advances, 6*(7). https://doi. org/10.1126/sciadv.aay1502.

[86] Johnson, E. C., Demontis, D., Thorgeirsson, T. E., Walters, R. K., Polimanti, R., Hatoum, A. S., Sanchez-Roige, S., Paul, S. E., Wendt, F. R., Clark, T., Lai, D., Reginsson, G. W., Zhou, H., He, J., Baranger, D. A. A., Gudbjartsson, D. F., Wedow, R., Adkins, D. E., Adkins, A. E.,… Agrawal, A. (2020). A large-scale genome-wide association study meta-analysis of cannabis use disorder. *Lancet Psychiatry, 7*(12), 1032-1045. https://doi.org/10.1016/s2215-0366(20)30339-4.

[87] Stephens, P. C., Sloboda, Z., Stephens, R. C., Teasdale, B., Grey, S. F., Hawthorne, R. D., & Williams, J. (2009). Universal school-based substance abuse prevention programs: Modeling targeted mediators and outcomes for adolescent cigarette, alcohol and marijuana use. *Drug and Alcohol Dependence, 102*(1-3), 19-29. https://doi. org/10.1016/j.drugalcdep.2008.12.016.

[88] Hollist, D. R., & McBroom, W. H. (2006). Family structure, family tension, and self-reported marijuana use: A research finding of risky behavior among youths. *Journal of Drug Issues, 36*(4), 975-998.

[89] Rusby, J. C., Light, J. M., Crowley, R., & Westling, E. (2018). Influence of parent–youth relationship, parental monitoring, and parent substance use on adolescent

substance use onset. *Journal of Family Psychology, 32*(3), 310-320. https://dx.doi. org/10.1037%2Ffam0000350.

[90] Kandel, D. B. (2001). *Parental influences on adolescent marijuana use and the baby boom generation: Findings from the 1979-1996 national household surveys on drug abuse*. U.S. Department of Health and Human Services, Substance Abuse and Mental Health Services Administration. https://files. eric.ed.gov/fulltext/ ED466906.pdf.

[91] Brook, J. S., Brook, D. W., Arencibia-mireles, O., Richter, L., & Whiteman, M. (2001). Risk factors for adolescent marijuana use across cultures and across time. *The Journal of Genetic Psychology, 162*(3), 357-374. https://doi. org/10.1080/ 00221320109597489.

[92] Borawski, E. A., Ievers-Landis, C. E., Lovegreen, L. D., & Trapl, E. S. (2003). Parental monitoring, negotiated unsupervised time, and parental trust: the role of perceived parenting practices in adolescent health risk behaviors. *Journal of Adolescent Health, 33*(2), 60-70. https://doi.org/10.1016/s1054-139x(03)00100-9.

[93] Vermeulen-Smit, E., Verdurmen, J., Engels, R., & Vollebergh, W. (2015). The role of general parenting and cannabis-specific parenting practices in adolescent cannabis and other illicit drug use. *Drug and Alcohol Dependence, 147*, 222-228. https://doi. org/10.1016/j.drugalcdep.2014.11.014.

[94] Schaps, E., & Solomon, D. (2003). The role of the school's social environment in preventing student drug use. *The Journal of Primary Prevention, 23*(3), 299-328. https://doi.org/10.1023/A:1021393724832.

[95] Ethier, K. A., Harper, C. R., & Dittus, P. J. (2018). School environment is related to lower health and safety risks among sexual minority middle and high school students. *Journal of Adolescent Health, 62*(2), 143-148. https://doi.org/10.1016/j. jadohealth.2017.08.024.

[96] Vogel, M., Rees, C. E., McCuddy, T., & Carson, D. C. (2015). The highs that bind: School context, social status and marijuana use. *Journal of Youth and Adolescence, 44*(5), 1153-1164. https://doi. org/10.1007/s10964-015-0254-8.

[97] Cornell, D., & Huang, F. (2016). Authoritative school climate and high school student risk behavior: A cross-sectional multi-level analysis of student self-reports. *Journal of Youth and Adolescence, 45*(11), 2246-2259. https://doi.org/10.1007/ s10964-016-0424-3.

[98] Sznitman, S. R., & Romer, D. (2014). Student drug testing and positive school climates: Testing the relation between two school characteristics and drug use behavior in a longitudinal study. *Journal of Studies on Alcohol and Drugs, 75*(1), 65-73. https://doi.org/10.15288/jsad.2014.75.65.

[99] Evans-Whipp, T. J., Plenty, S. M., Catalano, R. F., Herrenkohl, T. I., & Toumbourou, J. W. (2015). Longitudinal effects of school drug policies on student marijuana use in Washington state and Victoria, Australia. *American Journal of Public Health, 105*(5), 994-1000. https://dx.doi. org/10.2105%2FAJPH. 2014.302421.

[100] Mulla, M. M., Bogen, K. W., & Orchowski, L. M. (2020). The mediating role of school connectedness in the associations between dating and sexual violence

victimization and substance use among high school students. *Prev Med, 139*, 106197. https://doi.org/10.1016/j.ypmed.2020.106197.

[101] U.S. Department of Justice. (2000). *Promising strategies to reduce substance abuse: An OJP Issues and Practices Report.* https://www.ojp.gov/pdffiles1/ojp/183152.pdf.

[102] Fletcher, A., Bonell, C., Sorhaindo, A., & Rhodes, T. (2009). Cannabis use and 'safe' identities in an inner-city school risk environment. *International Journal of Drug Policy, 20*(3), 244-250. https://doi. org/10.1016/j.drugpo.2008.08.006.

[103] Education Development Center. (2017). *CAPT decision-support tools: Preventing youth marijuana use: Factors associated with use-using prevention research to guide prevention practice*. Substance Abuse and Mental Health Services Administration. http://www.ca-cpi.org/docs/Resources/SAMHSA/Preventing-Youth-Marijuana-Use.pdf.

[104] Van den Bee, M. B. M., & Pickworth, W. B. (2005). Risk factors predicting changes in marijuana involvement in teenagers. *JAMA Psychiatry, 62*(3), 311-319. https://doi.org/10.1001/archpsyc.62.3.311.

[105] Thornton, R. L., Glover, C. M., Cené, C. W., Glik, D. C., Henderson, J. A., & Williams, D. R. (2016). Evaluating strategies for reducing health disparities by addressing the social determinants of health. *Health Affairs, 35*(8), 1416-1423. https://doi. org/10.1377/hlthaff.2015.1357.

[106] National Conference of State Legislators. (2020, April 16). *State industrial hemp statutes*. https://www.ncsl.org/research/agriculture-and-rural-development/state-industrial-hemp-statutes.aspx.

[107] Cole, J. M. (2013, August 29). *Memorandum for all United States attorneys: Guidance regarding marijuana enforcement*. U.S. Department of Justice. https://www.justice.gov/iso/opa/resources/3052013829132756857467.pdf.

[108] National Conference of State Legislators. (2021, August 23). *State medical marijuana laws*. https://www.ncsl.org/research/health/state-medical-marijuana-laws.aspx.

[109] Ogden, D. W. (2009, October 19). *Memorandum for selected United States attorneys: Investigations and prosecutions in states authorizing the medical use of marijuana*. U.S. Department of Justice Archives. https://www.justice.gov/archives/opa/blog/memorandum-selected-united-state-attorneys-investigations-and-prosecutions-states.

[110] Lampe, J. R. (2019, October 9). *The Controlled Substance Act (CSA): A legal overview for the 116th Congress*. Congressional Research Service. https://sgp.fas.org/crs/misc/R45948.pdf.

[111] Maxwell, J. C., & Mendelson, B. (2016). What do we know about the impact of the laws related to marijuana? *Journal of Addiction Medicine, 10*(1), 3-12. https://dx.doi. org/10.1097%2FADM.0000000000000188.

[112] Svrakic, D. M., Lustman, P. J., Mallya, A., Lynn, T. A., Finney, R., & Svrakic, N. M. (2012). Legalization, decriminalization & medicinal use of cannabis: A scientific and public health perspective. *MO Med, 109*(2), 90-98. https://www.ncbi.nlm.nih. gov/pmc/articles/PMC6181739/.

Section 2. What Research Tells Us

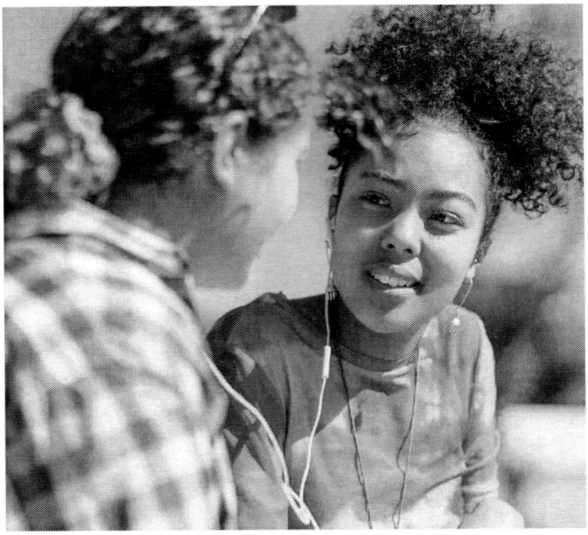

Substance use prevention programs seek to promote positive youth development and build social-emotional, refusal, self-efficacy, and other skills to reduce marijuana initiation and use. Environmental strategies aim to change or influence community conditions, systems, and policies. The interventions included in this section should not be considered in isolation. Prevention interventions are most effective when they are coordinated to complement and reinforce one another over time [1].

The programs and strategies included were selected after conducting a comprehensive environmental scan and in collaboration with subject matter experts. Eligible programs and policies were required to meet the following criteria:

- Be clearly defined and replicable
- Address the target outcome of reduction or prevention of marijuana use among youth (middle and high school students)
- Be currently in use
- Have accessible implementation supports

This section presents substance use prevention programs that show promise in reducing youth marijuana use or that are effective in reducing substance use in general. A table of prevention programs, with information on their intent, target populations, and key outcomes, is included. The section also discusses community interventions and environmental strategies. Although the environmental strategies presented are grounded in the tobacco and/or alcohol literature, some may also be effective in helping reduce youth marijuana use. States like New York, California, and Colorado are already in the early stages of implementing some of the interventions discussed.

Comprehensive Approaches to Prevention

Prevention is most effective when interventions are matched to the target population's level of risk and needs. To determine risk and needs, community coalitions and prevention organizations conduct a community needs assessment using available data to identify gaps in preventive efforts and the risk and protective factors that influence substance use.

Prevention interventions fall into three broad categories: [2]

1) *Universal prevention interventions* take the broadest approach and are designed to reach all individuals within a particular population by reducing risk factors and promoting protective factors. Universal prevention interventions may include policies/environmental strategies and programs that target individuals in schools, whole communities, or workplaces. Universal prevention interventions are likely to have the broadest impact in affecting populations of varied risk levels at once [3].
2) *Selective prevention interventions* target biological, psychological, or social risk factors that are more prominent among groups at high risk than among the wider population. They may also seek to increase protective factors. The audience for these interventions is often families, parents, or young people, or some combination. Examples include prevention education for youth groups or peer support groups for young adults with a family history of SUD.
3) *Indicated prevention interventions* target individuals who are already involved in risky behavior, such as substance use, that puts them at risk for SUD. These interventions include referrals to support services for youth who screen positive for substance use or violate substance use policies, or screening and consultation for families of youth admitted to hospitals with potential alcohol-related injuries.

Community coalitions can be essential partners active in selecting and implementing interventions within each of these categories. A strong prevention plan for a community combines programs and environmental strategies across the three categories to reach people with different risk levels and ensure a comprehensive prevention approach.

Research Opportunity

This evidence review identified research studies for alcohol, tobacco, and marijuana. Although the body of research around youth prevention with marijuana-related outcomes is growing, clinicians continue to face the challenge of limited evidence, particularly from well-designed randomized controlled trials (RCTs), when selecting programs to address youth marijuana use. The field would benefit from more research on youth marijuana use, prevention programs and environmental strategies, and the effectiveness of those strategies among diverse populations (inclusive of race, ethnicity, age, and sex).

Youth Substance Use Prevention Programs with Marijuana-Related Outcomes

There is an extensive body of literature demonstrating the effectiveness of substance use prevention programs for reducing youth tobacco, alcohol, and other drug use. Many of these interventions focus on positive youth development and building social-emotional, refusal, self-efficacy, and similar skills. The evidence behind these interventions has been reviewed extensively, including in the *Blueprints for Healthy Youth Development* and the *Surgeon General's Report on Alcohol, Drugs, and Health.*

Programs with a strong evidence base were further evaluated on whether they had been replicated, included fidelity supports, were in use or had been recently updated, and were not prohibitively expensive. These criteria were selected to ensure that diverse stakeholders across a variety of settings could feasibly implement the programs included in this chapter. These programs are potential options for families, schools, and communities seeking to prevent youth substance use.

Although some programs are designed to reduce youth marijuana use specifically, most are designed to address substance use in general. The programs listed in the table that are specifically designed to prevent marijuana use currently have limited research available; however, they may be promising in specifically preventing marijuana use among youth.

Promising Marijuana Use Prevention Interventions	Description	Primary Age and/or Grades	Expected Outcomes
Teen Marijuana Check-Up	A brief motivational enhancement intervention publicized as a non-pressured and confidential opportunity for the teen marijuana smoker to "take stock" of his/her use. The intervention is designed for in-school implementation and intended to elicit the teen's voluntary participation. Cost: It is estimated that the program costs approximately $100 per participant.	Grades 9 to 12	Reductions in quantity and frequency of marijuana use [4].
Cannabis/Marijuana Awareness and Prevention Toolkit	A theory-based and evidence-informed curriculum designed to be implemented by educators, parents, and/or community-based organizations. The curriculum is aimed at preventing middle and high school students from using marijuana. Cost: This program is available for free.	Middle and High School Students	Prevention of marijuana use (studies currently in progress).
SPORT	A single-session screening and brief intervention designed to promote positive healthy behaviors, such as engaging in physical exercise, while also preventing substance use. The creators of SPORT recently developed a new program "Marijuana Prevention Plus Wellness." This program is adopted from the original evidence-based SPORT program and is designed specifically to prevent marijuana use [5]. Cost: The module costs $499 per program (separate programs for high school, middle school, adolescent).	Ages 8 to 18; Elementary, Middle, and High School Students [5]	Prevention of marijuana use and promotion of healthy behaviors, such as engaging in physical activity [5].

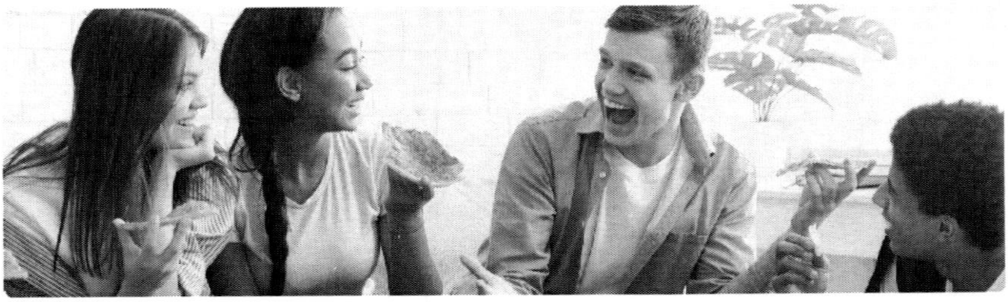

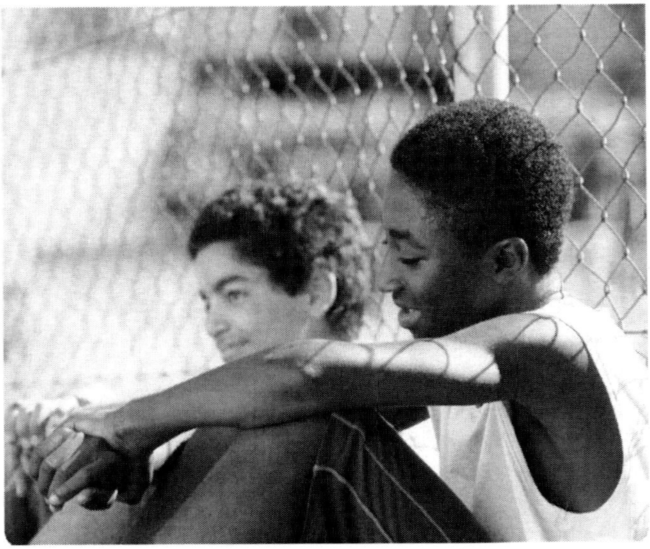

Broader substance use prevention programs may also have an impact on marijuana use in youth, either by addressing common risk and protective factors for marijuana or other substance use, or because they have a component of their larger program addressing marijuana use.

Each of the programs listed in the table below has demonstrated an impact on broader substance use-related outcomes and may have components that address marijuana specifically.

Additional detail on the evidence behind each of these programs can be found in the *Surgeon General's Report on Alcohol, Drugs, and Health.*

Substance Use Prevention Interventions	Description	Primary Age and/or Grades	Expected Outcomes
Family-Focused			
Familias Unidas	A program designed for Hispanic youth and families that targets risk factors, such as poor adolescent communication, and protective factors, such as parental involvement [6]. Cost: The Implementation Package costs $50,000 to train 10 participants. There are additional costs for more trainees.	Ages 12 to 18; Middle and High School Students [6]	Prevent substance use and risky sexual behaviors [6].
Guiding Good Choices	A five-session curriculum that supports parents in reducing the risk that their child will engage in substance use. Children attend one session that teaches substance use resistance skills. Parents attend the remaining four sessions and learn skills needed to reduce the risk that their child will engage in substance use [7]. Cost: A one-time group leader training is required. A 3-day on-site training for up to 12 participants is $4,200 plus travel. The Core Program Kit costs $881. Family Guides cost $13.99 per family.	Ages 11 to 14; Middle School Students [7]	Reduce drug use and related behavioral problems [7] Reduction in use and related behavioral problems, as found in a study with schools blocked on school size and a proportion of students in lower income households [7].
Strengthening Families Program	A program that reduces substance use and behavior problems among youth by engaging youth and their families in skills training sessions. Sessions are designed to enhance protective factors, such as family relationships, parenting skills, and youth social and emotional skills [8]. Cost: Estimates for the total program for one course of 10 families is $13,800, plus an additional $2,200 for 6 and 12 month boosters.	Ages 10 to 14; Middle and High School Students [8]	Reduce risk factors for later alcohol and drug use, mental health problems, and delinquency [8].

Substance Use Prevention Interventions	**Description**	**Primary Age and/or Grades**	**Expected Outcomes**
School-Focused			
All Stars	A student-centered program designed to delay the onset of risky behaviors among youth. The curriculum includes group activities, games, art projects, video making, small group discussions, partner work, and a parent component [9]. Cost: A package ranges from $4-10 per student; teachers' manuals are $100 each.	Ages 10 to 19; Elementary, Middle, and High School Students [9]	Delay the onset of risky behaviors. Specific behaviors targeted by the program include use of tobacco, marijuana, opioids, and inhalants, fighting and bullying, and early sexual activity [9].
Keepin' It Real	A substance use prevention and social and emotional competency enhancing program, in which lessons are based on real stories of adolescents and designed to be highly interactive. There are three versions of the program: multicultural, rural, and Spanish [10]. Cost: It is $300 to purchase the program, plus $7 per student.	Ages 11 to 19; Middle and High School Students [10]	Prevent substance use. Enhance social and emotional competencies [10].
LifeSkills Training	A classroom-based universal prevention program that teaches personal self-management, social, and information and resistance skills related to drug use [11]. Cost: Full curriculum sets range from $265-$645 for one teacher's manual and 30 student guides depending on grade level.	Ages 9 to 19; Elementary, Middle, and High School Students [11].	Prevent substance use and violent behaviors [11].
Good Behavior Game	Also called the PAX Good Behavior Game, this program is a set of strategies to help students learn important self-management skills while collaborating to make their classroom a peaceful and productive learning environment [12]. Cost: Each staff person implementing the program is required to purchase the standard kit ($199 per kit) or the PLUS kit ($249 per kit). Training ranges	Ages 5 to 11; Elementary School Students [12]	Increase capacity for self-regulation. Improve academic performance. Reduce alcohol and other illicit drug use. Improvement in health outcomes [13].

Substance Use Prevention Interventions	Description	Primary Age and/or Grades	Expected Outcomes
	from $2,500-$13,000 depending on number of training days needed.		
PreVenture	Prevents substance use among at-risk youth by introducing motivational pathways and coping skills tailored to each youth's personality profile [14]. Cost: There is no cost to participate, but facilitators must be trained ($780) and their certification renewed each year ($120).	Ages 13 to 19; High School Students [14]	Promote positive mental health outcomes and prevent substance use, including delayed initiation and reduced frequency of marijuana use [14].
Project Alert	Designed to instill negative attitudes and beliefs about drug use, while also equipping youth with the skills needed to say no to drugs. The program curriculum takes the form of short, fast-paced lessons that can be easily incorporated into the school day [15]. Cost: This program is available for free.	Ages 11 to 14; Middle School Students15	Reduce substance use. Foster anti-drug attitudes and beliefs. Improve drug resistance skills [15].
Project Towards No Drug Abuse	A drug prevention program designed for at-risk youth, providing instruction in motivation activities to not use drugs, skills in self-control, communication, and resource acquisition, and decision-making strategies [16]. Cost: Initial training and technical assistance costs $2,100 plus trainer travel costs for a two-day training for up to 25 teachers. An additional $200 per teacher's manual and $12 per student workbook.	Ages 14 to 19; High School Students [16]	Prevent problem behaviors, including alcohol, tobacco, and other drug use by positively affecting youth's decision-making, motivational factors, and skills such as social self-control [16]

Substance Use Prevention Interventions	Description	Primary Age and/or Grades	Expected Outcomes
Community-Focused			
Communities that Care*	A program that guides communities through a five-stage process, beginning with catalyzing community members and assessing a community's risks and strengths. The goals of the program are to promote healthy youth development, improve youth outcomes, and reduce problem behaviors [17]. Cost: Estimated costs for the first year of the program are $127,000 and include training and technical assistance, a coordinator, and a youth survey.	Ages 10 to 17; Middle and High School Students [17]	Prevent problem behaviors, including substance use and delinquency [17].
PROSPER* *PROmoting* *Partnerships to Enhance Resilience*	An evidence-based delivery system designed to strengthen families, build youth skills, and reduce youth substance use, as well as other problem behaviors. Community teams composed of representatives from community service agencies, parents, youth, and other community members implement the system [18]. Cost: Estimated costs for the first year of the program are $149,000 and include implementation plans, trainings, staff, access to the data system, and data collection.	Ages 10 to 14; Middle School Students [18]	Prevent problem behaviors, including substance use. Promote positive youth development and strong families [18].
*Note that these programs can be considered processes for selecting and implementing the most appropriate substance use interventions for specific communities. They are often defined as frameworks to support the successful implementation of prevention programs in communities.			

Community-Level Interventions/Environmental Strategies

Community-level interventions focus on the entire population or a specific population segment within a country, state, county, or city. Environmental strategies attempt to change social norms and attitudes, systems, and economic conditions to influence behavior and reduce marijuana use.

> States considering legalizing marijuana may want to establish a minimum purchasing and use age of at least 21, comparable to the legal age to purchase alcohol and tobacco. This is of particular importance when considering that marijuana remains illegal at the federal level and research continues to demonstrate its negative impacts on the developing brain.

Laws, policies, and ordinances are examples of community-level, environmental interventions. There are several evidence-based prevention policies stakeholders can consider for preventing marijuana use in states where non-medical or medical marijuana use is legal. Given the increasing number of states that have legalized marijuana for adult use, many local and state governments are grappling with how to best regulate a newly legal marijuana market. Stakeholders can implement each of the environmental strategies discussed in this section at the state and/or local level, depending on the specific laws of each state. Community coalitions and state and local public health officials should be involved in determining which environmental strategies are most appropriate and supporting the implementation of those strategies.

This section provides insight into some of the options communities are implementing to prevent and reduce youth marijuana use. It draws on evidence from alcohol and tobacco use prevention efforts and examples from states implementing these strategies as part of their marijuana retail system. When available, the guide separately presents the evidence related to marijuana.

Currently, evidence on the impact of these environmental strategies to prevent youth marijuana use is limited because legalization of marijuana is relatively new.

States and localities are only recently able to regulate marijuana's sale, purchase, and marketing.

The environmental strategies discussed here are a sample of evidence-based approaches that may reduce youth marijuana use. Many are based on evidence from alcohol and tobacco studies showing that reducing access to and the availability of substances significantly impacts youth use of those substances. The policies described in this chapter include regulating the price, number and characteristics of retail outlets that sell marijuana, specific products permitted to be sold, and content and placement of marijuana marketing.

Environmental strategies in this chapter are summarized in the table below.

Strategy	Characteristics	Expected Outcomes
Regulation of the price of marijuana	• Increasing taxes (either by weight, THC content, or price). • Banning price promotions (such as coupons, two for one deals, and happy hours).	• Decrease in youth marijuana use. • Decrease in use of high potency marijuana products [19]. This study uses administrative records from the Washington State Liquor and Cannabis Board [19].
Regulation of marijuana retail outlets	• Limiting number and locations of retailers through licensing or zoning. • Limiting hours/days of sale. • Banning those under the age of 21 in dispensaries. • Regulating where marijuana and related products can be sold.	• Decrease in youth marijuana use, as reported in a study that includes data from a cross-section of 6th, 8th, and 11th graders in 35 Oregon counties [20].
Regulation of marijuana product manufacturing and packaging	• Banning marijuana products with added synthetic flavors and odors. • Banning THC-infused edibles likely to attract children and youth, such as candies, cookies, and beverages. • Banning THC-infused alcohol and tobacco products. • Requiring plain product packaging. • Requiring transparency on product labels, including THC and CBD content and ingredients. • Require prominent graphic marijuana warning labels with varied and rotating messaging.	• Reduction in youth marijuana initiation. • Reduction in youth marijuana use and use disorder. • Reduction in use of flavored edibles. • Increased health knowledge. • Increased motivation to quit. • Reduced brand awareness and identification. • Reduction in product appeal. • Increase in understanding of the risks of marijuana [21-23].
Limitations on marijuana advertising and marketing	• Banning marijuana advertising on television, radio, billboards, and social media. • If not banned, limiting advertising with youth audiences. • Removing marketing, promotion, and advertising dollars from admissible business expenses for state income tax calculations. • Funding public health media campaigns. • Prohibiting health and therapeutic claims.	• Increase in understanding the risks of marijuana. • Reduction in positive perceptions of marijuana use. • Decrease in youth marijuana use. • Reduction in advertising by marijuana retailers [24-25]. The Davis study uses data from 6th through 12th graders in seven communities [25].

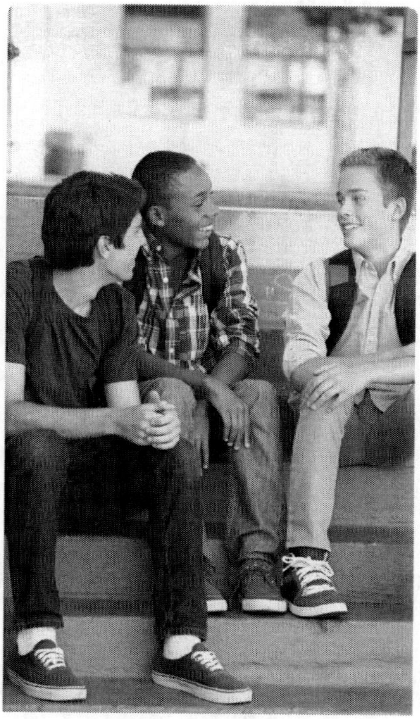

Price and Taxation of Marijuana

Like alcohol and tobacco, the cost of marijuana can be controlled by raising the price of the product through taxes and establishing a price floor (i.e., minimum price). Youth and young adults are particularly responsive to tax increases because they generally have limited disposable income; therefore, high prices deter purchase and use [26-28]. Based on studies about youth alcohol and tobacco use, increasing the cost of marijuana products by taxing them may be an effective marijuana use prevention and reduction intervention [29-30], though research on the effects of marijuana taxes on youth use are not currently available [31].

Raising alcohol and tobacco taxes is recommended as one of the best ways to reduce use, particularly among youth [32-33]. For example, increasing the price of cigarettes by 10 percent reduces adult smoking by only 2 percent, young adult (ages 20 to 25) smoking by 4 percent, and youth (ages 12 to 17) smoking by approximately 7 percent [34]. Data from 43 states found that for every dollar increase in the cigarette tax, there was a 2 percent reduction in smoking among 14- and 15-year-olds [35]. This study uses data from the 1999-2013 Youth Risk Behavior Surveys [35]. Similarly, a 10 percent increase in alcohol prices would be expected to result in a 3 to 10 percent decrease in alcohol consumption across the population [36, 32-33].

Revenue from increasing marijuana taxes may be earmarked specifically for prevention, treatment, counter-marketing, and research and evaluation to help continue efforts to protect the health and safety of youth. This revenue should supplement the funds that are already earmarked for these activities. For example:

- California uses tax revenue for a youth prevention, education, and treatment fund, as well as childcare and community reinvestment.
- Colorado uses tax revenue for education programs.
- Massachusetts uses tax revenue for public safety programs.
- Oregon uses tax revenue for drug misuse
- prevention and treatment programs.
- Maine plans to use its tax revenues for public health and public safety programs [37].

Importantly, any price strategy implemented should automatically account for inflation each year for the tax to not lose value over time.

In addition to taxation, banning price promotions, such as buy one get one free deals, happy hours, bulk purchases, or gifting marijuana products when non-marijuana products are sold and vice versa, can also help reduce youth marijuana use. This strategy has been shown effective in preventing use and misuse of alcohol and tobacco. For example, youth who live in counties with more coupons and price promotions are more likely to be current smokers than youth who live in counties with fewer coupons and price promotions [38-39]. The Kim study uses data from a representative sample of licensed tobacco retailers in New York [39].

Implementation Examples

- California has established a separate tax per ounce on marijuana flowers and leaves [40].
- Illinois [41] and New York [42] tax marijuana based on level of THC content.
- Washington has implemented a 37 percent excise tax on retail price, and bans discounts on marijuana, including coupons and sale/clearance products [43].

Regulation of Retail Outlets through Licensing and/or Zoning

There are two primary ways a jurisdiction or state can potentially limit the number and location of marijuana retailers: licensing and zoning [44].

Licensing regulates and affords certain rights to businesses and can be used to limit the number of marijuana establishments. Zoning rules are legal guides that determine where businesses can operate and determine where marijuana establishments can be located [44].

Licensing and zoning authority generally depends on the regulatory structure of the state and localities; and licensing can often be controlled through a public health entity, such as a local or state public health department. A state's regulatory structure, specifically the state's marijuana laws, will likely dictate how much authority localities have in passing licensing, zoning, or other ordinances. Licensing is often done at the state level but can also be combined with local licensing. Zoning is one of the strategies most frequently implemented by local city and county governments to regulate access to marijuana in response to their specific local data.

These policies should be considered in tandem. For example, pairing a zoning ordinance with density caps on retailers can help avoid clustering of numerous outlets within one small area, which has shown adverse effects for youth alcohol use [45-46], and can help prevent marijuana establishments from being disproportionately located in low income areas [47]. For marijuana outlets, a government-controlled distribution system may have the greatest potential to protect public health, as is the case for alcohol in 17 states and several other jurisdictions [48-49].

Implementation Examples

- Washington [50] and Oregon [51] do not allow marijuana outlets within 1,000 feet of any school or other sensitive areas.
- Nevada limits retail licensing based on population size at the county level. For example, a county with a population between 100,000 and 699,999 may have up to 20 licensed retailers, whereas counties with 55,000 to 99,999 people may have four, and counties with populations of less than 55,000 may license two retailers [52].

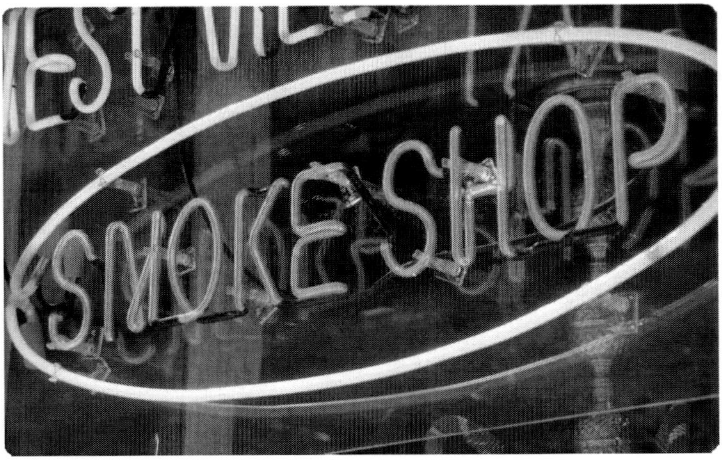

Restricting Youth Access to Marijuana in Retail Establishments

States and jurisdictions can limit marijuana retailer hours and the manner of marijuana delivery to reduce youth access. The Community Preventive Services Task Force[4] recommends limiting the hours of alcohol sale in on-premise settings based on evidence that it reduces excessive alcohol consumption and related harms [29, 53]. Local and state governments can take a similar approach in regulating marijuana and some have already done so.

Additionally, allowing youth into marijuana establishments may create numerous challenges, including requiring age verification at the point of sale in addition to the point of entry, and normalizing marijuana use for youth. Allowing access to marijuana establishment only to people 21 and older can help prevent these challenges.

Relatedly, states have reduced youth exposure to marijuana products by mandating that only marijuana is sold in explicitly licensed dispensaries and establishments; other products, such as sodas, snacks, alcohol, or tobacco are not to be sold in these establishments. Similarly, prohibiting marijuana sales in grocery stores and other retail establishments will decrease availability of, and youth access to, the product.

---

[4] The Community Preventive Services Task Force is an independent panel of public health and prevention experts who come together to provide evidence-based findings and recommendations on community-based health promotion and disease prevention interventions.

Implementation Examples

- Colorado has restricted the hours that marijuana retailers can be open from 8 a.m. to midnight [54].
- All states currently require anyone entering marijuana establishments to be at least 21 years old, except for those with a medical recommendation.

Banning Products and Packaging That Attract Youth

Marijuana products with added synthetic flavors and odors (such as fruit and candy) may be particularly attractive to youth. These products, typically flavored for inhalation, include vapes and flavored wrappers for combusted products like blunts. Additionally, strains and products may be named as if they were flavored (e.g., mango vapes, Cherry Pie, Pineapple Haze, Peanut Butter Cup) even if they are not, which may be just as effective at attracting youth. THC-infused foods and beverages, such as candies, cookies, sodas, and teas may also have packaging that mimics existing food or beverage products commonly marketed to youth. States that have legalized non-medical marijuana have considered banning these products. Products attractive to youth should be prohibited using clear, detailed, and enforceable regulations.

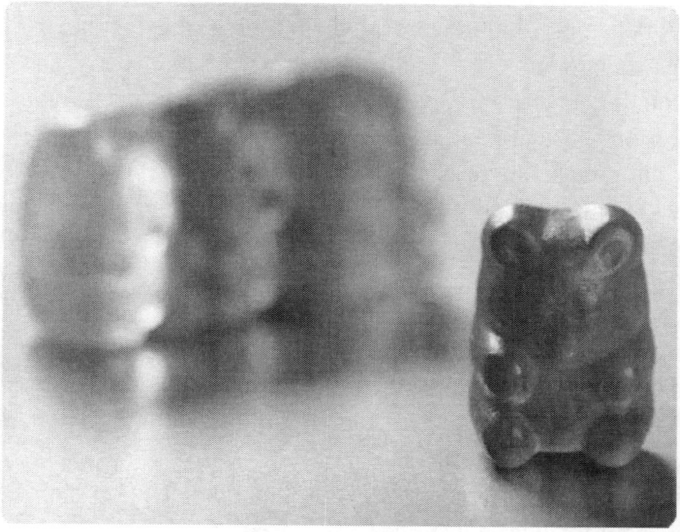

Additionally, marijuana products with high potency pose increased health risk to youth [55-56], including increase in frequency of use, likelihood of marijuana dependence, and risk of an anxiety disorder and psychosis [57-58]. Regulating the products that are sold and how they are packaged may help prevent youth initiation or reduce current use. Research on flavored tobacco bans found a decrease in adolescent tobacco use after passage of this policy, including reductions in the probability of being a smoker and the number of cigarettes smoked [59].

Implementation Examples

- Contra Costa County, California has prohibited flavored marijuana products for combustion or inhalation and banned vaping products to protect youth.60 Michigan, Oregon [61], and four California cities have banned THC-infused beverages [61].
- Connecticut limits flower potency to 30 percent THC and concentrates to 60 percent, and prohibits the addition of flavors, terpenes, and other additives to marijuana unless pre-approved [62].

Regulating Marijuana Packaging

Marijuana product packaging with cartoon images or imagery appeals to youth. For example, children are drawn to food packaging that includes color, novel shapes, products that smell sweet, fruity, or like candy, and cartoons or promotional characters [63]. The imagery on products serves as brand identification for youth and as marketing at in-store displays [22]. Efforts to reduce youth-appealing marketing and the implementation of plain packaging laws for tobacco products have led to reductions in youth tobacco use [64-65].

The Dunlop study used data from adult smokers in New South Wales, Australia [64]. Packaging can be regulated to reduce youth access by requiring it to be tamper-resistant, child-resistant, opaque, and resealable. They can be made less attractive to children and youth by restricting names, flavors, images of people, animals, cartoon figures, bright colors, logos, and branding [66], and prohibiting products and packaging that imitate non-marijuana products (such as candy, chips, or granola bars) [22].

Additionally, marijuana packaging, particularly on edibles, can be mandated to include nutrition facts and serving sizes, ingredient lists, expiration dates, and lot numbers. Regulations can explicitly prohibit false statements or health claims on packaging labels.

Finally, clear and large warning labels identifying the harms of marijuana use should be placed on the marijuana packaging, as is done with both tobacco and alcohol products.

Implementation Examples

- Alaska and Massachusetts have mandated opaque, plain packaging for marijuana products [67-68]. Hawaii has done the same for medical marijuana [69].
- Indiana, Utah, Texas, and Florida require a QR code that allows consumers to look up batch numbers, potency, and other ingredients [70-73].
- Canada requires prominent rotating warning labels on a yellow background. For example: "WARNING: Adolescents and young adults are at greater risk of harms from cannabis. Daily or near-daily use over a prolonged period of time can harm brain development and function" [74].
- California requires that all marijuana products include a warning label. The label must read: "WARNING: This product can expose you to marijuana smoke, which is known to the state of California to cause cancer, birth defects, and other reproductive harm" [75].

Limiting Marijuana Advertising and Marketing

There is a substantial body of literature that shows that increased exposure to alcohol and tobacco marketing leads to increases in youth use of these products [76-78]; similar findings are emerging in marijuana marketing, as well [79].

A recent report found that 69 percent of U.S. consumers do not understand the difference between THC and CBD [65]. Additionally, technical names for THC analogs (e.g., Delta-8, Delta-10, and THC-O acetate) can further confuse consumers. Transparency on marijuana product labels can help consumers distinguish between CBD products that do and do not have THC elements, preventing potentially harmful levels of THC in the bloodstream, particularly among youth [64-65].

Reducing youth exposure to marijuana marketing may help prevent or reduce marijuana use among youth and young adults. Strategies include banning advertising on television, radio, billboards, and social media, and limiting advertising with youth audiences, such as advertising on billboards or other forms of media. For example, advertising can be prohibited in venues where more than 10 or 15 percent of the audience are youth between the ages of 12 and 20 [80-81].

Additional strategies include reducing misleading information about the harmfulness of marijuana products by prohibiting health-related claims on any marijuana advertisements, and removing marijuana marketing, promotion, and advertising dollars from admissible business expenses for tax purposes.

Implementation Examples

- Colorado has instituted a policy that retail marijuana establishments cannot advertise on television, radio, print media, or websites where more than 30 percent of the audience is under the age of 21 [82]. Other states may consider lower thresholds, such as 10 to 15 percent.
- Mono County and the city of Palm Springs in California do not allow health or therapeutic claims on marijuana products or their marketing.

Funding Public Health Media Campaigns

To counteract the marketing and advertising campaigns of the marijuana industry, states and communities can develop public health media campaigns to promote science-based messages about youth marijuana use, leading to reductions in youth use and shifts away from positive attitudes.

These campaigns are most effective when used in conjunction with other environmental strategies, such as taxes [21]. Public health prevention campaigns, such as the Truth Campaign, that discuss the harms of certain products have been effective in preventing and reducing youth substance use [25].

Social Media

While paid advertisements for marijuana products are prohibited on social media platforms, such as Facebook, Instagram, and Twitter, there is still substantial marijuana marketing through other channels, such as social media influencers sharing posts of the product. Influencers are people who have built a reputation for their knowledge on a specific product or lifestyle, and who will often share brands or products with their followers, encouraging them to purchase those products. Studies have found that pro-marijuana content is prevalent on social media frequently seen by youth and young adults [83]. One in three youth in states with legal recreational marijuana have been found to engage (such as liking or following) with marijuana brands on social media [84]. This engagement poses a challenge to parents, communities, and stakeholders, as exposure to marijuana marketing is linked with increased use [85].

The role of state and local governments in regulating advertising on social media is challenging. States such as Rhode Island have taken innovative approaches to reduce marijuana marketing by third parties on social media, requiring that if any third party uses a marijuana brand's trademark, brand, name, location, or other characteristics on social media, the company must notify the Department of Business Regulation. The marijuana company must also send a cease-and-desist notice to the third party [86].

Additionally, parents and community coalitions can work directly with social media platforms to discourage marketing of these products by third parties.

References

[1] McMorris, B. J., Hemphill, S. A., Toumbourou, J. W., Catalano, R. F., & Patton, G. C. (2007). Prevalence of substance use and delinquent behavior in adolescents from Victoria, Australia and Washington State, United States. *Health Educ Behav, 34*(4), 634-650. https://doi. org/10.1177%2F1090198106286272.

[2] Institute of Medicine. (1994). *Reducing risks for mental disorder: Frontiers for preventive intervention research* (P. J. Mrazek, & R. J. Haggerty, Eds.). The National Academic Press. https://pubmed.ncbi.nlm.nih.gov/25144015/.

[3] Frieden, T. R. (2010). A framework for public health action: The health impact pyramid. *American Journal of Public Health, 100*(4), 590-595. https://dx.doi.org/10.2105%2FAJPH.2009.185652.

[4] Budney, A. J., Roffman, R., Stephens, R. S., & Walker, D. (2007). Marijuana dependence and its treatment. *Addict Sci Clin Pract, 4*(1), 4-16. https://dx.doi.org/10.1151%2Fascp07414.

[5] Prevention Plus Wellness. (2021). *Marijuana prevention plus wellness.* https://preventionpluswellness.com/products/sport-marijuana-awareness-program.

[6] University of Miami Miller School of Medicine Department of Public Health. (n.d.). *Familias Unidas*. https://familias-unidas.info/.

[7] Blueprints for Healthy Youth Development. (2018). *Guiding Good Choices (GGC)*. https://www.blueprintsprograms.org/guiding-good-choices-ggc/.

[8] Kumpfer, K. (2020). *Strengthening Families Program*. https://strengthening familiesprogram.org/.

[9] All Stars. (2021). *All Stars Core*. https://www. allstarsprevention.com/all-stars-core.html.

[10] Real Prevention. (n.d.). *Keepin' it real*. https://real-prevention.com/keepin-it-real/.

[11] Botvin LifeSkills Training. (n.d.). *Program Structure*. https://www.lifeskills training.com/program-structure/.

[12] Blueprints for Healthy Youth Development. (2021). *Good Behavior Game*. https://www. blueprintsprograms.org/programs/20999999/good-behavior-game/.

[13] PAXIS Institute. (2021). *PAX Good Behavior Game*. https://www.paxis.org/pax-good-behavior-game.

[14] Venture Lab. (n.d.). *Preventure*. https://www. conrodventurelab.com/projets/ preventure.

[15] Project Alert. (2021). *Substance abuse prevention for grades 7 & 8*. https://www.projectalert.com/.

[16] University of Southern California Institute for Prevention Research. (2021). *Project Towards No Drug Abuse*. https://tnd.usc.edu/.

[17] University of Washington. (2021). *The Center for Communities that Care*. https://www.communitiesthatcare.net/.

[18] Prosper. (2021). *PROSPER Partnerships*. http://helpingkidsprosper.org/.

[19] Hansen, B., Miller, K., & Weber, C. (2017). The taxation of recreational marijuana evidence from Washington state. *NBER Working Paper Series, 23632*. https://www.nber.org/system/files/working_papers/w23632/revisions/w23632.rev 0.pdf.

[20] Paschall, M. J., & Grube, J. W. (2021). Recreational marijuana availability in Oregon and use among adolescents. *Am J Prev Med, 58*(2), 63-69. https://dx.doi.org/10.1016%2Fj.amepre.2019.09.020.

[21] Wakefield, M. A., Loken, B. & Hornik, R. C. (2010). Use of mass media campaigns to change health behaviour. *The Lancet, 376*(9748), 1261-1271. https://dx.doi.org/10.1016%2 FS0140-6736(10)60809-4.

[22] Orenstein, D. G., & Glantz, S. A. (2018). Regulating cannabis manufacturing: Applying public health best practices from tobacco control. *Journal of Psychoactive Drugs, 50*(1), 19-32. https://dx.doi.org/10.1080%2F02791072. 2017.1422816.

[23] National Center for Chronic Disease Prevention and Health Promotion (US) Office on Smoking and Health. (2012). *Preventing tobacco use among youth and young adults: A report of the Surgeon General*. https://www.ncbi.nlm.nih. gov/books/NBK99237/.

[24] Jacobs, L. G. (2017). Regulating marijuana advertising and marketing to promote public health: Navigating the constitutional minefield. *Lewis & Clark Review, 21*(4), 1081-1133.

[25] Davis, K. C., Farrelly, M. C., Messeri, P., & Duke, J. (2009). The impact of national smoking prevention campaigns on tobacco-related beliefs, intentions to smoke and smoking initiation: Results from a longitudinal survey of youth in the United States. *Int. J. Environ. Res. Public Health, 6*(2), 722-740. https://dx.doi.org/10.3390%2Fijerph6020722.

[26] Van Ours, J. C. (2007). Cannabis use when it's legal. *Addictive Behaviors, 32*(7), 1441-1450. https://papers.ssrn.com/sol3/papers.cfm?abstract_ id=670141.

[27] Pacula, R. L., & Lundberg, R. (2014). Why changes in price matter when thinking about marijuana policy: A review of the literature on the elasticity of demand. *Public Health Review, 35*(2), 1-18. https://dx.doi.org/10.1007%2FBF03391701.

[28] Gruber, J., & Zinman, J. (2001). Youth smoking in the U.S.: Evidence and implications. In J. Gruber (Ed.), *Risky behavior among youths: An economic analysis* (pp. 69-120). University of Chicago Press. https://www.nber.org/system/files/chapters/c10687/c10687.pdf.

[29] Community Preventive Services Task Force. (2009). *Alcohol - Excessive consumption: Maintaining limits on hour of sale*. https://www.thecommunityguide.org/findings/alcohol-excessive-consumption-maintaining-limits-hours-sale.

[30] Wagenaar, A. C., Tobler, A. L., & Komro, K. A. (2010). Effects of alcohol tax and price policies on morbidity and mortality: A systematic review. *Am J Public Health, 100*(11), 2270-2278. https://dx.doi. org/10.2105%2FAJPH.2009.186007.

[31] Chaloupka, F. J., Yureki, A., & Fong, G. T. (2012). Tobacco taxes as a tobacco control strategy. *Tobacco Control, 21*, 172-180. https://doi.org/10.1136/tobaccocontrol-2011-050417.

[32] World Health Organization. (2017). *Tobacco taxes in WHO member states.* https://www.who.int/tobacco/global_report/2017/technical_note_III.pdf.

[33] Chisholm, D., Doran, C., Shibuya, K., & Rehm, J. R. (2006). Comparative cost-effectiveness of policy instruments for reducing the global burden of alcohol, tobacco and illicit drug use. *Drug and Alcohol Review, 25*, 552-563. https://doi.org/10.1080/09595230600944487.

[34] Chaloupka, F. J., & Warner, K. E. (1999). The Economics of Smoking. *NBER Working Paper Series, 7047*. 10.3386/w7047.

[35] Hawkins, S. S., Bach, N., & F.Baum, C. (2016). Impact of tobacco control policies on adolescent smoking. *Journal of Adolescent Health, 58*(6), 679-685. https://dx.doi.org/10.1016%2Fj. jadohealth.2016.02.014.

[36] Elder, R., Lawrence, B., Aneeqah, Ferguson, Naimi, T. S., Brewer, R. D., Chattopadhyay, S. K., Toomey, T. L., & Fielding, J. E. (2010). The effectiveness of tax policy interventions for reducing excessive alcohol consumption and related harms. *Am J Prev Med, 38*(2), 217-229. https://dx.doi. org/10.1016%2Fj.amepre.2009.11.005.

[37] Urban Institute. (2021). *Marijuana taxes.* https://www.urban.org/policy-centers/cross-center-initiatives/state-and-local-finance-initiative/state-and-local-backgrounders/marijuana-taxes#:~:text=Marijuana%20purchases%20are%20also%20subject,and%20%240.35%20per%20 marijuana%20seed.

[38] Pacula, R. L., Kilmer, B., Wagenaar, A. C., Frank J. Chaloupka, & Jonathan P. Caulkins. (2014). Developing public health regulations for marijuana: Lessons

from alcohol and tobacco. *Am J Public Health, 104*(6), 1012-1028. https://dx.doi.org/10.2105%2FAJPH.2013.301766.

[39] Kim, A. E., Loomis, B. R., Busey, A. H., Farrelly, M. C., Willett, J. G., & Juster, H. R. (2013). Influence of retail cigarette advertising, price promotions, and retailer compliance on youth smoking-related attitudes and behaviors. *Journal of Public Health Management and Practice, 19*(6), E1-9. https://doi.org/10.1097/phh.0b013e3182980c47.

[40] California Department of Tax and Fee Administration. (2020). *Tax guide for cannabis businesses*. https://www.cdtfa.ca.gov/industry/cannabis.htm.

[41] Illinois Revenue. (n.d.). *Cannabis taxes*. https://www2.illinois.gov/rev/research/taxinformation/other/Pages/Cannabis-Taxes.aspx.

[42] Newman, G., & Peleg, S. (2021). Tax issues and the New York Regulation and Taxation Act. *The National Law Review, XI*(90). https://www.natlawreview.com/article/tax-issues-and-new-york-marijuana-regulation-and-taxation-act.

[43] Washington State Liquor and Cannabis Board. (2020). *Marijuana Tax Reporting Guide*. https://lcb. wa.gov/taxreporting/marijuana-tax-reporting-guide.

[44] ChangeLab Solutions and National Policy & Legal Analysis Network. (2012). *Healthy planning policies: A compendium from California general plans*. https://www. changelabsolutions.org/sites/default/files/Healthy_Planning_Policies_Compendium_FINAL_%28CLS-20120530%29_090925.pdf.

[45] Grubesic, T. H., & Pridemore, W. A. (2011). Alcohol outlets and clusters of violence. *International Journal of Health Geographics, 10,* 30. https://dx.doi.org/10.1186%2F1476-072X-10-30.

[46] Reboussin, B. A., Song, E.-Y., & Wolfson, M. (2011). The impact of alcohol outlet density on the geographic clustering of underage drinking behaviors within census tracts. *Alcoholism: Clinical and Experimental Research, 35*(8), 1541-1549. https://dx.doi.org/10.1111%2Fj.1530-0277.2011.01491.x.

[47] Trangenstein, P. J., Sadler, R. C., Morrison, C. N., & Jernigan, D. H. (2020). Looking back and moving forward: The evolution and potential opportunities for the future of alcohol density measurement. *Addiction Research & Theory, 29*(2), 117-128. https://doi.org/10.1080/16066359.2020.1751128.

[48] Silver, L. D., Naprawa, A. Z., & Padon, A. A. (2020). Assessment of incorporation of lessons from tobacco control in city and county laws regulating legal marijuana in California. *JAMA Network Open, 3*(6), e208393-e208393. https://doi.org/10.1001/jamanetworkopen.2020.8393.

[49] Hahn, R. A., Middleton, J. C., Elder, R., Brewer, R., Fielding, J., Naimi, T. S., Toomey, T. L., Chattopadhyay, S., Lawrence, B., & Campbell, C. A. (2012). Effects of alcohol retail privatization on excessive alcohol consumption and related harms: A community guide systematic review. *Am J Prev Med, 42*(4), 418-427. https://doi.org/10.1016/j. amepre.2012.01.002.

[50] Municipal Research and Services Center (MRSC). (2019). *Marijuana Regulation in Washington State*. http://mrsc.org/getdoc/8cd49386-c1bb-46f9-a3c8-2f462dcb576b/Marijuana-Regulation-in-Washington-State.aspx.

[51] Oregon Health Authority. (n.d.) *Medical Marijjuana Dispensary Directory*. https://www.oregon. gov/oha/ph/diseasesconditions/chronicdisease/medical marijuanaprogram/pages/dispensary-directory.aspx.

[52] State of Nevada. (2020). 2020 Nevada Revised Statutes, Chapter 678B-Licensing and Control of Cannabis. https://law.justia.com/codes/nevada/2020/chapter-678b/.

[53] Community Preventive Services Task Force. (2008). *Alcohol-Excessive consumption: Maintaining limits on days of sale*. https://www.thecommunity guide.org/findings/alcohol-excessive-consumption-maintaining-limits-days-sale.

[54] State of Colorado. (n.d.). *Laws about marijuana use*. https://www.colorado. gov/pacific/marijuana/laws-about-marijuana-use#:~:text=Limited%20hours%20 of%20sale%3A,you%20head%20to%20a%20retailer.

[55] U.S. Department of Health and Human Services. (2019). *U.S. Surgeon General's advisory: Marijuana use and the developing brain*. https://www.hhs.gov/surgeongeneral/reports-and-publications/addiction-and-substance-misuse/advisory-on-marijuana-use-and-developing-brain/index.html.

[56] Stuyt, E. (2018). The problem with the current high potency THC marijuana from the perspective of an addiction psychiatrist. *Missouri Medicine, 115*(6), 482-486.

[57] Di Forti, M., Morgan, C., Dazzan, P., Pariante, C., Mondelli, V., Marques, T. R., Handley, R., Luzi, S., Russo, M., Paparelli, A., Butt, A., Stilo, S. A., Wiffen, B., Powell, J., & Murray, R. M. (2009). High-potency cannabis and the risk of psychosis. *Br J Psychiatry, 195*(6), 488-491.

[58] Hines, L. A., Freeman, T. P., Gage, S. H., Zammit, S., Hickman, M., Cannon, M., Munafo, M., MacLeod, J., & Heron, J. (2020). Association of high-potency cannabis use with mental health and substance in adolescence *JAMA Psychiatry, 77*(10), 1044-1051. https://dx.doi. org/10.1001%2Fjamapsychiatry.2020.1035.

[59] Courtemanche, C. J., Palmer, M. K., & Pesko, M. F. (2017). Influence of the flavored cigarette ban on adolescent tobacco use. *Am J Prev Med, 52*(5), e139-e146. https://dx.doi.org/10.1016%2Fj. amepre.2016.11.019.

[60] Getting It Right From the Start. (2021). *Examples of what your neighbors are doing to protect youth, public health, and socail equity*. https://gettingitrightfromthestart.org/wp-content/uploads/2021/02/Best-Practices-in-Action-Map_2-2-21.pdf.

[61] Oregon Liquor Control Commission. (2020). *Non-cannabis additives in inhalable cannabinoid products: Rationale for rulemaking*. https://www.oregon.gov/olcc/Docs/commission_agendas/2020/Non-Cannabis-Addtives-in-Inhalable-Cannabinoid-Products.pdf.

[62] Visit New England. (2021). *Marijuana in Connecticut*. https://www.visit connecticut.com/state/marijuana-in-connecticut/.

[63] University of Washington. (2016). Factors that might attract children to marijuana edibles. *Science Daily*. https://www.sciencedaily.com/releases/2016/08/ 160825141908.htm.

[64] Dunlop, S. M., Dobbins, T., Young, J. M., Perez, D., & Currow, D. C. (2014). Impact of Australia's introduction of tobacco plain packs on adult smokers' pack-related perceptions and responses: results from a continuous tracking survey. *BMJ Open, 4*(12), e005836. https://dx.doi. org/10.1136%2Fbmjopen-2014-005836.

[65] Hammond, D., Wakefield, M., & Durkin, E. B. (2013). Tobacco packaging and mass media campaigns: Research needs for Articles 11 and 12 of the WHO Framework Convention on Tobacco Control. *Nicotine Tob Res, 15*(4), 817-831. https://doi.org/10.1093/ntr/nts202.

[66] Story, M., & French, S. (2004). Food advertising and marketing directed at children and adolescents in the US. *Int J Behav Nutr Phys Act, 1*(1), 3. https://doi.org/10.1186/1479-5868-1-3.

[67] State of Alaska. (2021). Section 3 Alaska Adminstrative Code § 306.345 - Packaging and labeling. https://casetext.com/regulation/alaska-administrative-code/title-3-commerce-community-and-economic-development/part-19-alcoholic-beverage-control-board/chapter-306-marijuana-control/article-3-retail-marijuana-stores/section-3-aac-306345-packaging-and-labeling.

[68] Massachusetts Cannabis Control Commission 935 Mass. Reg. 500.150 - Edibles (2021). https://casetext.com/regulation/code-of-massachusetts-regulations/department-935-cmr-cannabis-control-commission/title-935-cmr-500000-adult-use-marijuana/section-500150-edibles.

[69] Hawaii Administrative Rules, Medical Marijuana Dispensaries, Publ. L. No. 11-850-92 - Packaging and labeling for retail sale (2015). https://health. hawaii.gov/opppd/files/2015/06/11-850.pdf.

[70] Indiana Code § 24-4-21-4 (2018). Packaging requirements. https://law.justia.com/codes/indiana/2018/title-24/article-4/chapter-21/section-24-4-21-4/.

[71] Utah Publ. L. No. R68-26-5 - Label Requirements (2020). https://ag.utah.gov/wp-content/uploads/2020/11/R68-26.pdf.

[72] Texas Publ. L. No. §300.402 - Packaging and Labeling Requirements (2020). https://www.law. cornell.edu/regulations/texas/25-Tex-Admin-Code-300-402.

[73] State of Florida. (2019). Florida State Senate Bill No. CS/CS/SB 1020: State hemp program. https://www.flsenate.gov/Session/Bill/2019/01020.

[74] Government of Canada. (2019). *Cannabis health warning messages.* https://www.canada.ca/en/health-canada/services/drugs-medication/cannabis/laws-regulations/regulations-support-cannabis-act/health-warning-messages.html.

[75] State of California. (1986) Safe Drinking Water and Toxic Enforcement Act, Proposition 65. https://oehha.ca.gov/proposition-65.

[76] Jernigan, D., Noel, J., Landon, J., Thornton, N., & Lobstein, T. (2017). Alcohol marketing and youth alcohol consumption: A systematic review of longitudinal studies published since 2008. *Addiction, 12*(Suppl 1), 7-20. https://doi.org/10.1111/add.13591.

[77] Sargent, J. D., Cukier, S., & Babor, T. F. (2020). Alcohol marketing and youth drinking: Is there a causal relationship, and why does it matter? *Journal of Studies on Alcohol and Drugs, Supplement*, Suppl 19, 5-12. https://dx.doi.org/10.15288%2Fjsads.2020. s19.5.

[78] Soneji, S., Barrington-Trimis, J. L., & Wills, T. A. (2017). Association between initial use of e-cigarettes and subsequent cigarette smoking among adolescents and young adults: A systematic review and meta-analysis. *JAMA Pediatrics, 171*(8), 788-797. https://dx.doi. org/10.1001%2Fjamapediatrics.2017.1488.

[79] Ayers, J. W., Caputi, T. L., & Leas, E. C. (2019). The need for federal regulation of marijuana marketing. *JAMA, 321*(22), 2163-2164. https://doi.org/10.1001/jama.2019.4432.

[80] Jernigan, D. H. (2011). Framing a public health debate over alcohol advertising: The Center on Alcohol Marketing and Youth 2002–2008. *Journal of Public Health Policy, 32*, 165-179. https://doi. org/10.1057/jphp.2011.5.

[81] U.S. Department of Health and Human Services. (2015). *E-cigarette use among youth and young adults: A report of the Surgeon General*. https://e-cigarettes.surgeongeneral.gov/documents/2016_ SGR_Full_Report_non-508.pdf.

[82] Colorado Marijuana Rules, Publ.. L. No. 1 CCR 212-3 (2020). https://www.sos.state.co.us/CCR/GenerateRulePdf.do?ruleVersionId=9303&fileName=1%20CCR%20212-3.

[83] Moreno, M. A. (2019) Study: Higher Social Media Engagement with Marijuana Marketing Linked to Higher Rates of Use. *School of Medicine and Public Health University of Wisconsin-Madison*. https://www.med.wisc.edu/news-and-events/2019/october/megan-moreno-marijuana-marketing-and-usage/.

[84] Cavazos-Rehg, P., Krauss, M., & Bierut, L. J. (2016) Marijuana-Related Posts on Instragram *Prevention Science, 17*, 710-720. https://pubmed.ncbi.nlm.nih.gov/27262456/.

[85] Krauss, M., Sowles, S. J., Sehi, A., et al. (2017) Marijuana advertising exposure among current marijuana users in the *U.S. Drug and Alcohol Dependence, 174*, 192-200. https://www.ncbi.nlm. nih.gov/pmc/articles/PMC5436304/.

[86] State of Rhode Island and Providence Plantations. (2020). Office of Cannabis Regulation - Advertising Guide. Department of Business Regulation, State of Rhode Island. https://dbr.ri.gov/documents/news/medical_marijuana/Advertising.pdf.

Section 3. Guidance for Selecting and Implementing Evidence-Based Policies and Programs

Before a state, community, school, or organization selects an intervention to prevent marijuana use among youth, it is important to assess its appropriateness for the setting and context in which it will be implemented. This section provides a framework to use when implementing prevention interventions and includes recommendations for addressing implementation challenges for the policies and programs described in Sections 2 and 4.

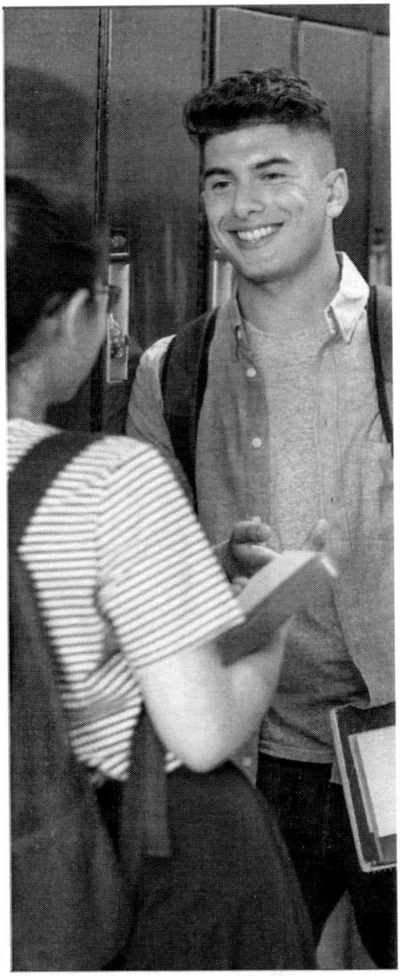

Using the Strategic Prevention Framework

Several frameworks and guidelines provide insight into how to plan for, select, and implement programs and policies that will meet prevention needs and produce desired outcomes. SAMHSA's Strategic Prevention Framework (SPF) provides a comprehensive, five-step approach for understanding and addressing youth marijuana use prevention within states and communities:

1) *Assessment* - Identify prevention needs using qualitative and quantitative data, such as incidence and prevalence of marijuana use among youth and factors that influence marijuana use.
2) *Capacity* - Determine what resources the state, community, or implementing organization has and what is needed to prevent and reduce marijuana use among youth (i.e., the human, organizational, state, community, or financial resources available).
3) *Planning* - Develop a comprehensive implementation plan that includes goals, objectives, strategies, programs, and policies to address the marijuana prevention priorities identified in steps 1 and 2.
4) *Implementation* - Implement programs and policies, using available guides and manuals for the interventions selected in step 3.
5) *Evaluation* - Evaluate the implementation process and assess whether the program or policy is having the intended effect (see more in Section 5).

A guiding principle underlying this framework is cultural competence, including using a population-based definition of community that lets the community define itself, engaging culturally competent evaluators, and including the target population in all aspects of prevention planning. Additionally, sustainability is a guiding principle: sustaining funding, processes that have engaged members of the target population, and the overall programs or strategies that improve the specified outcomes for the target population.

States and communities should continually assess their needs, which is especially necessary with a rapidly evolving issue like marijuana use. The population engaged in marijuana use may change over time, as may the marijuana products young people use, or the amount and types of marijuana advertisements and retail establishments. Regular needs assessments will ensure communities are implementing the best possible interventions for their specific circumstances and are not overly relying on previously implemented programs and policies. As laws related to legalization, decriminalization, and regulation continue to evolve, marijuana use will change in response to these policy changes. Marijuana use is also likely to be influenced by the marijuana industry's marketing strategies [1-2]. By conducting regular needs assessments, states and communities can ensure they are implementing the most appropriate interventions and can make revisions, adaptations, or changes, as needed.

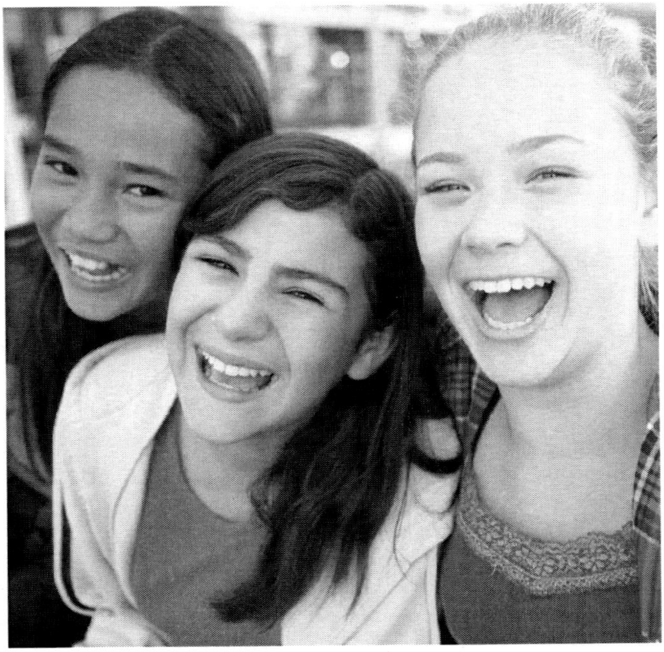

An overarching consideration when selecting and implementing policies to prevent marijuana use among young people is that, despite it being illegal, youth are at increased risk of marijuana use as these products become increasingly accessible in states that have legalized or decriminalized adult use. Given decades of research showing the direct effects adult markets have on youth, this section includes discussion on the challenges of and strategies for regulating marijuana use in the adult market [3].

Key Considerations for Prevention Program and Policy Implementation

Stakeholder Engagement

Challenge

- Gaining support from school administrators, school district officials, health administrators, healthcare professionals, child advocacy groups, parent associations, and city or county officials to implement a marijuana prevention policy or program is critical to success. Every intervention needs one or more champions.

Strategy

- Identify the most relevant champions for each community. Champions may include parents, educators, community members, and youth themselves, who can all educate policy and decision makers about evidence-based prevention strategies. These stakeholders should be engaged in the process early and often for the best effect. Appeals to stakeholders and potential champions should include a mix of current data, ideally from the local community, on marijuana use in the community or schools, along with personal stories from youth and parents who have been affected by marijuana use and its associated harms.

Financing

Challenge

- Obtaining and sustaining program funding for materials, training resources, and staff efforts is a common challenge. Often, limited funding is available for prevention efforts and resources are stretched thin. Environmental and regulatory strategies may have the advantage of being low cost, or even of generating revenue in the case of taxes.

Strategies

- From the very beginning of any intervention planning, it is important to estimate costs and develop a budget, being sure to include time and costs related to relationship development, capacity building, staff training, evaluation, and other necessary implementation components. A comprehensive plan should address and allocate resources to implement, maintain, and evaluate the program over time.
- When implementing environmental strategies, it is important to estimate the costs associated with educating relevant stakeholders on the specific policy change. This education may involve the city, county, or state needing to purchase new signage, provide information packets or educational outreach to marijuana producers or retailers on changes, or develop new enforcement organizations.

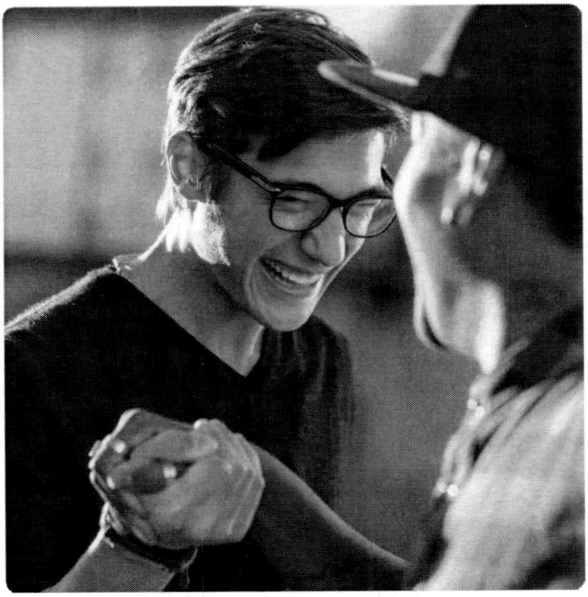

Key Considerations for Implementing Programs to Prevent Marijuana Use among Youth

Once a state, community, or organization has selected a program or policy to address marijuana use, stakeholders can use several strategies to support implementation efforts and address potential challenges and barriers.

Tailoring Interventions

Challenge

- Given the scarcity of data on marijuana-specific prevention programs, the effectiveness of these interventions among various populations or among individuals with different demographic characteristics is limited. Since marijuana use rates vary in communities by demographics, such as age, race/ethnicity, and sexual orientation, programs may require some adaptation to have the intended impact.

Strategy

- The U.S. Department of Health and Human Services has developed National Standards for Culturally and Linguistically Appropriate

Services (CLAS) [4]. The principal standard of CLAS is to "provide effective, equitable, understandable, and respectful quality care and services that are responsive to diverse cultural health beliefs and practices, preferred languages, health literacy, and other communication needs." CLAS includes 15 standards that should each be evaluated when selecting and implementing an intervention [4]. Communities should review and implement the CLAS principles when tailoring prevention programs, and be sure to rigorously evaluate how the revisions may have affected intended program outcomes.

Adaptation vs. Fidelity

Challenge

- As communities consider implementing programs or policies, stakeholders may have questions about how to adapt the model to their specific circumstances, while still maintaining fidelity to the core elements of the intervention. Fidelity is the degree to which a program delivers an intervention as intended and must be maintained for desired outcomes.

Strategies

- There is a large body of implementation science research that examines the tension between adaptation and fidelity, and the importance of balancing the two [5-6]. One approach is to develop intervention-specific descriptors for the components essential for fidelity, and what adaptations may be allowed [5]. Another approach is to develop hybrid prevention programs that include adaptation from the beginning, while also working to maximize fidelity of the intervention [6].
- SAMHSA recommends all programs conduct the following steps when considering adaptation:
  1) Identify and understand the theory of the program.
  2) Obtain or conduct a core components analysis of the program.
  3) Assess fidelity adaptation concerns for the implementation site.
  4) Consult with the program developer, as needed.
  5) Consult with the organization or community where the intervention will be implemented.

6) Develop an overall implementation plan based on steps one through five [7].

- To ensure adapted programs or policies are implemented with their core elements upheld, program implementers need to collect rigorous data to assess the adapted intervention for fidelity to the program. When the implemented program is not able to maintain fidelity to the established program, a rigorous evaluation of the adapted intervention provides evidence for the field on the impact of the intervention for reducing marijuana use among youth and young adults.

Staff Training

Challenge

- It is vital that staff are properly trained for successful program implementation and to build program capacity. However, this may be difficult to achieve due to staff turnover and limited time for existing staff to become familiar with the program.

Strategy

- When preparing to implement an intervention, organizations and communities must ensure staff have access to ongoing support and training on the program. Additionally, it is valuable to know broader marijuana regulatory and policy context to understand the environment in which the program is operating. Throughout the life of the program, additional staff training may be necessary to ensure continued program success.

Key Considerations for Implementing Policies to Address Marijuana Use among Youth

Getting a policy enacted and passed takes political will, persistence, and knowledge of the policy process. Key stakeholders include the local, state, or federal agencies that will be responsible for regulating and reporting requirements, the elected officials who will vote on the policy, and any public officials or state/local board members and engaged community members who will implement the new policy.

Additionally, when developing a policy, community members should be empowered to provide leadership and help drive policy change. It is critical to engage a host of partners, such as public health and policy/legislative experts, parents, educators, law enforcement, and youth. These individuals can help craft not only the policy language, but also determine the best communications and media strategies to promote political will and raise public awareness. When working with a government to implement a policy, whether it is at the city, county, state, or federal level, there are three important activities to keep in mind:

1) *Public Awareness* - Any rule change will require educating the public and/or the specific organizations affected. For example, if a city prohibits the sale of flavored marijuana products, city officials must inform marijuana retailers and the broader public about this change.
2) *Regulations* - If a new policy affects existing structures or systems, new procedures will need to be established. In the example of implementing zoning laws, policy makers will need to determine how licenses will be tracked and how often new licenses will be provided to those who apply for them. In the state of Washington, the Washington State Liquor and Cannabis Board (WSLCB) administers licenses and enforces zoning regulations. Prior to granting a marijuana license, WSLCB is required to notify local authorities when an entity applies for a marijuana license within their jurisdiction. Upon notification, the locality has 20 days to respond with an approval, objection, or no response to the licensing request. WSLCB also provides guidance documents that may help those seeking a marijuana license to comply with local zoning regulations [8].
3) *Enforcement* - Nearly all policies require some level of monitoring or enforcement. Cities that pass ordinances limiting what and where marijuana products may be sold will need to ensure retailers have the correct license and will need to maintain consistent enforcement of that new policy. The Commonwealth of Massachusetts created the Cannabis Control Commission (CCC), a five-member organization assigned with ensuring the marijuana industry is safe, responsible, and successful. The CCC monitors and enforces marijuana policy through inspections, audits, and issuance of fines and penalties [9].

In addition to these common factors, there are several challenges that must be considered when implementing policies to prevent marijuana use among youth and young adults. Some of these challenges, and strategies to address them, are discussed below.

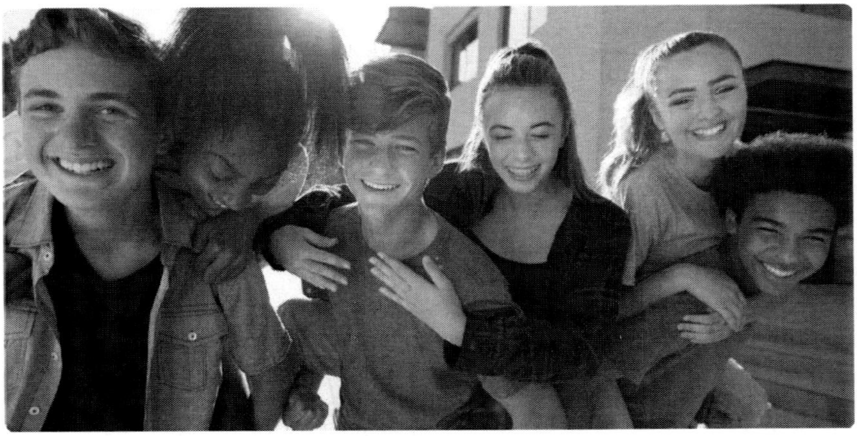

State Preemption

Challenge

- Currently, most states that have legalized marijuana for adult use provide localities the authority to implement their own policies on marijuana sales that may be more restrictive than state requirements. Localities may even opt out of state laws and ban marijuana operations within their localities completely [10]. However, the legislative landscape around marijuana is rapidly evolving, and state and local policy makers should remain aware of the larger state and federal regulatory environments in which they operate.

Strategies

- If needed, legal experts on marijuana policy can help a jurisdiction better understand potential preemption issues (i.e., when cities and counties are banned from passing marijuana control policies that are stronger than the state policy equivalent) and existing nuances or gray areas in the law, as well as encourage lawmakers to enact policies to protect from preemption. The ability for jurisdictions to pass more restrictive policies that are responsive to their local needs is critical, and numerous entities, including the Centers for Disease Control and Prevention (CDC), Healthy People 2030, the National Association of County and City Health Officials, and the U.S. Surgeon General, have noted that preemption laws do not advance public health priorities.

- The Alcohol Policy Information System maintains an updated list of whether localities have authority to regulate adult marijuana sales within each state.

Evolving Community Needs

Challenge

- The marijuana landscape is continually evolving, and the most appropriate program or policy for the state or community may change over time.

Strategy

- Regularly collecting and analyzing data on youth marijuana use behavior will help determine what products are being used, where they are obtaining their products, and if certain subgroups are using marijuana at higher rates than others. Stakeholders engaged in prevention efforts, including parents and youth, can also provide first-hand information about marijuana use patterns and behaviors within the state/community. Regularly assessing these data will ensure the state/community is implementing the best interventions for their specific needs.

Marijuana Product Diversity

Challenge

- There is a wide variety of marijuana products currently available in states with legal adult use, and new products are rapidly being developed and marketed. From marijuana-infused drinks, such as colas and fruit punches, to pill-like marijuana "capsules," there are many ways to consume marijuana [11]. Hemp-derived psychoactive cannabinoids, such as Delta 8-THC, are also increasingly available on the market. Policies focused only on the prevention of smoking of marijuana, such as smoke-free laws, may exclude these other products, and, therefore, may neglect to prevent marijuana use in a large portion of a state or by the community's youth.

Strategy

- Communities can work with public health and legal experts to determine if the policies being considered should explicitly include all products, or only those that are most used by youth, such as edibles. Continuous monitoring of the evolving product market is critical to determine what products youth are using most, and if and how they should be regulated.

Industry Influence

Challenges

- As the marijuana industry is continually growing, favorable legislation and strong lobbying are leading to a boom in the commercialization of marijuana products. The marijuana industry spent a record $4 million on federal lobbying in 2020 [12, 13]. By 2025, the legal marijuana market is projected to double to $41.5 billion [14].
- Increasing commercialization of substances can lead to greater youth exposure and use. The marijuana industry marketing their products as "wellness" products and "fun" edibles, such as marijuana gummies and chocolates, introduces additional challenges in reducing youth use [15-16].

Strategies

- As state and community leaders, parents, and other stakeholders collaborate to pass and implement policies to prevent marijuana use, they must be aware of industry strategies and messaging, and prepare counter messaging to gain support for public health policies.
- A vast majority of Americans agree that youth should not be exposed to marijuana products [17]. Those focusing on the prevention of marijuana use among youth can use this belief to engage diverse stakeholders and implement policies to restrict marketing to youth and thwart the portrayal of marijuana as a wellness product. A comprehensive prevention strategy should also include media

campaigns that promote messages to counter industry influence and reach youth who are most susceptible to industry advertising.

Implementation Guides and Manuals

Policy implementation is complex, but detailed guidance for implementing policies is limited, especially in comparison to family, classroom, or community-based programs, which often have prescribed curricula. Below are several tools and resources to help stakeholders implement the strategies described in Section 2, with specific implementation guides provided where possible. Overarching guidance is also included, as many of the recommendations and suggestions are similar across all programs and policies.

Interventions

Programs

- Cannabis/Marijuana Awareness and Prevention Toolkit resources
- SPORT step-by-step implementation directions
- Strengthening Families Program training opportunities
- All Stars teaching manual
- Keepin' It Real teaching manual
- LifeSkills Training planning workbook, fidelity checklist, and curriculum alignment tools
- Good Behavior Game manual
- Training and resources for PreVenture facilitators
- Project Alert Implementation Tips and Teen Leader Trainer's Manual
- Project Towards No Drug Abuse implementation manual
- Communities that Care implementation guide
- PROSPER training for state partners through Iowa State University

Regulating Marijuana Prices

- Overview of marijuana taxes by the Urban Institute, including what the options are and how states have implemented tax policies
- A briefing book on how marijuana taxes work from the Urban Institute and the Brookings Institution

Regulating Marijuana Retailers

- Tobacco Retailer Density, a guide from ChangeLab Solutions on implementing place-based strategies
- Strategizer 55: Regulating Alcohol Outlet Density by the Community Anti-Drug Coalitions of America (CADCA) and the Center on Alcohol Marketing and Youth is an action guide on how to regulate outlets; though not specific to marijuana, many of the strategies and activities are similar
- A guide on options to regulate marijuana, originally developed by for California to reduce youth use, written by Alcohol Policy Consultations

Regulating Marijuana Marketing

- "Model Ordinance Regulating Local Cannabis Retail Sales and Marketing in California" from the Public Health Institute

Regulating Marijuana Products

- Numerous states have specific packaging and labeling policies, including Massachusetts, Oregon, Michigan, and Washington

Tools to Support Policy Interventions

- Information on policy communication and the legislative process by CADCA
- Resources developed by the National Conference of State Legislatures that outline state legislative processes and the marijuana policies in effect in different states
- The Campaign for Tobacco-Free Kids has developed guides for media and policy campaigns; toolkits can be utilized by state or local governments
- The Network for Public Health Law helps identify policy approaches that will advance the goals of an organization or community and has a series of resources on preventing substance use and making healthier communities
- The Prevention Technology Transfer Center Network has an abundance of substance use prevention resources and tools, including webinars and trainings

References

[1] D'Amico, E. J., Miles, J. N., & Tucker, J. S. (2015). Gateway to curiosity: Medical marijuana ads and intention and use during middle school. *Psychology of Addictive Behaviors, 29*(3), 613-619. https://dx.doi.org/10.1037%2Fadb0000094.

[2] Fiala, S. C., Dilley, J. A., Firth, C. L., & Maher, J. E. (2018). Exposure to marijuana marketing after legalization of retail sales: Oregonians' experiences, 2015–2016. *American Journal of Public Health, 108*(1), 120-127. https://doi.org/10.2105/ajph.2017.304136.

[3] Jernigan, D., Noel, J., Landon, J., Thornton, N., & Lobstein, T. (2008). Alcohol marketing and youth alcohol consumption: A systematic review of longitudinal studies published since 2008. *Addiction, 112*(Suppl 1), 7-20. https://doi.org/10.1111/add.13591.

[4] Department of Health and Human Services. (n.d.). *National CLAS Standards*. https://thinkculturalhealth.hhs.gov/clas.

[5] Pérez, D., Stuyft, P. V., Zabala, M. D. C., Castro, M., & Lefèvre, P. (2016). A modified theoretical framework to assess implementation fidelity of adaptive public health interventions. *Implementation Science, 11*(91). https://doi.org/10.1186/s13012-016-0457-8.

[6] Castro, F. G., Barrera Jr., M., & Martinez Jr., C. R. (2004). The cultural adaptation of prevention interventions: Resolving tensions between fidelity and fit. *Prev Sci, 5*(1), 41-45. https://doi.org/10.1023/b:prev.0000013980.12412.cd.

[7] Substance Abuse and Mental Health Services Administration. (2019). *A guide to SAMHSA's Strategic Prevention Framework*. https://www. samhsa.gov/sites/default/files/20190620-samhsa-strategic-prevention-framework-guide.pdf.

[8] Washington State Liquor and Cannabis Board. (2020). *Washington State Liquor and Cannabis Board*. https://lcb.wa.gov/.

[9] Cannabis Control Commission. (2021). *Cannabis Control Commission*. https://mass-cannabis-control. com/.

[10] Alcohol Policy Information System (APIS). (n.d.). *Alcohol Policy Information System (APIS)*. https://alcoholpolicy.niaaa.nih.gov//.

[11] Pierre, J. (2018). *Coca, Cola, and Cannabis: Psychoactive Drugs as Beverages*. https://www. psychologytoday.com/za/blog/psych-unseen/201810/coca-cola-and-cannabis-psychoactive-drugs-beverages.

[12] Open Secrets Center for Responsive Politics. (2021). *Marijuana: Lobbying, 2020*. https://www.opensecrets.org/federal-lobbying/industries/summary?cycle=2021&id=N09.

[13] Mulcahy, S. (2020, April 6). The cannabis industry spent more on lobbying than ever before in 2019. What's next is unclear. *Cannabis Wire*. https://cannabiswire.com/2020/04/06/the-cannabis-industry-spent-more-on-lobbying-than-ever-before-in-2019-whats-next-is-unclear/.

[14] Montoya, Z., Conroy, M., Vanden Heuvel, B., Pauli, C. S., & Park, S.-H. (2020). Cannabis contaminants limit pharmacological use of cannabidiol. *Frontiers in Psychiatry, 11,* 571832. https://dx.doi. org/10.3389%2Ffphar.2020.571832.

[15] Friese, B. (2017). "Is marijuana even a drug?" A qualitative study of how teens view marijuana use and why they use it. *Journal of Psychoactive Drugs, 49*(3), 209-216. https://dx.doi.org/10.1080% 2F02791072.2017.1290854.

[16] Krauss, M. J., Sowles, S. J., Stelzer-Monahan, H. E., Bierut, T., & Cavazos-Rehg, P. A. (2017). "It takes longer, but when it hits you it hits you!": Videos about marijuana edibles on YouTube. *Substance Use & Misuse, 52*(6), 709-716. https://doi.org/10.1080/10826084.2016.1253749.

[17] Larkin, P. (2018). Marijuana edibles and "gummy bears." *Buffalo Law Review, 66*(2), 313-383.

Section 4. Examples of Interventions for Prevention of Marijuana Use Among Youth

This section highlights efforts made in three communities to prevent marijuana use among youth:

- Ventura County, California
- Boulder County, Colorado
- Indian River County, Florida

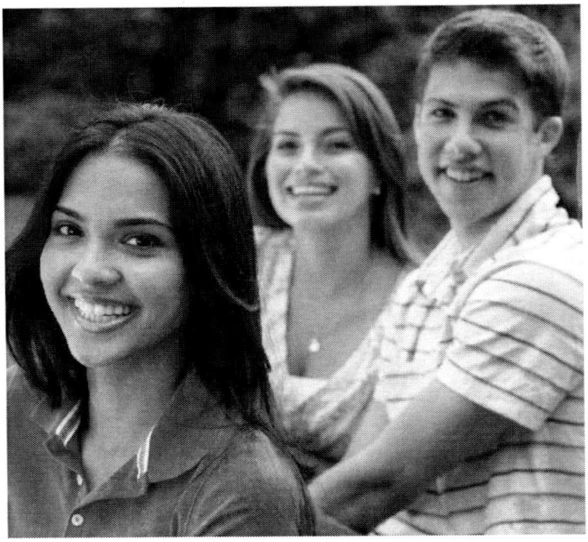

These case examples describe practical applications of programs and policies as part of comprehensive community-based strategies to prevent youth marijuana use across the social-ecological model (SEM) (e.g., individual, school, and community levels). The environmental strategies and programs to prevent marijuana use build on, or are expansions of, long-standing tobacco and alcohol control efforts. Understanding the context in which communities are implementing marijuana use prevention strategies is critical to comprehend the broader, multi-level prevention strategies affecting youth in each county and state regulatory structure.

To be included in this section, examples had to meet the following criteria:

- Involve the implementation of one or more of the policies or programs included in Section 2
- Have evidence of causal impact on reducing marijuana use or be based on an established program or theory of change
- Be implemented as part of a comprehensive prevention strategy

Specific information about the programs and environmental strategies featured in this section was gathered from experts and through an environmental scan, including a review of published journal articles, state policies and regulations, and resources and publications from state and federal government agencies and nonprofit organizations.

Environmental Strategies and Programs Described in Section 2:

- Cannabis/Marijuana Awareness and Prevention Toolkit (CAPT)
- Communities That Care
- LifeSkills Training
- Project ALERT
- SPORT
- Strengthening Families Program
- Price policies
- Licensing and zoning policies

California

Prevention Strategies in Ventura County, California

Background

California was the first state to legalize medical marijuana in 1996 and one of the first states to legalize marijuana for non-medical adult use in 2016. Prior to the legalization of marijuana for non-medical adult use, local communities had taken steps to regulate medical marijuana to protect the health, welfare, and safety of all residents [1]. These early local community efforts provided an opportunity to build regulatory and monitoring infrastructures that reduced challenges that arose later from legalization of marijuana for non-medical adult use. California has a growing portfolio of prevention programming in place because of statewide policy requiring that a portion of the marijuana tax revenue be used to promote youth prevention efforts at state and local levels.

Community Featured: Ventura County, California
Prevention Programs: Project ALERT; Project Towards No Drug Abuse (TND), Cannabis/Marijuana Awareness and Prevention Toolkit (CAPT)
Environmental Strategies: Regulation of marijuana products, price policies, regulation of retail outlets, limiting marijuana marketing, zoning ordinances

Ventura County, located in Southern California, is home to 846,249 residents, 23 percent of whom are under the age of 18 [2]. In Ventura County, officials engaged local stakeholders and experts to strategically advance public health and safety measures in response to the changing marijuana policy landscape [1].

According to data from the California Healthy Kids Survey (CHKS), current state and local marijuana use trends among youth have remained unchanged since legalization, despite a decline observed prior to legalization.

Grade Level	Past 30-Day Marijuana Use			
	California		Ventura County	
	2016	2019	2016	2019
7th Graders	2%	4%	3%	4%
9th Graders	10%	10%	8%	10%
11th Graders	16%	16%	16%	15%

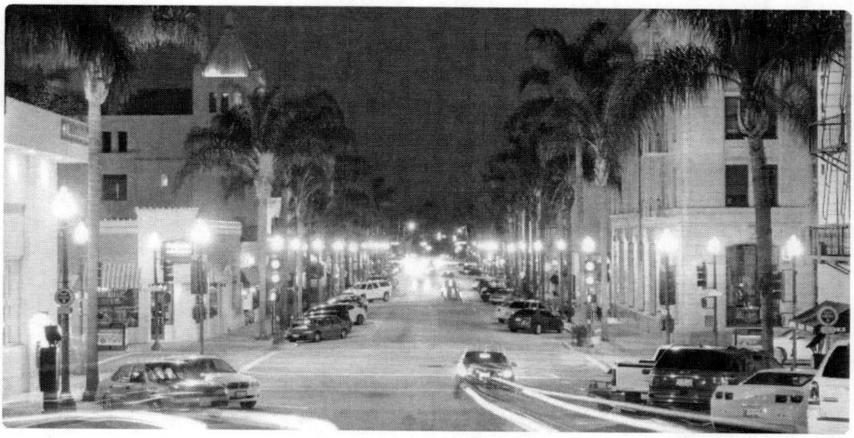

At a Glance
California Marijuana Policies

Non-Medical Adult Use: Legal
Medical Use: Legal
Decriminalized: Yes

The use and possession of marijuana is legal for adults aged 21 and over in California. Individuals who are between the ages of 18 and 21 are permitted to use medical marijuana, provided it is obtained through authorized channels.

Regulatory Structure: In California, marijuana is licensed and regulated by the Department of Food and Agriculture (cultivation), the Department of Public Health (manufacturing), and the Bureau of Cannabis Control (distribution, testing, and retailing), although in 2021 these entities are being combined into a single regulatory agency.

Retail Policies: Retail outlets cannot be within 600 feet of schools unless the community agrees to a smaller distance. There are no state limits on the number of retailers, although many local ones exist. Posting of health warnings is not required in dispensaries but small warnings are required on packaging (in 6-point font). There are no limits on flavored products or potency except for an edible dose of 10mg. Onsite consumption is allowed if locally authorized.

Taxes and Pricing: Sales taxes are imposed at the cultivation stage on products produced and transferred and an excise tax of 15 percent of the value of retail marijuana is also applied. Retail sales are subject to state (7.25 percent) and local (0 to 2.75 percent) sales taxes, depending on the community. There is no minimum price, and certain discounts (but not free product) are allowed unless locally prohibited. State tax revenue is used for administration, law enforcement, youth prevention and education, and criminal justice programming efforts, as well as for childcare.

Local Regulations: Local communities that do not want marijuana sold must specifically prohibit its commerce, otherwise the state recognizes it as permitted and will issue licenses. If permitted, local communities can license businesses along with state licensing, tax locally, tax based on potency, restrict products allowed for sale or marketing (such as flavored products or beverages), require additional warnings, prohibit discounts, or set other regulations. Although local communities can ban the sale of marijuana, they cannot prohibit possession or personal cultivation.

Marijuana Prevention Initiatives in Ventura County

Programs

Ventura County has 20 school districts serving approximately 140,000 students in kindergarten through 12th grade [3]. Several Ventura County school districts have implemented marijuana prevention programs, including Project Towards No Drug Abuse (TND), the Cannabis/Marijuana Awareness and Prevention Toolkit (CAPT), and Project ALERT. More detailed information on two of these programs is included below [4-5].

Project ALERT. Project ALERT was implemented in the Simi Valley Unified School District (SVUSD). In SVUSD, Project ALERT is taught in the required science course, with all 11 core lessons taught in 7th grade and the three booster lessons taught in 8th grade, as designed. All teachers complete a log of the lessons delivered to students. Schools within the county, including the SVUSD, are beginning to track changes in marijuana use using data from CHKS. These data can be used to support the need for continued prevention work and curriculum focused on educating students about the dangers of substance use. Every two years, the district administration and individual school principals in SVUSD collaborate with the county evaluator to review the district's data and evaluate areas of strength and needed improvement. Both these data and related discussions drive their programming.

Cannabis/Marijuana Awareness and Prevention Toolkit (CAPT). CAPT has been implemented in schools, youth groups, and after-school programs in Ventura County. CAPT consists of a free, online set of lessons and activities to teach youth about marijuana. Implementation of CAPT can vary, as schools and other educators can decide the curriculum; however, there is a three-lesson suggested curriculum. The program is free, and the toolkit developer (Stanford University) provides free training to those implementing it. Stanford also provides online/remote learning lessons, activities, and quizzes to accompany the program and will work with schools to evaluate the effectiveness of the toolkit within individual programs.

Environmental Strategies

Environmental strategies governing the sale and marketing of marijuana have been implemented at the county level and within individual cities. These strategies include smoke-free policies and policies related to marketing, taxes, and retailer restrictions. Ventura County has been able to implement these environmental strategies because California gives local communities the authority to establish their own marijuana regulations that are more restrictive than state policy.

In Ventura County, a measure allowing for the commercial cultivation, processing, and distribution of marijuana in pre-existing structures within unincorporated areas was passed in November 2020 and implemented on January 1, 2021. This measure opened areas of the county to the cultivation of marijuana outside of Oxnard, Port Hueneme, and Ojai (three of the ten incorporated towns in the county), increasing the amount of product produced locally. However, retail marijuana can still only be sold in storefronts in Oxnard, Port Hueneme, and Ojai, while Thousand Oaks only allows medical storefront sales [6].

These cities limit hours and do not allow onsite consumption. Ojai, Oxnard, and Thousand Oaks capped the number of retailers. However, in 2020, recreational delivery was allowed in these four cities and in the unincorporated areas of the county, including medical delivery only in Oxnard, whereas six cities prohibited delivery. Thousand Oaks is the only city in the county to have banned billboards and requires the sale of medical marijuana to be by appointment.

No product restrictions, such as bans on flavored products, vaping products, or high potency products, are in place. Ventura County reflects the complicated nuances of regulation in California, with varying degrees of legalization and legal access, ranging from relatively high availability of marijuana outlets to complete bans on marijuana sales.

Studies are underway in California to examine the effects of local policy variation on marijuana use during pregnancy and by youth, including in Ventura County.

Lessons Learned

Planning and Research: SVUSD reviews their prevention programming annually to determine fidelity (defined as the degree to which a program delivers an intervention as intended; must be maintained for desired outcomes), and administers pre- and post-tests or holds focus groups for students who have completed programming to assess for acceptability and effectiveness.

Prevention: Overall school-based intervention and education programs appear to be in use. Environmental, systems, and policy change approaches focused on public health protection and reducing youth use where the product is legal may be less extensively used, although a full ban continues in place in a significant part of the county. For example, although Ventura County, Oxnard, and the City of Ventura ban flavored tobacco products, no such ban exists for flavored marijuana sales or delivery where retail sale is allowed.

Staffing: SVUSD identifies and appoints dedicated staff to lead initiatives, including an onsite teacher at each school who is trained in the program and can serve as a leader and liaison for specific programming activities.

Research and Data: Exploring how price and tax policies (e.g., increasing taxes over time) can help shape the market and affect youth marijuana use is critical and relies on the collection of data to better understand the relationship between youth use, harms, and price. The natural experiment underway in California with varying degrees of legalization, taxation, and regulation across the state provides a valuable setting for future research.

Colorado

Prevention Strategies in Boulder County, Colorado

Background

In late 2012, Colorado became the first state to legalize marijuana for non-medical adult use [7-9]. Since then, policies and the impacts of legalized marijuana relevant to health, politics, culture, and law enforcement have been closely monitored. The state collects and frequently reports on legalization data related to public safety, public health, youth use, and other key indicators. Key findings from the most recent report, published in 2018, include:

- The rate of serious marijuana-related crimes has remained unchanged from pre-legalization levels [10].
- Rates of hospitalization with possible marijuana exposures increased steadily from 2000 through 2015, from 803 hospitalizations per 100,000 before commercialization of marijuana (2000-2009) to 2,696 hospitalizations per 100,000 after commercialization (2014-2015) [10].
- Rates of suicide increased post-legalization, as did rates of suicide with marijuana present [10].
- In the 2016-2017 school year, marijuana use was the most common reason for school expulsions and law enforcement referrals [10].

Community Featured: Boulder County, Colorado
Prevention Programs: Communities That Care (CTC)
Environmental Strategies: Regulation of retail outlets, limiting marijuana marketing, zoning ordinances

The proportion of high school students reporting having used marijuana ever in their lifetime or in the past 30-days remained statistically unchanged from 2005 to 2017 [10]. A more recent report on health outcomes after marijuana legalization in Colorado, published in 2021, found that the ways Colorado youth are using marijuana is changing, with an increase in the proportion of youth dabbing and vaping marijuana between 2015 and 2019, and a small decrease in smoking marijuana [11]. The report also noted that the rate of past 30-day marijuana use is continuing to increase among Colorado adults [11].

Boulder County, Colorado, is located along the Northern Front Range and is home to 300,000 people, of whom just under 19 percent are under the age of 18. Upon legalization of marijuana in Colorado, the Boulder County Healthy Futures Coalition, a group of organizations and individuals dedicated to reducing substance use in the county, made prevention of marijuana use among youth a priority.

	Changes in Marijuana Use Prevalence			
Grade Level	**Colorado [11]**		**Boulder County [12-13]**	
	2013	**2019**	**2013**	**2019**
High school	20%	20%	20%	24%

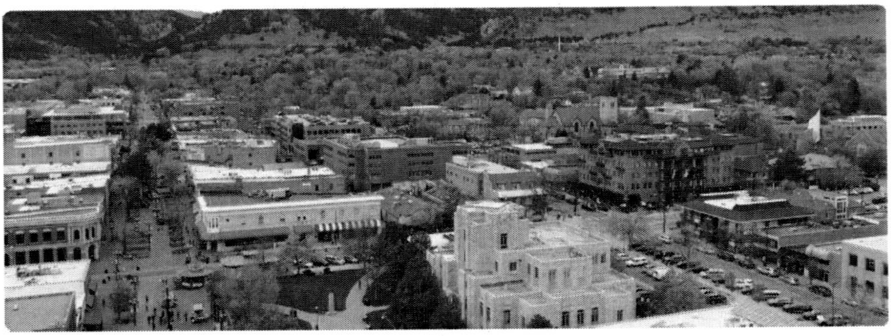

At a Glance
Colorado Marijuana Policies

Non-Medical Adult Use: Legal
Medical Use: Legal
Decriminalized: Yes

The use and possession of marijuana is legal for adults aged 21 and over in Colorado. Individuals who are between the ages of 18 and 21 are permitted to use medical marijuana, provided it is obtained through authorized channels.

Regulatory Structure: The Colorado Department of Public Health and Environment is responsible for the inspection of retail marijuana testing facilities, and the Colorado Department of Agriculture oversees the cultivation of marijuana and hemp. The Marijuana Enforcement Division of Colorado's Department of Revenue is assigned with licensing and regulating the medical and retail marijuana industries.

Retail Policies: Only licensed retailers can sell marijuana products. Retail dispensaries cannot be within 1,000 feet of schools unless the community agrees to a smaller distance, or an existing retailer is grandfathered in. Dispensaries can only be open between the hours of 8 a.m. and midnight. Products must be child-proof and in resealable packaging that is clearly labeled with key information, including health warnings. In June 2021 the legislature adopted new rules to respond to increasing THC potency, including serving size information on labels and restrictions on the amount of concentrates that can be purchased at one time.

Taxes and Pricing: Retail marijuana is subject to a 10 percent sales tax on top of the state's 2.9 percent standard tax rate. There is also a 15 percent excise tax on the wholesale price of retail marijuana between cultivators and businesses. However, these taxes do not apply to medical marijuana.

Local Regulations: Local communities are able, but not required, to set their own additional laws and regulations as they pertain to non-medical adult marijuana use.

Marijuana Prevention Initiatives in Boulder County

Programs

Nederland, a town located in Boulder County, Colorado, highlights challenges facing towns even in counties that have committed to substance use prevention. While Boulder County itself has made substance use prevention a priority, the town of Nederland has historically experienced challenges with and limitations in providing prevention programming. To address the need for prevention programming locally, and to align with Boulder County priorities, a local nonprofit organization, TEENS, Inc., worked with the state health department to implement Communities That Care (CTC) in Nederland.

A group of Nederland community members formed a CTC coalition to address substance use and other problem behaviors among local youth [14]. The Nederland coalition continues to be hosted by TEENS, Inc., which serves as the fiscal sponsor/contractor to the state, and has representation across key sectors, including local government, businesses, schools, law enforcement, faith-based organizations, media, health care, service providers, community members, parents, family, and youth [14].

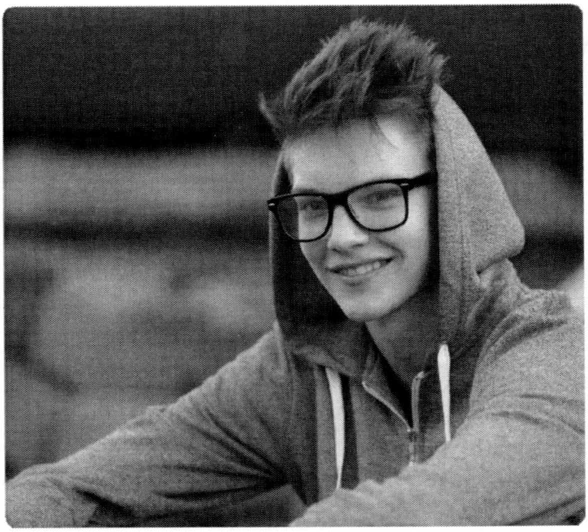

The CTC coalition used data from the Healthy Kids Colorado Survey to identify three primary risk and protective factors in Nederland to consider in their prevention efforts. These three risk and protective factors were: individual-level favorable attitudes toward substance use (risk); community opportunities for prosocial involvement (protective); and community laws and norms favorable to substance use (risk). Goals and strategies were set for each risk and protective factor. The coalition also implemented a series of programs intending to improve community opportunities for prosocial involvement.

Environmental Strategies

Nederland has implemented a series of environmental strategies to regulate access to marijuana, namely zoning ordinances, marketing restrictions, and point of sale sign requirements. In Boulder County, marijuana regulations are determined at the city or town level in incorporated towns [15], while unincorporated areas are subject to the county's marijuana policies [15]. For example, one county-wide regulation requires that marijuana dispensaries located in business, commercial, or transition zones be at least 500 feet away from other dispensaries in the same zone [16].

Nederland requires marijuana outlets to be located within specifically zoned areas, such as neighborhood commercial, general commercial, and the central business district. Manufacturing and testing facilities have separate zoning requirements, as well. Marijuana outlets are banned only if within 100 feet of a licensed childcare facility or a school. Nederland also has specific sign requirements for marijuana outlets, including a notice that the premise is a marijuana outlet and banning signs that have flashing lights, advertise marijuana, or include pictorial representations of marijuana other than the one provided by the town [17].

Since its initiation, the CTC coalition has worked on implementing additional environmental strategies in Nederland. For the goal of addressing community laws and norms that are substance use risk factors, the coalition is working to build community support for ordinances, regulations, and requirements for establishments selling alcohol or marijuana. The identification of specific risk and protective factors led to the passing of several regulations, including an ordinance capping the number of dispensary locations at the current level (four) and a resolution for the town government to opt out of allowing licenses for establishments that allow the use of marijuana onsite in the community. In addition, the work of the CTC coalition led to the creation of a public review zoning process for any marijuana-related commercial establishments.

While the work of the CTC coalition in Nederland has successfully led to the implementation of environmental strategies, there are no data available yet on the impact of these strategies on marijuana use among youth.

Lessons Learned

Advocacy: Because CTC is about maintaining a high-capacity coalition over the long term, securing stakeholder support prior to implementing evidence-based interventions is vital for program success and sustainability.

Collaboration: As demonstrated in Nederland, coalitions should be composed of members representing a diverse group of stakeholders from both the public and private sectors, including government, business, education, health care, media, criminal justice, and invested community members.

Costs and Funding Sources: Coalitions are often funded by the county or state or by grants to form and assess their local conditions but often lack funding to implement appropriate interventions. Prioritizing how to use existing funds and identifying opportunities to secure new funds will optimize the ability of coalitions to implement evidence-based interventions. Engagement from numerous community sectors can help in identifying and obtaining new sources of funding. Coalitions may also need to seek a fiscal agent to support their work.

Leadership: Coalitions need strong leadership that is well-versed in the areas of prevention, local government, policy and legislation, and administration to build relationships with partners in different sectors and promote engagement.

Planning and Research: Coalitions or other stakeholders trying to determine the most appropriate prevention interventions should first conduct a readiness assessment. A readiness assessment will help to determine the local conditions that may facilitate implementation, subsequently minimizing potential challenges that may occur during the implementation process. Coalitions can review existing data or collect their own data as part of this initial assessment.

Political Support: When attempting to pass an ordinance that would prohibit marijuana retail establishments in the community, Nederland's CTC coalition found that public safety and/or public resource messaging may be more effective than public health messaging to secure support for a marijuana use prevention initiative.

Flexibility: Coalitions are not always driving policy change in their community and need to be agile and responsive to community activities that are also working toward the implementation of environmental strategies. Based on Nederland's experience, community coalitions need the flexibility to both lead and support substance use prevention work if it aligns with the mission and goals of their organization.

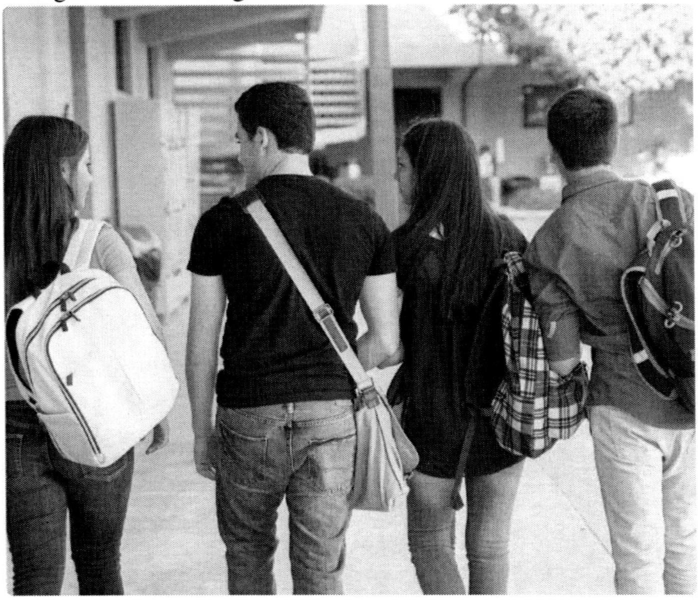

Florida

Prevention Strategies in Indian River County, Florida

Background

Legislation permitting the use of medical marijuana in Florida was passed in 2016. Initially, medical marijuana was legalized only for use in terminally ill patients (those with less than a year to live); however, a constitutional amendment was passed later the same year that expanded access to medical marijuana for individuals with certain chronic conditions. In 2017, legislation was passed that allowed medical marijuana only in the form of oils, pills, sprays, edibles, and other non-combustible consumption formulations. In March 2019, smokable medical marijuana became an approved route of consumption for medical marijuana [18]. However, recreational marijuana sale, possession, and use remain illegal in Florida.

Community Featured: Indian River County, Florida
Prevention Programs: Strengthening Families Program, LifeSkills Training, SPORT Prevention Plus Wellness
Environmental Strategies: Regulation of marijuana products, regulation of retail outlets, limiting marijuana marketing, zoning ordinances

Indian River County sits on the Atlantic coast of Florida and has a population of just over 130,000 people, with approximately 14 percent under the age of 18. Since the legalization of medical marijuana in Florida, the rate of youth marijuana use has increased among middle school students but remains consistent among high school students. However, the rate of synthetic marijuana use among high schoolers more than doubled, from 0.8 percent in 2016 to nearly two percent in 2020, while remaining constant at one percent statewide [19].

Grade Level	Changes in Marijuana Use			
	Florida [19]		Indian River County [19]	
	2016	2020	2016	2020
High school	17%	16%	18%	17%
Middle school	3%	4%	2%	4%

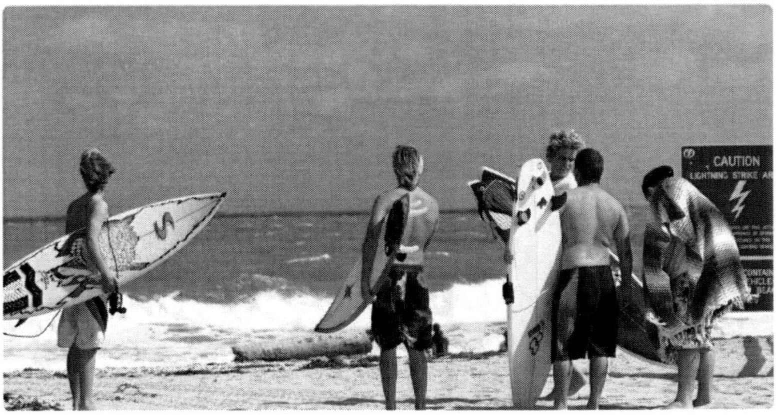

At a Glance
Florida Marijuana Policies

Non-Medical Adult Use: Illegal

Medical Use: Legal

Decriminalized: Not decriminalized statewide, but varies by community

Medical marijuana is legal in the state of Florida for individuals aged 18 or older with a qualifying medical condition. Individuals under the age of 18 may be permitted to use medical marijuana in a combustible form if they have a terminal condition. They must also have parental approval and a recommendation from two physicians to obtain a medical marijuana card. All patients and caregivers must have a Medical Marijuana Use Registry identification card, and only qualified physicians can order low-THC cannabis, medical marijuana, or cannabis delivery devices for their patients.

Regulatory Structure: The Florida Department of Health is the governing agency for medical marijuana in Florida. Specifically, the department's Office of Medical Marijuana Use oversees the statewide Medical Marijuana Use Registry, licenses Florida businesses to cultivate, process, and dispense medical marijuana to qualified patients, and certifies marijuana testing laboratories.

Retail Policies: Only licensed medical marijuana treatment centers are permitted to grow, process, and dispense marijuana, and patients may purchase it from only these treatment centers.

Taxes and Pricing: There is no excise tax or sales tax on medical marijuana or medical marijuana delivery devices.

Local Regulations: Local communities can ban marijuana dispensaries entirely. If communities allow dispensaries, they must be zoned no more strictly than pharmacies, and the number cannot be limited. A dispensary cannot be within 500 feet of a school (unless the community grants a special permit). Per state law, cities and/or counties are unable to set local taxes for medical marijuana or set permitting fees.

Marijuana Prevention Initiatives in Indian River County

Programs

Limited resources for marijuana prevention programming are available at the state level. Most of Florida's youth-focused prevention is focused on substance use in general and not on marijuana specifically. Indian River County offers both school and community-based prevention programs through the *Substance Awareness Center of Indian River County* [20]. Some of the prevention programs available to youth include (but are not limited to): the Strengthening Families Program, SPORT Prevention Plus Wellness, and LifeSkills Training. More details about these three programs are included below.

Strengthening Families Program. The Strengthening Families Program is offered in Indian River County through a five-agency collaborative. This program provides weekly group sessions for the entire family, free of charge, that focus on three life skills courses: parenting skills, youth social/life skills, and family life skills.[21] Results from this program on marijuana outcomes in Indian River have not been published.

LifeSkills Training. The LifeSkills Training (LST) prevention program is offered to approximately 5,000 Indian River County students each year in 5th, 6th, 7th, and 8th grades by five trained facilitators. During the summer months, the program is implemented through summer camps offered at the Boys and Girls Clubs and other youth organizations [22].

Indian River County has implemented LST in:

- 5th grade at all 13 county elementary schools for eight weeks, partnering with local police departments
- 6th grade in two schools for 16 weeks
- 7th grade in two schools for 10 weeks

- 8th grade for five weeks in two schools
- Seven summer camps

Since implementation in 2012, over 10,000 students have received at least some LST courses, and students reported significant improvements in health knowledge, anti-drug attitudes, and life and refusal skills. Among 5th to 8th grade students, past 30-day marijuana use decreased from 12 percent in 2008 to 9 percent in 2018 [22].

SPORT Prevention Plus Wellness. SPORT Prevention Plus Wellness has been implemented in all county middle schools (6th to 8th grade). Organizations that implement SPORT Prevention Plus Wellness are provided with pretest and posttest surveys to evaluate program implementation fidelity and effectiveness; however, no statewide analysis of the program has been conducted. Anticipated outcomes of the SPORT program include reduction of favorable attitudes toward marijuana use, improved commitment to school, altered interactions with friends who use marijuana, and decreased marijuana use.

Environmental Strategies

Most marijuana policy in Florida is set at the state level, although local jurisdictions were able to enact their own policies before a preemption law limiting local authority was passed in 2017. Once this law was passed, the existing community-level medical marijuana zoning regulations were made irrelevant. Ultimately, cities and counties are given the authority to permit or prohibit the presence of medical marijuana dispensaries in their community but have limited ability to implement other regulatory policies.

However, bans can be nuanced. For example, county bans apply only to unincorporated areas of the county, so incorporated cities and towns can still allow medical marijuana, as is the case in Indian River County. Any medical marijuana regulation enacted by a city or county must be equivalent to pharmacy regulations, given that medical marijuana is regulated as a medication.

Lessons Learned

Education: Educating policy makers about the adverse effects of marijuana on the developing brain is essential to garner their support for regulations/statutes related to preventing marijuana use among youth.

There is also a need for national and statewide education campaigns focused specifically on preventing youth marijuana use. Such campaigns have demonstrated an ability to influence youth behavior and choices. Campaigns can also help alter existing social norms, perception of harm, and attitudes around youth marijuana use.

Enhanced Enforcement Activities: Communities should ensure adequate resources are available for monitoring and enforcing existing marijuana policies. Although agencies may have the authority to monitor and enforce state policy, they may not have the necessary staffing or financial support to do so. A proactive approach to monitoring and enforcement is also preferred to one that is driven by public complaints and observations.

Planning and Research: Collecting data on key medical marijuana use indicators, such as physicians making recommendations/referrals for medical marijuana, the types of products being recommended, patient demographics, and the number of patients who receive recommendations/referrals, allows community prevention coalitions, health departments, and prevention organizations to understand their local conditions and help policy makers determine the most effective policy solutions.

Product Classification: By classifying medical marijuana in the same way as prescription drugs dispensed at pharmacies, communities in Florida do not have the option of limiting the availability of marijuana without also limiting the availability of pharmacies, thus reducing access to the medications and resources available at pharmacies. Other states do not tie their classification of marijuana to other medicinal products, allowing for targeted marijuana regulation [23-24].

References

[1] Rae Hanstad Consulting. (2014). *Marijuana in Ventura County: A gateway for discussion.* Ventura County Behavioral Health Department. https://www.counties.org/sites/main/files/file-attachments/ventura_co_gateway_for_discussion.pdf.

[2] Health Matters in Ventura County. (2021). *Summary Data for County: Ventura.* http://www. healthmattersinvc.org/demographicdata.

[3] Ventura County Office of Education. (2021). *School Districts in Ventura County.* https://www.vcoe.org/School-Districts-in-Ventura-County.

[4] Goldstein, R., & Sumner, D. A. (2019). California cannabis regulation: An overview. *California Agrilculture, 73*(3), 101-102. https://doi.org/10.3733/ca.2019a0021.

[5] State of California. (2018). Medicinal and Adult Use Cannabis Regulation and Safety Act, California Publ. L. No. 26000-26260. https://leginfo.legislature.ca.gov/faces/codes_displayexpandedbranch.xhtml?tocCode=BPC&division=10.&title=&part= &chapter=&article=.

[6] County of Ventura. (2021, March 24) *Cannabis in Ventura County*. https://www.ventura.org/cannabis/.

[7] Healy, J. (2019, June 30). Reefer madness or pot paradise? The surprising legacy of the place where legal weed began. *The New York Times*. https://www.nytimes.com/2019/06/30/us/marijuana-colorado-legalization.html.

[8] Coolican, J. P. (2019, March 9). A green wave of pot. *StarTribune*. https://www.startribune.com/colorado-offers-a-picture-of-what-marijuana-legalization-might-look-like-in-minnesota/506709502/.

[9] The Associated Press. (2017, August 25). Letter to Sessions: The Colorado way on pot is 'a model for other states'. *CPR News*. https://www.cpr.org/2017/08/25/letter-to-sessions-the-colorado-way-on-pot-is-a-model-for-other-states/.

[10] Colorado Department of Public Safety. (2018). *Colorado Division of Criminal Justice publishes report on impacts of marijuana legalization in Colorado*. https://publicsafety.colorado.gov/press-release/colorado-division-of-criminal-justice-publishes-report-on-impacts-of-marijuana.

[11] Colorado Department of Public Health and Environment. (2020). *Healthy Kids Colorado Survey and Smart Source Information*. https://cdphe. colorado.gov/hkcs.

[12] Boulder County. (2013). *2013 Boulder Valley School District High School Youth Risk Behavior Survey (YRBS) Process and Data Tables*. https://assets.bouldercounty.org/wp-content/uploads/2017/03/hkcs-2013-county-hs-tables.pdf.

[13] University of Colorado. (2019). *Healthy Kids Colorado Survey: High school district level report survey results*. https://assets.bouldercounty.org/wp-content/uploads/2020/09/hkcs-results-bvsd-high-school-2019-version-1.pdf.

[14] Teens, Inc. (n.d.). *Communities That Care*. https://teensinc.org/prevention/.

[15] Boulder County. (2021). *Marijuana licensing*. https://www.bouldercounty.org/records/licenses/marijuana-licensing/.

[16] Boulder County. (2019). *Checklist for new marijuana licenses & permits*. https://assets.bouldercounty.org/wp-content/uploads/2019/07/ml-New-Application-Checklist.pdf.

[17] City of Nederland. (2020). Code of Ordinances, Chapter 18-Building Regulations, Article V-Signs. https://library.municode.com/co/nederland/codes/code_of_ordinances?nodeId=CH18BURE_ARTVSI.

[18] Florida Health Medical Quality Assurance. (n.d.). *Medical use of marijuana in a form for smoking*. https://flhealthsource.gov/mum/.

[19] Rothenbach Research and Consulting, LLC, & Florida Department of Children & Families Office of Substance Abuse & Mental Health. (2020). *2020 Florida Youth Substance Abuse Survey State Report*. https://www.myflfamilies.com/service-programs/samh/prevention/fysas/2020/docs/2020%20Statewide%20FYSAS%20Report%20per%20 Section%20C2-2.3.pdf.

[20] Substance Awareness Center of Indian River County. (n.d.). *Prevention works!* https://sacirc.org/prevention/.

[21] Castletc. (2014, February 26). New dates announced for Castle's Strengthening Families program. *TC Palm.* https://archive.tcpalm.com/news/new-dates-announced-for-castles-strengthening-families-program-ep-350996701-341964281.html/.

[22] Botvin LifeSkills Training. (2019, April 1). *Indian River County Florida and Botvin LifeSkills Training - Prevention is a partnership*. https://www.lifeskillstraining.com/indian-river-county-florida-and-botvin-lifeskills-training-prevention-is-a-partnership/.

[23] Michigan Department of Licensing and Regulatory Affairs. (2020). *Marihuana Licenses.* https://www.michigan.gov/documents/mra/2019-67_LR_Marihuana_Licenses_694519_7.pdf.

[24] State of Pennsylvania. (2021). *Pennsylvania Medical Marijuana Program.* https://www.health.pa.gov/topics/programs/Medical%20Marijuana/Pages/Medical%20Marijuana.aspx.

Section 5. Resources for Evaluation and Quality Improvement

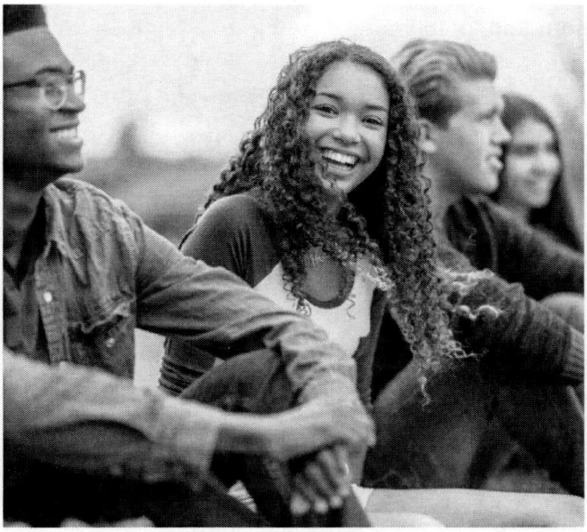

The primary purposes of evaluating public health strategies are: [1]

1) *Assess implementation:* Was the intervention implemented as intended and what factors are influencing the intervention's success?
2) *Determine effectiveness:* Did the intervention achieve its goals and objectives and expected outcomes?

3) *Evaluate efficiency:* Were resources such as budget and timeframe used appropriately?
4) *Measure cost-effectiveness:* Did the benefits, or outcomes, resulting from the intervention exceed the costs of implementing it?
5) *Assess attribution:* Can progress on goals and objectives be attributed to the intervention, as opposed to other environmental or organizational factors?

Program and policy evaluation answers critical questions about whether an intervention is producing the intended outcomes, and why or why not. Evaluation can also show how a program or policy benefits individuals and be helpful in securing additional funding by providing evidence of program/policy effectiveness. In addition, information gathered through evaluation can be used to encourage dissemination and adoption of the intervention to other communities.

This section provides an overview of approaches to evaluate the implementation and outcomes of interventions to prevent marijuana use among youth and young adults. The section also includes information on implementing a continuous quality improvement (CQI) process, which allows for rapid evaluation to improve interventions quickly based on the results. Finally, it includes specific evaluation resources, including potential outcomes to track.

Types of Evaluations and Study Designs

Evaluation is best planned and initiated:

- Before a program or policy is implemented to determine its feasibility (formative evaluation)
- During implementation (process evaluation)
- After the intervention has been delivered (short-term and long-term outcomes and impact evaluation)

Each of these evaluation types is useful in judging an intervention's effectiveness in preventing marijuana use among youth and young adults. However, when considering policy evaluation, it is important to remember there is no concrete end date—the changes from a policy may not be observable for a period of years, and immediate outcomes (e.g., reductions in the number of marijuana outlets) may differ from long-term outcomes (e.g., reductions in youth marijuana use).

Both qualitative and quantitative methods, as well as community participatory approaches, are important when evaluating programs and policies.

Although it is often omitted when planning and implementing an intervention, evaluation is an integral part of the implementation process and should be considered from the start.

Formative evaluation assesses the readiness of an organization or community to implement the intervention, articulates a theory of change, and determines the extent to which an intervention can be evaluated in a reliable and credible fashion.

Process (implementation) evaluation collects data about an intervention's implementation. This evaluation enables program managers and policy makers to assess whether an intervention was implemented as planned, and whether and to what extent it reached the intended audience.

Outcome evaluation collects baseline data and data at defined intervals (e.g., annually) during and after full implementation of the intervention to assess short- and long-term outcomes related to the targeted behaviors. These outcomes of interest should be collected from program participants or community members. These outcome data provide program managers and policy makers with information to assess changes or improvements in attitudes and behaviors that can be associated with the intervention.

Impact evaluation assesses an intervention's effectiveness in achieving its ultimate goals. Impact evaluations determine the extent to which changes in outcomes can be attributed to the newly implemented intervention. Conducting impact evaluations of policy implementation can be challenging; it often takes many years to see changes in behavior that may be associated with a specific policy. These evaluations typically require either strong data collected before policy passage to do a pre/post comparison, or data from a similar jurisdiction which has not implemented the policy to compare the two jurisdictions to each other. Stakeholders and funders should be aware that an impact evaluation of the policy may not be feasible without additional funding and resources.

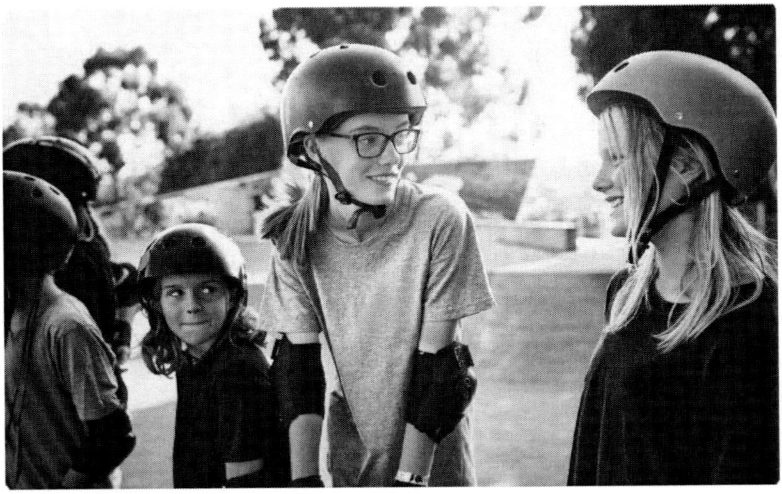

Continuous Quality Improvement (CQI)

What is CQI?

CQI involves a systematic process of assessing program or practice implementation and short-term outcomes and then involving program staff in identifying and implementing improvements in service delivery and organizational systems to achieve better treatment outcomes. CQI helps assess fidelity, the degree to which a program delivers a practice as intended.

CQI differs from process evaluation in that it involves quick assessments of program performance, timely identification of problems and potential solutions, and implementation of small improvements to enhance treatment quality. CQI is usually conducted by internal staff. Process evaluation involves longer-term assessments and is best conducted by an external evaluator.

Why use CQI?

CQI takes a broader look at the systems and environment in which programs or policies operate. Because of the pivotal role it plays in performance management, organizations or stakeholders implementing new programs or policies to prevent marijuana use among youth or young adults are encouraged to implement CQI procedures.

What are the steps involved in CQI?

Although steps in the CQI process may vary based on objectives, typical CQI steps are:

- Identify a problem or issue needing improvement and a target improvement goal
- Analyze the problem and its root causes
- Develop an action plan to correct the root causes of the problem,
- including specific actions to be taken
- Implement the actions in the action plan
- Review the results to confirm that the issue and its root causes have been addressed and short- and long-term prevention outcomes have improved
- Repeat these steps to identify and address other issues as they arise

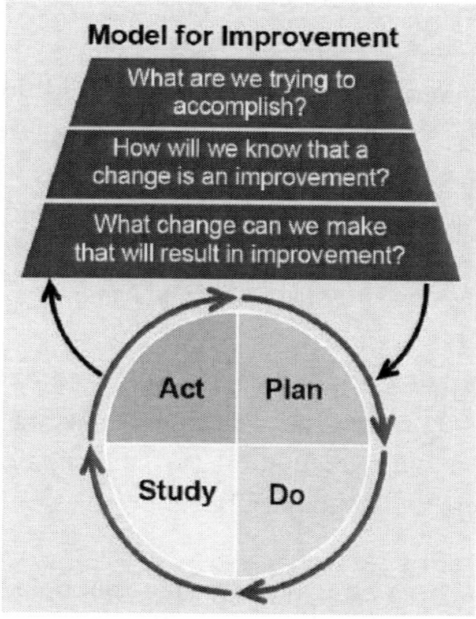

Institute for Healthcare Improvement. (n.d.). Science of improvement: Testing changes. http://www.ihi.org/resources/Pages/HowtoImprove/ScienceofImprovementTestingChanges.aspx

New Jersey Department of Children and Families. (n.d.). Five Stages of Continuous Quality Improvement. https://www.nj.gov/dcf/about/divisions/opma/CQI%20framework.pdf

NIATx National Program Office. (n.d.). What is NIATx? https://www.niatx.net/what-is-niatx/

U.S. Department of Health & Human Services Office of Adolescent Health. (n.d.). Continuous Quality Improvement, Part 1: Basics for Pregnancy Assistance Fund Programs. https://www.hhs.gov/ash/oah/sites/default/files/cqi-intro.pdf

Outcomes

An important but often challenging step in the process of implementing programs and policies is determining whether they have yielded desired outcomes. An *outcome* is the change an intervention is intended to accomplish through the implementation of a program or policy.

Regardless of which evaluation design is best for an intervention, it may take time to realize some of the intended outcomes. *Short-term effects* of a program or policy may be seen immediately, such as changes in knowledge, beliefs, or perceptions, while long-term outcomes may take much longer.

Long-term outcomes include change in behavior, such as reductions in initiation and prevalence of marijuana use. Additionally, the nature of marijuana use may change over time as programs and policies are implemented, or as new marijuana products are added to the market. Collecting data on the patterns of marijuana use, including what products are being sold or used, how they are being used, and by whom, will help communities conduct their regular needs assessments, as described in Section 3.

Given changing patterns of marijuana use and new regulatory policies, there are several key data elements communities need to collect to understand marijuana prevention and reduction efforts. Stakeholders working to prevent marijuana use among youth should: [2]

- Collect data on existing policies at the national, state, local, tribal, and territorial levels
- Examine how marijuana products are marketed in their community to understand the potential impact of future regulation
- Track patterns of marijuana sales and use in populations at high risk, such as racial/ethnic, gender identity, and sexual orientation minorities

Provided below is a list of potential outcomes, illustrative outcome indicators, and sources of survey questions that may be used to evaluate interventions to prevent marijuana use among youth.

Outcome	Illustrative Indicators	Examples of Sources of Survey Questions
Short-Term Outcomes		
Knowledge of the harms of marijuana use, strengthened social norms	Level of perceived harm of marijuana products among youth and young adults	Monitoring the Future Study
Perceived social norms on marijuana use	Proportion of youth and young adults who overestimate the marijuana use rate among their peers	National Survey on Drug Use and Health
Policy and enforcement efforts	Proportion of jurisdictions with public policies that establish a fee on each marijuana product sold	State or local policy tracking systems
	Proportion of jurisdictions with comprehensive policies that require retail licenses to sell marijuana	
	Enforcement intensity measured by citations/warnings given to retail establishments	Local or state law enforcement or licensing entities maintaining citation data
Price of marijuana products	Amount of marijuana product taxes and fees	NIAAA Alcohol Policy Information System
Exposure to marijuana marketing	Density of stores selling marijuana products	Government bodies/organizations licensing marijuana retailers
Availability of marijuana products	Number and content of marijuana advertisements	State marijuana regulatory bodies
Long-Term Individual- and Population-Level Outcomes and Impacts		
Initiation of marijuana use	Proportion of youth and young adults who report never having tried a marijuana product	National Survey on Drug Use and Health Youth Risk Behavior Surveillance Survey Behavioral Risk Factor Surveillance System
Marijuana use prevalence	Prevalence of marijuana use among youth and young adults	National Survey on Drug Use and Health Youth Risk Behavior Surveillance Survey Behavioral Risk Factor Surveillance System
Sales of marijuana products	Sales of flavored products reported in a community Percent of marijuana sales composed of high potency products	Tax data, commercial market databases, retail establishments

Sources of National Data on Marijuana Use Among Youth and Young Adults

	National Survey on Drug Use and Health (NSDUH) [3]	Monitoring the Future Survey (MTF) [4]	Youth Risk Behavior Surveillance System (YRBSS) [5]	Behavioral Risk Factor Surveillance System (BRFSS) [6]	Population Assessment of Tobacco and Health (PATH) [7]	National Health and Nutrition Examination Survey (NHANES) [8]
Sponsoring Agency or Organization	Substance Abuse and Mental Health Services Administration	National Institute on Drug Abuse	Centers for Disease Control and Prevention	Centers for Disease Control and Prevention	Food and Drug Administration; National Institutes of Health	Centers for Disease Control and Prevention
Type of Survey	Cross-sectional	Cross- sectional and longitudinal	Cross-sectional	Cross-sectional	Longitudinal	Cross- sectional
Mode of Survey Administration	Audio, computer-assisted self-interview	School- based, self-administered questionnaire	School-based, self-administered questionnaire	Telephone surveys	Home-based interview	Interviews and physical examinations
Ages/Grades	≥12 years	8th and 10th grades (since 1991) and 12th grade (since 1975); college students; young adults	9th to 12th grades	≥18 years	≥12 years	All ages
Level of Data Available	National, state, sub-state regions	National, regional	National, state, district	National and state, as well as counties and metropolitan/micropolitan areas for some data	National, state, census region	National

Several publicly available datasets that include measures on marijuana are detailed below. Communities wanting more localized data should look to see what surveillance measures their county and state public health departments are already collecting at the county or census tract levels. Communities should additionally consider whether there is an appropriate community they can compare their data against to conduct an impact evaluation. Depending on the data available, this may be a similar city or county, or stakeholders may compare their community data to state averages.

Qualitative Data

Throughout an evaluation, it is important to engage those implementing the program or policy and those affected by it. Hearing the voices of key stakeholders through qualitative data collection, such as interviews or focus groups, provides necessary context, and allows evaluators to gain a deeper understanding of the story behind the quantitative data collected.

Qualitative data may be collected from youth who use marijuana to better understand attitudes and perceptions of marijuana, such as why they use the product and how, and during and after an intervention has been implemented to learn their perspectives on what is and is not working. Interviews can also be conducted with those who implement the intervention to understand what is going well and what may need to be changed in future versions. If survey data show that an increase in tax policy is affecting one demographic group differently than others, focus groups may help stakeholders understand why these differences are occurring.

Qualitative data collection efforts should be considered at the beginning of any evaluation, and reconsidered at the end, to help provide context for quantitative study findings [9].

As findings from the evaluation emerge, corrections should be made, as needed, to improve the intervention and initiatives to prevent youth marijuana use. Results should also be shared with stakeholders and the broader community. Disseminating the findings will contribute to the growing body of evidence on effective strategies to prevent marijuana use among youth and young adults, allowing other organizations and communities to benefit from knowledge gained during the evaluation.

Evaluation Resources

- Overarching Policy Evaluation Guidance
    - SAMHSA's Strategic Prevention Framework and Selecting the Best Fit guidance includes assistance on how coalitions and prevention planners can evaluate programs and environmental strategies.
    - A guide on the Introduction to Process Evaluation developed by CDC, which focuses on Tobacco Use Prevention and Control, defines process evaluation, and describes the rationale, benefits, key data collection components, and program evaluation management procedures.
    - CADCA's Evaluation Primer: Setting the Context for a Community Anti-Drug
    - Coalition Evaluation specifically addresses coalition evaluation.
    - The National Institutes webpage on evaluation of Health provides guidance on qualitative evaluation methods.
- Overarching Program Evaluation Guidance
    - A Framework for Program Evaluation from the Program Guide on the Introduction to Program Evaluation for Public Health Programs, developed by CDC, is intended to assist managers and staff of public, private, and community public health programs plan, design, implement, and use comprehensive evaluations.
    - Examples of evaluation measures was developed by the Rural Health Information Hub includes process and outcome measures meant to keep a project team working towards the same goal.
    - The Performance and Evaluation Office (PPEO) at CDC framework summarizes essential elements of program evaluation.
    - Introduction to Program Evaluation for Public Health Programs is a self-study guide from CDC that includes worksheets and checklists for implementing the steps in CDC's Framework for Program Evaluation.
- Quality Improvement and Continuous Performance Monitoring
    - Roadmap to a Culture of Quality Improvement is a guide to the quality improvement process for local health departments developed by the National Association of County & City Health Officials (NACCHO).

- The National Network of Public Health Institutes developed a webinar on "CQI: Building a Performance Management System to Strengthen Quality Improvement," with speakers from the Macomb County Health Department.

References

[1] Centers for Disease Control and Prevention. (2012). *Introduction to program evaluation for public health programs: A self study guide*. https://www.cdc.gov/eval/guide/index.htm.

[2] Illinois Department of Human Services. (2019). *Marijuana prevention strategies resource guide*. http://www.dhs.state.il.us/OneNetLibrary/27896/documents/Cannabis_Prevention_Strategies.pdf.

[3] Substance Abuse and Mental Health Services Administration. (2020). *Key substance use and mental health indicators in the United States: Results from the 2019 National Survey on Drug Use and Health*. https://www. samhsa.gov/data/sites/default/files/reports/rpt29393/2019NSDUHFFRPDFWHTML/2019NSDUHFFR090120.htm.

[4] National Institute on Drug Abuse. (2019, December 18). *Monitoring the Future 2019 survey results: Overall findings*. https://www.drugabuse.gov/drug-topics/trends-statistics/infographics/monitoring-future-2019-survey-results-overall-findings.

[5] Centers for Disease Control and Prevention. (2020). *Youth Risk Behavior Surveillance—United States, 2019*. https://www.cdc.gov/mmwr/volumes/69/su/pdfs/su6901-H.pdf.

[6] Centers for Disease Control and Prevention. (2019). *Behavioral Risk Factor Surveillance System (BRFSS)*. https://www.cdc.gov/brfss/.

[7] National Institutes of Health. (2020). *PATH Population Assessment of Tobacco and Health*. https://pathstudyinfo.nih.gov/.

[8] Centers for Disease Control and Prevention. (2021). *National Health and Nutrition Examination Survey*. https://www.cdc.gov/nchs/nhanes/index.htm.

[9] Commonwealth of Massachusetts. (2021). Massachusetts Cannabis Control Commission 935 Mass. Reg. 500.150-Edibles. https://casetext. com/regulation/code-of-massachusetts-regulations/department-935-cmr-cannabis-control-commission/title-935-cmr-500000-adult-usemarijuana/section-500150-edibles.

Appendix: Acknowledgments

This publication was developed with a significant contribution from Alicia Sparks, PhD, MPH and Lynn Silver, MD, MPH, FAAP. This guidance is based on the thoughtful input of SAMHSA staff and the Technical Expert

Panel on Reducing Marijuana Use Among Youth from October 2020 through June 2021. A series of guide development meetings was held virtually over a period of several months. Three expert panel meetings were convened during this time.

SAMHSA Staff

Aida Balsano, PhD Center for Substance Abuse Prevention*
Christine Cichetti National Mental Health and Substance Use Policy Laboratory*
Thomas Clarke, PhD National Mental Health and Substance Use Policy Laboratory
Tanya Geiger, PhD, MPH National Mental Health and Substance Use Policy Laboratory*
Donelle Johnson, PhD, MHSA National Mental Health and Substance Use Policy Laboratory*
Nelia Nadal, MPH Center for Substance Abuse Prevention*
Krishnan Radhakrishnan, MD, PhD, MPH National Mental Health and Substance Use Policy Laboratory

Technical Expert Panel

Debbie Berndt Parent Movement 2.0
Jessica Cotto, MPH National Institute on Drug Abuse (NIDA), National Institutes of Health (NIH)
Deepak Cyril D'Souza, MD Yale University School of Medicine, VA Connecticut Healthcare System (VACHS)
Amy B. Goldstein, PhD National Institute on Drug Abuse (NIDA), National Institutes of Health (NIH)
Sion Kim Harris, PhD, CPH Center for Adolescent Behavioral Health Research (CABHRe), Boston Children's Hospital, Harvard Medical School
Kristin M. Holland, PhD, MPH Centers for Disease Control and Prevention
Katia Howlett, PhD, MPP, MBA National Institute on Drug Abuse (NIDA), National Institutes of Health (NIH)
David Jernigan, PhD Boston University School of Public Health, CityHealth

Rich Lucey Drug Enforcement Administration
LaTrice Montgomery, PhD University of Cincinnati College of Medicine
Rosalie Liccardo Pacula, PhD University of Southern California Sol Price School of Public Policy
Rebecca Ramirez, MPH Public Health Consultant
Gillian Schauer, PhD, MPH Alcohol and Drug Abuse Institute (ADAI)
Lynn Silver, MD, MPH, FAAP Public Health Institute and University of California San Francisco*
Ryan Treffers, JD Pacific Institute for Research and Evaluation
Ryan Vandrey, PhD Johns Hopkins University School of Medicine

Contract Staff

Amy Berninger, MPH Abt Associates
Anna Garner Abt Associates
Margaret Gwaltney, MBA Abt Associates*
Caroline Kupersmith Abt Associates
Daniel Jefferson Smith Abt Associates
Alicia C. Sparks, PhD, MPH Abt Associates*
Sarah Steverman, PhD, MSW Abt Associates*
Korrin L. Bishop Korrin Bishop Writing & Editing
*Members of Guide Planning Team

Chapter 5

DAWN and Marijuana*

Center for Behavioral Health Statistics and Quality

The Drug Abuse Warning Network (DAWN) is a nationwide public health surveillance system administered by the Substance Abuse and Mental Health Services Administration's (SAMHSA's) Center for Behavioral Health Statistics and Quality. As of October 15, 2020, data are being abstracted from 49 hospitals. Ultimately, the system will include at least 50 non-Federal general hospitals with 24-hour emergency departments (EDs), consisting of 10 sentinel hospitals and 40 probability-sampled hospitals. Data are abstracted directly from hospital electronic health records. DAWN captures data on ED visits related to recent substance use and misuse, such as alcohol use, illicit drug use, suicide attempts, and nonmedical use of pharmaceuticals.

DAWN data can be used to monitor substance misuse trends and serve as an early warning system to identify new psy- choactive substances. Since hospital recruitment is incomplete and the data are *unweighted*, this profile provides only preliminary results that are not generalizable to the US; caution must therefore be exercised in interpreting the data presented here.

This profile presents data on ED visits related to marijuana use. The information provided below summarizes *unweighted* data abstracted from 4/1/2019 to 10/15/2020. The data on alcohol presented here include ED visits related to underage (less than 21 years old) alcohol use and adult (ages 21 years and older) alcohol use in combination with other substances since the abstraction of ED visits for adults involving only alcohol was not yet complete.

---

* This is an edited, reformatted and augmented version of Center for Behavioral Health Statistics and Quality, dated December 2020.

In: Marijuana
Editor: Charles M. Edmond
ISBN: 979-8-88697-869-8

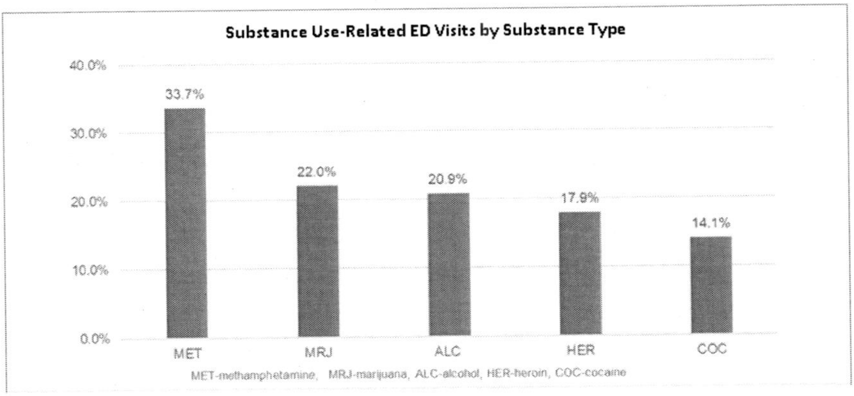

This graph shows substance use-related ED visits by substance type, focusing on the most common illicit sub- stances and alcohol. Marijuana (22%) was the second most common substance involved in substance-related ED visits.

Marijuana Use-Related ED Visits by Age

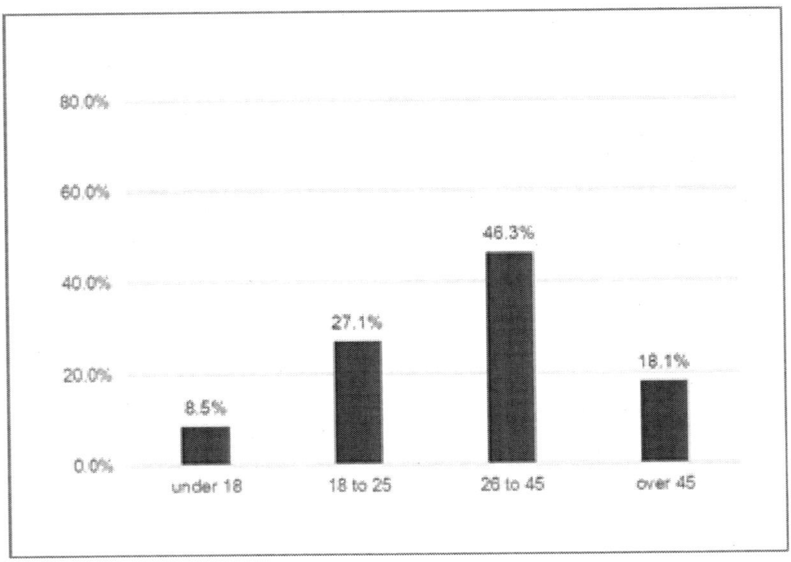

Patients aged 26 to 45 accounted for 46.3% of mar- ijuana-related ED visits, and patients aged 18 to 25 accounted for 27.1%, the second largest proportion of these visits.

Marijuana Use-Related ED Visits by Gender

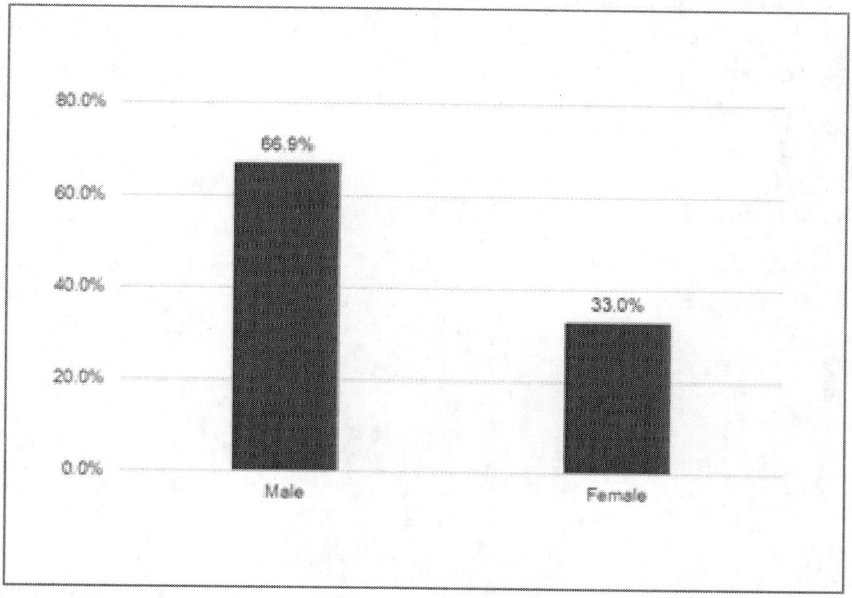

Two-thirds of marijuana-related ED visits involved male patients (66.9%); about one-third of the visits (33%) involved female patients.

Marijuana Use-Related ED Visits to Total ED Visits by Community Type

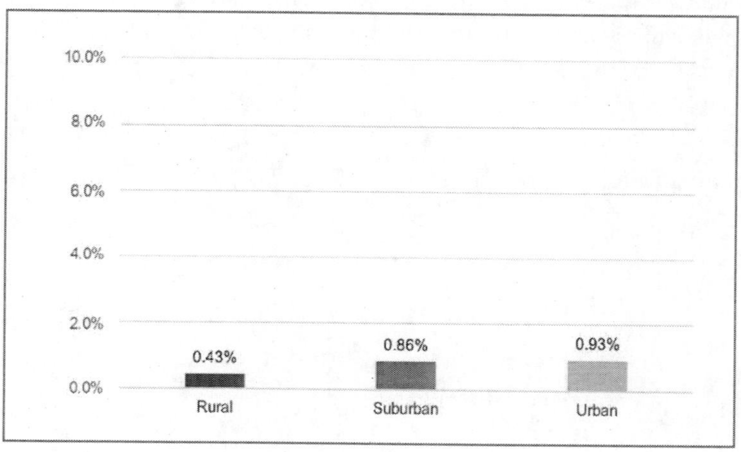

This graph shows the percentage of marijuana- related ED visits to total ED visits by community type. In this graph, the denominator is total ED visits within each community type. Marijuana-related ED visits were a higher proportion of all ED visits in urban (0.93%) and suburban (0.86%) communities as compared to rural (0.43%) communities.

Marijuana Use-Related ED Visits by Disposition

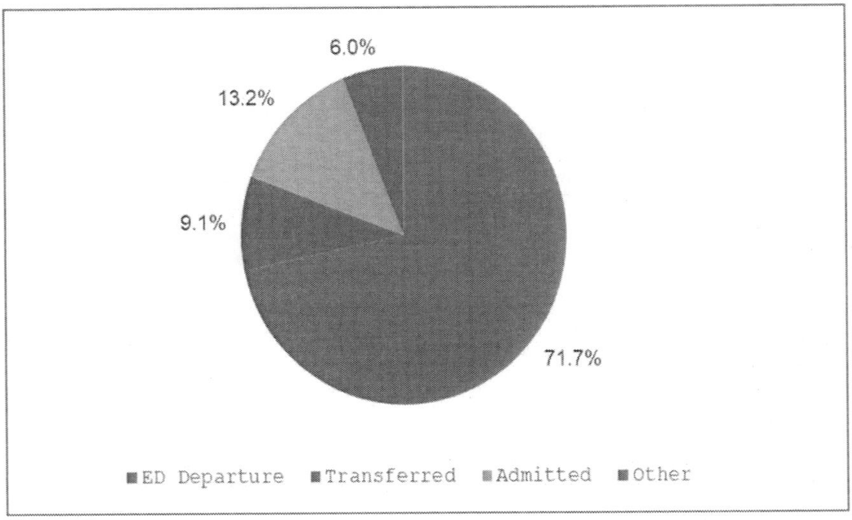

Over seventy percent (71.7%) of marijuana-related ED visits resulted in the patient's release from the ED, such as departing the ED for home or receiving a referral for substance use and/or psychiatric treatment. Remaining dispositions included admission to the hospital (13.2%), transfer to another facility (9.1%) and other outcomes (6%), such as *left against medical advice.*

For more information, please call (240) 276-1250.

Index

E

F

H

I

L

M

N